ADVANCES IN

Pediatrics

Editor-in-Chief
Carol D. Berkowitz, MD, FAAP, FACEP

Chief, Division of General Pediatrics,
Department of PediatricsAurora,
Harbor-UCLA Medical Center,
Distinguished Professor of Pediatrics,
David Geffen School of Medicine at UCLA,
Torrance, California

ELSEVIER

PHILADELPHIA LONDON TORONTO MONTREAL SYDNEY TOKYO

ADVANCES IN Pediatrics

VOLUMES 1 THROUGH 67 (OUT OF PRINT)

VOLUME 68

Advances in the Surgical Management of Esophageal Atresia, by*Alexis N. Bowder* and *Dave R. Lal*

Trends in Pediatric Recreational Drug Use and Ingestions, by*Raymen R. Assaf* and *Kelly D. Young*

Editor: Kerry Holland
Developmental Editor: Diana Ang

Reprints: For copies of 100 or more of articles in this publication, please contact the Commercial Reprints Department, Elsevier Inc., 360 Park Avenue South, New York, NY 10010-1710. Tel: 212-633-3874; Fax: 212-633-3820; E-mail: reprints@elsevier.com.

Printed in the United States of America.

Editorial Office:
Elsevier
1600 John F. Kennedy Blvd,
Suite 1800
Philadelphia, PA 19103-2899

International Standard Serial Number: 0065-3101
International Standard Book Number: 13: 978-0-323-98685-4

ADVANCES IN
Pediatrics

CONTRIBUTORS

HEATHER AGAZZI, PhD, Professor, Department of Pediatrics, University of South Florida, Tampa, Florida, USA

PARUL BHATIA, MD, Associate Professor, Pediatrics (Clinician-Educator), Department of Pediatrics, Keck School of Medicine of USC, Children's Hospital Los Angeles, Los Angeles, California, USA

JESSICA L. BORELLI, PhD, Associate Professor, Department of Psychological Science, University of California, Irvine, Irvine, California, USA

ADRIENNE BRUCCOLERI, DNP, Department of Pediatrics, University of South Florida Morsani College of Medicine, Tampa, Florida, USA

AILEEN CANNON, MD, Department of Pediatrics, University of South Florida Morsani College of Medicine, Tampa, Florida, USA

FRANK AYESTARAN CASSAINI, MD, Department of Pediatrics, Division of Pediatric Nephrology, Assistant Professor, University of South Florida Health, St Petersburg, Florida, USA

DYLAN K. CHAN, MD, PhD, FAAP, Associate Professor, Department of Otolaryngology–Head and Neck Surgery, University of California, San Francisco, San Francisco, California, USA

ANNA M. CHENG, MD, Department of Pediatrics, University of Texas Southwestern Medical Center, Dallas, Texas, USA

SUKJOO CHO, MD, Department of Pediatrics, University of South Florida Morsani College of Medicine, Tampa, Florida, USA

AMELIA T. COLLINGS, MD, Department of Surgery, Indiana University School of Medicine, Indianapolis, Indiana, USA

MELINDA DANOWITZ, DO, Divisions of Endocrinology and Diabetes, and Pediatric Endocrinology, Children's Hospital of Philadelphia, Philadelphia, Pennsylvania, USA

SARAH DICKINSON, PhD, Assistant Professor, Department of Pediatrics, University of South Florida, Tampa, Florida, USA

ARIA FALLAH, MD, MSc, FRCSC, Department of Neurosurgery, David Geffen School of Medicine, University of California, Los Angeles, Los Angeles, California, USA

CLAUDIA GAVIRIA-AGUDELO, MD, Assistant Professor Pediatrics, Pediatric Infectious Diseases, University of South Florida Morsani College of Medicine, Tampa, Florida, USA

MEGAN GOSS, MD, Pediatrics Resident Physician, UC Irvine/CHOC Children's Hospital of Orange County, Orange, California, USA

ADDA GRIMBERG, MD, Professor, Department of Pediatrics, Perelman School of Medicine, University of Pennsylvania, Scientific Director, Diagnostic and Research Growth Center, Children's Hospital of Philadelphia, The Hub for Clinical Collaboration, Division of Endocrinology, Philadelphia,Pennsylvania, USA

SARAH C. HAYNES, PhD, MPH, Assistant Professor, Department of Pediatrics, UC Davis School of Medicine, UC Davis Center for Health and Technology, Sacramento, California, USA

KATRIN JARADEH, BS, Medical Student, School of Medicine, University of California, San Francisco, San Francisco, California, USA

VINCENT JORIS, MD, Department of Neurosurgery, Sainte-Justine University Hospital Centre, Montréal, Quebec, Canada

LORRAINE I. KELLEY-QUON, MD, MSHS, Division of Pediatric Surgery, Children's Hospital Los Angeles, Department of Surgery, Keck School of Medicine of USC, Department of Population and Public Health Sciences, University of Southern California, Los Angeles, California, USA

ANDREA LAFNITZEGGER, DO, Resident Physician, Year 2, University of South Florida Morsani College of Medicine, Tampa, Florida, USA

JAKE LESSER, MD, Medical School Graduate, University of South Florida Health, Tampa, Florida, USA

JAMES P. MARCIN, MD, MPH, Professor, Department of Pediatrics, UC Davis School of Medicine, UC Davis Center for Health and Technology, Sacramento, California, USA

DEBORAH McCURDY, MD, Clinical Professor, Department of Pediatrics, Division of Allergy/Immunology/Rheumatology, David Geffen School of Medicine, University of California, Los Angeles, Mattel Children's Hospital, Los Angeles, California, USA

SAGARIKA NALLU, MD, Director of Pediatric Sleep Medicine, Department of Pediatric Neurology, University of South Florida Morsani College of Medicine, Tampa, Florida, USA

MARISSA NEWMAN, Student, University of California, Los Angeles, Los Angeles, California, USA

MARJORIE ODEGARD, MD, Division of Pediatric Surgery, Children's Hospital Los Angeles, Department of Surgery, Keck School of Medicine of USC, Los Angeles, California, USA

SAIDA OMAROVA, MD, Department of Pediatrics, University of South Florida Morsani College of Medicine, Tampa, Florida, USA

TAPAN PADHYA, MD, Chair, Department of Otolaryngology–Head and Neck Surgery, University of South Florida Morsani College of Medicine, Tampa, Florida, USA

VALERIE PANZARINO, MD, Department of Pediatrics, Division of Pediatric Nephrology, Associate Professor, University of South Florida Health, Tampa, Florida, USA

ASHLEY M. PERRY, MD, Department of Pediatrics, University of South Florida Morsani College of Medicine, Tampa, Florida, USA

REBECCA M. PLANT, MD, Assistant Professor, Department of Pediatrics, University of South Florida, Tampa, Florida, USA

JOSEPH PUCCIO, MD, Department of Pediatrics, University of South Florida Morsani College of Medicine, Tampa, Florida, USA

JULIE REMS-SMARIO, EdD, Early Language and Education Programs Consultant, California School for the Deaf, California Department of Education, CORE, Fremont, California, USA

JUAN FELIPE RICO, MD, Associate Professor, Division of Hematology/Oncology, Department of Pediatrics, University of South Florida Morsani College of Medicine, Tampa, Florida, USA

NATHAN S. RUBALCAVA, MD, Section of Pediatric Surgery, Department of Surgery, University of Michigan, Mott Children's Hospital, Ann Arbor, Michigan, USA; Department of Surgery, Creighton University Health Science Campus, Phoenix, Arizona, USA

BETH RYMESKI, DO, Cincinnati Children's Hospital Medical Center, Cincinnati, Ohio, USA

THUSA SABAPATHY, MD, FAAP, Assistant Clinical Professor of Pediatrics, University of California, Irvine School of Medicine, The Center for Autism and Neurodevelopmental Disorders, Santa Ana, California, USA

PAUL SAENGER, MD, Professor of Pediatrics, NYU Langone Health–Long Island, Mineola, New York, USA

ABHAY VARUN SHARMA, MD, Department of Otolaryngology–Head and Neck Surgery, University of South Florida Morsani College of Medicine, Tampa, Florida, USA

ELIZABETH E. SLOAN, MD, Instructor, Department of Pediatrics, Division of Rheumatology, Scottish Rite for Children and Children's Health, The University of Texas Southwestern Medical Center, Dallas, Texas, USA

CHARLES H. SONG, MD, Chief of Pediatric Allergy and Immunology, Harbor-University of California, Los Angeles, Torrance, California, USA

K. ELIZABETH SPECK, MD, MS, FACS, Section of Pediatric Surgery, Department of Surgery, University of Michigan, Mott Children's Hospital, Ann Arbor, Michigan, USA

ROBIN STEINBERG-EPSTEIN, MD, FAAP, Clinical Professor of Pediatrics, Chief, Division of Developmental Behavioral Pediatrics, University of California, Irvine School of Medicine, The Center for Autism and Neurodevelopmental Disorders, Santa Ana, California, USA

MARGARET STEINER, MD, Pediatric Endocrine Fellow, NYU Langone Health–Long Island, Mineola, New York, USA

FARN-HSUAN TSENG, MD, PGY3, Harbor-University of California, Los Angeles, Torrance, California, USA

PRIYA VAIDYANATHAN, MD, Associate Professor of Pediatrics, Department of Pediatric Endocrinology, Children's National Hospital, Washington, DC, USA

CARRIE WANG, BA, University of South Florida Morsani College of Medicine, Tampa, Florida, USA

ALEXANDER G. WEIL, MD, FRCSC, Department of Neurosurgery, Sainte-Justine University Hospital Centre, Montreal, Quebec, Canada

WENDY WEISS, DO, Department of Pediatrics, University of South Florida Morsani College of Medicine, Tampa, Florida, USA

ADVANCES IN
Pediatrics

CONTENTS VOLUME 69 • 2022

The accelerated uptake of telemedicine during the coronavirus disease 2019 pandemic has resulted in valuable experience and evidence on the delivery of telemedicine for pediatric patients. The pandemic has also highlighted inequities and opportunities for improvement. This review discusses lessons learned during the pandemic, focusing on provider-to-patient virtual encounters. Recent evidence on education and training, developing and adapting clinical workflows, patient assessment and treatment, and family-centered care is reviewed. Opportunities for future research in pediatric telemedicine are discussed, specifically with regard to engaging pediatric patients, improving and measuring access to care, addressing health equity, and expanding the evidence base.

Helping Our Toddlers, Developing Our Children's Skills: Innovative Behavioral Management Training for Pediatric Residents

Heather Agazzi, Sarah Dickinson, and Rebecca M. Plant

This article describes the implementation of a behavioral management training program into pediatric and combined medicine-pediatric residencies at a large urban academic medical center in southwest Florida. We describe 2 modalities for training residents in effective behavioral modification strategies immediately useable in pediatric practice. Results indicate that residents significantly increased their knowledge of effective, evidence-based strategies and continued to use them 6 to 12 months following completion of the training.

Childhood Hearing Health and Early Language Exposure: A Culturally Sensitive Approach

Parul Bhatia, Julie Rems-Smario, Katrin Jaradeh, and Dylan Chan

Implementation of the universal newborn hearing screening has changed the landscape for children born deaf or hard of hearing, and with this, pediatricians must be knowledgeable about the screening and referral process, state protocols, and how to support patients and their families in their unique journeys. Early access to language–spoken, signed, both–forms the foundation for successful outcomes for the development of fluent language. For children using spoken language, early access to sound is critical and can often be achieved with the assistance of hearing devices, even in the newborn period. For all language modalities, state-funded Deaf mentor programs allow families to have meaningful exposure to the Deaf community. The authors come from different professions in the health care and education fields, including General Pediatrics, Otolaryngology Head and Neck Surgery, and the state Department of Education, and use different languages, including spoken and American Sign Language.

A Pediatrician's Guide to Working with Children on the Autism Spectrum in Coronavirus Disease 2019 and Beyond: Retrospect and Prospect
Thusa Sabapathy, Megan Goss, Jessica L. Borelli, and Robin Steinberg-Epstein

The COVID-19 pandemic is an unprecedented event with devastating effects on children and families, highlighting and broadening disparities in the care of children with developmental disabilities, while simultaneously catalyzing innovation. Children are vulnerable to the impacts of COVID-19, resulting in increased stress, anxiety, isolation, and health challenges, further amplified in autistic children and children with other neurodevelopmental disabilities. These children are uniquely vulnerable due to communication impairments, comorbid medical disorders, reduced adaptability, and reliance on therapeutic interventions. Abrupt reduction in services and access to care during the pandemic compromised physical and mental health and led to missed intervention opportunities at critical times. It is important to examine the effects that the pandemic triggered, address deficiencies, and recognize new opportunities to improve systems of care to prepare for unforeseen futures.

Brain Surgery for Medically Intractable Epilepsy

Vincent Joris, Alexander G. Weil, and Aria Fallah

This review covers the broad topic of brain surgery in the treatment of pediatric intractable epilepsy. The authors review the latest advancements in the presurgical workup as well as the mandatory tests needed to explore the epilepsy workup in these children. They describe the different types of epilepsy from a surgical standpoint (temporal, extratemporal, multifocal, and hemispheric epilepsies) and various surgical procedures that can be proposed depending on the clinical scenario: lesionectomies, lobectomies, hemispherectomies, neuromodulation, and palliative surgeries. They also describe the key differences of the pediatric patient as compared with the adult patient in such pathologic conditions.

Chronic and Recurrent Sinusitis in Children, as Manifestation of Immune Dysfunction and Atopic Background

Farn-Hsuan Tseng, Marissa Newman, and Charles H. Song

Rhinosinusitis in children, as in adults, can be classified by duration (acute, recurrent, and chronic) and by cause (viral, bacterial, and inflammatory) and needs to be treated accordingly after careful investigation which include through clinical history, laboratory tests, and, if necessary, nasal endoscopy and imaging studies.

Management of Pediatric Obstructive Sleep Apnea After Failed Tonsillectomy and Adenoidectomy

Abhay Varun Sharma, Tapan Padhya, and Sagarika Nallu

Pediatric obstructive sleep apnea (OSA) represents a different entity from its adult counterpart and therefore requires a different therapeutic approach. Adenotonsillectomy (AT) is the primary treatment of pediatric OSA, and evidence shows it is very effective. However, there is a growing understanding that residual OSA is common, and next steps for patients who fail primary AT are less certain. This article reviews current methods of evaluating and treating these complex patients.

The Antiphospholipid Syndrome in the Pediatric Population

Elizabeth E. Sloan and Deborah McCurdy

Pediatric antiphospholipid syndrome (APS) is characterized by autoantibodies directed against protein complexes on cellular membranes and leads to a prothrombotic, proinflammatory state. A child with APS may present with venous, arterial, or small vessel thrombosis. Other manifestations of APS include nonthrombotic manifestations, such as hematologic and neurologic symptoms. APS may be a primary condition or related to other autoimmune diseases. If APS-related thrombosis is unrecognized, the child may suffer recurrent thrombotic events after the withdrawal of anticoagulation. Thus, it is important to consider APS as a cause of thrombosis in children. Appropriate testing confirms the diagnosis and directs further care.

Pediatric Chronic Kidney Disease

Valerie Panzarino, Jake Lesser, and Frank Ayestaran Cassaini

Chronic kidney disease (CKD) in children has a significant impact on morbidity, mortality, and quality of life. The degree of renal dysfunction should be calculated using pediatric-specific formulas and the degree of CKD staged; this allows for appropriate dosing of medications based on renal function and monitoring for progression and comorbid conditions including metabolic acidosis, bone disease, anemia, cardiovascular complications, malnutrition and electrolyte abnormalities, growth failure, and psychosocial issues. Treatment strategies include treating the underlying disease and using general renal protective measures. Effective management of these complex issues requires a specialized multidisciplinary team approach.

Advances in Hemophilia A Management

Sukjoo Cho, Ashley M. Perry, Anna M. Cheng, Carrie Wang, and Juan Felipe Rico

Hemophilia A is an inherited insufficiency of Factor VIII (FVIII), one of the critical clotting factors. The gold standard for the management of moderate-to-severe hemophilia A is prophylaxis using regular replacement therapy with clotting factor concentrates. Compared with conventional treatment, extended half-life products reduce the burden of frequent factor replacement injections. Of note, up to 30% of patients with hemophilia A receiving prophylactic factor infusions develop "inhibitors," neutralizing anti-FVIII autoantibodies. Therapeutic options for patients with hemophilia A and inhibitors include the immune tolerance induction (ie, eradication of inhibitors) and the management of acute bleeds with bypassing agents and/or emicizumab. Emicizumab is a biphasic monoclonal antibody mimicking activated FVIII, approved for patients with hemophilia A with/without inhibitors. Gene therapy is an emerging therapy for hemophilia A, essentially curing patients with hemophilia A or transforming them to a milder phenotype by establishing continuous endogenous expression of FVIII after one-time treatment.

Genital Herpes Simplex Virus—An Updated Review

Saida Omarova, Aileen Cannon, Wendy Weiss, Adrienne Bruccoleri, and Joseph Puccio

The herpes virus was named by the Greek physician Hippocrates who called it herpes because the lesions appeared near each other and were vesicular. Alphaherpesvirinae, Betaherpesvirinae, and Gammaherpesvirinae are subfamilies of the human herpes virus family. The Alphaherpesvirinae subfamily includes the simplex viruses–HSV-1 and HSV-2–and varicellovirus–varicella zoster virus. There are more than 200 members of the Herpesviridae family capable of infecting different species, 8 of which are known to cause disease in humans. The simplex viruses can cause lifelong genital infections, and despite the prevalence of HSV-1 and HSV-2 infections in the United States decreasing in the past 20 years, infections with these viruses continue to contribute to significant clinical and psychological morbidities.

Vaccine Hesitancy in Pediatrics

Andrea Lafnitzegger and Claudia Gaviria-Agudelo

Vaccine hesitancy is a growing complex and multifaceted phenomenon. It encompasses a wide spectrum of context-dependent attitudes and beliefs. Multiple factors influence parental decision-making including knowledge, sources of information, risk perception, trust, and individual experiences among others. This review focuses on describing the most common reasons that contribute to vaccine hesitancy among parents. Social media and the Internet have been described as major elements that can negatively influence parental decision-making regarding vaccines. The next focus is describing effective interventions that clinical providers can apply.

Nonconfrontational and open discussions along with trusting and strong relationships between parents and providers seem to create a solid foundation toward vaccine acceptance. In addition, motivational interviewing is a helpful tool that has proven to be effective during these discussions. Ultimately, an individualized approach tailored to a specific community will likely be most effective in addressing vaccine hesitancy.

Turner Syndrome: An Update
Margaret Steiner and Paul Saenger

Turner syndrome is the most common sex chromosome abnormality in women. Infertility and short stature are the most striking findings seen in these patients. Unfortunately, many girls are still being diagnosed too late and therefore early diagnosis and treatment key. Turner syndrome affects many systems of the body; therefore, a comprehensive approach is key for therapeutic intervention.

Clinical Indications for Growth Hormone Therapy

Melinda Danowitz and Adda Grimberg

Growth hormone (GH) is an injectable medication originally used to replace the deficiency of the hormone, but has expanded to treating conditions that may reduce growth and adult height even when the body maintains endogenous GH production. In the United States, there are 8 Food and Drug Administration (FDA)-approved indications for pediatric GH therapy: GH deficiency, Prader–Willi Syndrome, small for gestational age (SGA) without catch-up growth, idiopathic short stature, Turner syndrome, *SHOX* gene haploinsufficiency, Noonan Syndrome, and chronic renal insufficiency. We characterize the growth patterns and effects of GH treatment in each of these indications. We also review patterns of growth that warrant referral to a pediatric endocrinologist, as well as safety updates. This review is intended to guide practitioners on the initial evaluation and management of patients with short stature, and the indications for GH therapy.

Update on Pediatric Hyperthyroidism

Priya Vaidyanathan

Typical symptoms which should lead to suspicion of hyperthyroidism are unintentional weight loss, tachycardia, and palpitations, heat intolerance, and hyperactivity. It is diagnosed by suppressed thyroid-stimulating hormone (TSH) with elevated thyroid hormone (TH) levels. Graves' disease (GD) due to antibodies stimulating the TSH receptor is the leading cause, and first-line treatment is with methimazole (MMI). Emerging data suggest MMI treatment, up to 8 years is effective and safe in improving the rate of remission. Radioactive iodine (RAI) and thyroidectomy offer definitive treatment and induce permanent hypothyroidism. Thyroid storm is a life-threatening condition with systemic decompensation and hyperpyrexia. Neonates of mothers with current or past GD are at risk for neonatal hyperthyroidism (NH). Appropriate identification and follow-up of at-risk neonates will reduce complications.

Updates on the Management of Pilonidal Disease
Amelia T. Collings and Beth Rymeski

This article reviews the current practices and evidence on the management of pilonidal disease in the pediatric population. Medical management, use of laser epilation, and minimally invasive surgical options are highlighted with a brief review of more invasive surgical options for refractory disease.

Current Management of Adhesive Small Bowel Obstructions in Children
Nathan S. Rubalcava and K. Elizabeth Speck

Adhesive small bowel obstructions are a common cause of morbidity in children who underwent prior abdominal surgery. The concept of partial versus complete bowel obstruction is outdated and lacks precision to be clinically useful. Identifying patients with indications for immediate operative intervention is critical and must be recognized to limit morbidity. Clinical protocols and contrast challenge algorithms have attempted to identify patients that will resolve their bowel obstruction nonoperatively; there has been slow uptake in the pediatric patient population versus adults until recently. Incorporating predictive models and standardized contrast challenge protocols will help reduce interpractitioner variability and improve clinical outcomes.

Postoperative Opioid Prescribing, Use, and Disposal in Children

Marjorie Odegard and Lorraine I. Kelley-Quon

This article provides an overview of postoperative opioid prescribing, use, and disposal patterns in children and also identifies gaps in knowledge and areas for improvement. We present evidence that there is a need to tailor prescriptions to specific procedures to reduce the number of excess, unused prescription opioid pills in the home. We also explain the need to provide culturally competent care when managing a child's pain after surgery. Finally, we discuss the need for widespread provider and caregiver education about safe prescription opioid use, storage, and disposal.

Advances in Pediatrics 69 (2022) xxv–xxvii
ADVANCES IN PEDIATRICS

PREFACE

Emerging from the Pandemic: Taking Up Where We Left Off with Newer Modalities, Assessment, and Treatment

Carol D. Berkowitz, MD

During the past year, COVID-19 continued to be a prominent topic for lectures, conferences, and webinars. The medical environment was transformed into a virtual arena, where audiences were able to hear speakers from around the nation without their need to travel. Resident and fellow recruitment also became virtual, leading to increased numbers of applicants, some of whom had limited clinical opportunities during medical school. Even in-person patient contact dropped, especially initially, and telemedicine replaced the in-person visit. Increasingly sophisticated virtual medical encounters continue to be offered, using video interviews. We now face new challenges, including the need for evidence-based guidelines and concerns about equity, where computer and internet access may be marginal. Many children were taught virtually, which was particularly challenging for children with special needs. The absence of in-person visits impacted the ability of physicians to do developmental screening and assess for autism. Therapeutic services for autistic children were severely impacted. Overall approaches to disruptive behaviors in children by "HOT DOC" (Helping Our Toddlers, Developing Our Children's Skills), a community-based group invention, was less accessible during the pandemic. The program was successfully taught to pediatric residents, providing them with practical training to help families. Among other children with special health care needs are deaf or hard of hearing (DHH [the preferred terminology]) individuals. Public awareness of the deaf culture was showcased by the academy award-winning movie "CODA" (Children of Deaf Adults).

While there has been a plethora of new drugs to treat epilepsy, some children remain drug-resistant, and brain surgery provides a reduced seizure burden and increased quality of life. Early referral to a pediatric epilepsy center is recommended as a means to reduce the risk of a secondary epileptic focus. Chronic sinusitis and obstructive sleep apnea (OSA) each involve both medical and surgical management. If chronic sinusitis persists after nasal irrigation, nasal or systemic steroids and/or antibiotics, adenoidectomy, and FESS

https://doi.org/10.1016/j.yapd.2022.05.001
0065-3101/22/© 2022 Published by Elsevier Inc.

(functional endoscopic sinus surgery) need to be considered. The Childhood Adenotonsillectomy Trial reported that adenotonsillectomy (T and A) had a beneficial effect on OSA, but there are times when OSA is not relieved by a T and A, and other anatomical findings, such as craniofacial anomalies, have to be considered.

Chronic childhood diseases are a testimony to improved care so that children grow into adolescents and adulthood. Antiphospholipid syndrome is a rare pediatric disorder that may be life-threatening. While the symptoms are suggestive of lupus, any child with thrombosis should be screened for antiphospholipid syndrome. Managing children with advanced stage kidney disease has improved the longevity and quality of life of these children. Like other chronic conditions, these children are best managed by a multidisciplinary team that also manages the comorbid conditions, including bone disease, anemia, growth failure, and psychosocial issues. Hemophilia A is an inherited insufficiency of Factor VIII and is sometimes referred to as the "Royal Disease." Queen Victoria was a carrier, and the condition was thought to contribute to the Russian Revolution of 1917. Replacement factor and newer therapeutic options, including emicizumab, a biphasic monoclonal antibody, could have changed the course of history had they been available back then!

Ultimately, the ability of children to return to in-person school was assisted by the development of COVID-19 vaccines and the eventual approval the vaccine for children older than 5 years. As with other vaccines, there was vaccine hesitancy, with some parents choosing not to vaccinate their children often based on misinformation that was in the media. The issue of vaccine hesitancy was addressed by the World Health Organization, who convened a working group in 2012. In the absence of in-person visits, many children fell behind on their immunizations. With the return to in-person visits, this gap is still being filled. It is hoped we will not see a resurgence of some of the diseases that vaccines had virtually eliminated, such as polio and measles. Unfortunately, there is not a vaccine for all diseases, and genital herpes simplex virus (HSV) is still a problem, especially for pregnant women and their newborn infants. Fortunately, there are nucleoside analogues that reduce the frequency and severity of primary and episodic HSV infection.

Short statue has always been high on the list of conditions that pediatricians manage. While short statue is a frequent component of Turner syndrome, it has become apparent that the spectrum of Turner syndrome is much broader than the classic image of the short girl with primary amenorrhea and a shield-like chest. In fact, a retrospective study of 522 women with Turner syndrome reported that 16% had spontaneous menarche and 3 had become pregnant. Growth hormone is part of the management of Turner syndrome as well as a host of other entities, such as Prader-Willi syndrome, Noonan syndrome, and chronic renal insufficiency. Just as the use of growth hormone has advanced, the treatment of hyperthyroidism has also changed, with methimazole being first-line therapy, and the use of methimazole for up to 8 years in children is associated with remission. Pilonidal cysts are best managed by a minimally invasive approach, including an endoscopic procedure with removal of pits and sinuses. While one always expects that surgery is needed in all cases of small bowel obstructions, the advice now is to distinguish between those requiring urgent surgical management and those who qualify for initial nonoperative care. When operative management is critical, postoperative care is equally important. Pain management in children is just as important as in adults and requires the same level of attention and expertise. Physicians should be cognizant of unconscious bias in pain management strategies when caring for minority children and their families. Opiates may not be used by families after discharge, and families need to be advised about safe storage and disposal.

Though it may feel as though time has stood still for the past 2½ years, newer treatments, approaches, and management have continued during this time. *Advances in Pediatrics* remains in the forefront of bringing together a wide range of topics with which pediatricians deal on a daily basis, virtually or in-person.

Carol D. Berkowitz, MD
Division of General Pediatrics
Department of Pediatrics
Harbor-University of California
Los Angeles Medical Center
David Geffen School of Medicine at UCLA
1000 West Carson Street
Torrance, CA 90509, USA

E-mail address: Cberkowitz52@gmail.com

Advances in Pediatrics 69 (2022) 1–11

ADVANCES IN PEDIATRICS

Pediatric Telemedicine

Lessons Learned During the Coronavirus Disease 2019 Pandemic and Opportunities for Growth

Sarah C. Haynes, PhD, MPH*, James P. Marcin, MD, MPH

Department of Pediatrics, UC Davis School of Medicine, UC Davis Center for Health and Technology, 4610 X Street, Suite 2300, Sacramento, CA 95817, USA

Keywords

• Telemedicine • Telehealth • Virtual visits • Video visits • Pediatrics

Key points

- Educational resources that incorporate the most recent evidence on pediatric telemedicine care are needed to promote consistency across providers, increase provider confidence, and improve quality of care.
- Patient-generated data, including remote patient monitoring, could improve the quality of virtual visits, but issues with measurement quality and parent self-efficacy must be addressed.
- Rigorous studies examining specific practices within telemedicine delivery and use are needed to develop evidence-based guidelines around virtual care for pediatric conditions.
- A focus on equity is essential for ensuring that telemedicine interventions do not widen health disparities.

INTRODUCTION

The coronavirus disease 2019 (COVID-19) pandemic has resulted in a dramatic and rapid increase in the adoption and implementation of telemedicine services, including in pediatrics [1–4]. Many pediatric providers that previously had not offered telemedicine services quickly adopted telemedicine and have continued to provide services well after the start of the pandemic. This shift presents opportunities to expand our understanding of the impact of telemedicine on access to care, quality of care, and health care costs on a broader scale.

*Corresponding author. *E-mail address:* shaynes@ucdavis.edu

https://doi.org/10.1016/j.yapd.2022.04.002
0065-3101/22/

The pandemic has changed the way that patients and caregivers, providers, and health systems think about telemedicine. A prepandemic review of the pediatric telemedicine landscape identified licensing requirements, provider interest, lack of resources to train providers, and reimbursement issues as the main challenges facing pediatric telemedicine programs [5]. The Public Health Emergency forced the resolution of many of these challenges, making telemedicine a necessary part of patient care as shelter-in-place orders and other infection prevention measures discouraged in-person encounters. Given that telemedicine will remain a mainstay of pediatric care, the field now faces the challenge of improving the delivery of telemedicine for pediatric patients to ensure that all patients have access to high-quality care [3]. Identifying evidence-based practices and understanding how these practices can be implemented and scaled are the next steps toward meeting this challenge.

Since the start of the pandemic in spring 2020, new research has been published, providing insights into promising practices for pediatric telemedicine, adoption by parents and providers, and barriers and facilitators to telemedicine use. These studies bring to the field great diversity in terms of patients, providers, settings, and specialties; they use larger amounts of data than were possible to collect prepandemic and are pragmatic, based in real-world settings. Understanding the lessons learned is important for optimizing telemedicine delivery going forward. With this in mind, the objectives of this review are to (1) summarize recent evidence on the delivery of telemedicine for pediatric patients with an emphasis on lessons learned during the pandemic and (2) highlight opportunities in telemedicine delivery and research.

MODELS OF CARE WITHIN PEDIATRIC TELEMEDICINE

Telemedicine encompasses several different models of technology-enabled health care services:

- "Provider-to-provider" telemedicine services allow communication between 2 providers (with or without the patient) and typically involve consultations in real time over video with pediatric subspecialists to primary care providers practicing in communities where specialists may not be available [6,7]. Before the pandemic, these types of consultations had been used for many pediatric subspecialists including cardiology, ophthalmology, nephrology, dermatology, neurology, endocrinology, and emergency medicine [8].
- Provider-to-patient telemedicine services or virtual visits allow for direct encounters over real-time video from the providers to the patient or family, often in the convenience of their homes. This model of care has seen the greatest increase in use since the beginning of the pandemic [3].
- School-based telemedicine services allow children to receive care through telemedicine at their local school while in the presence of a school nurse or other school personnel. School-based telemedicine services have been used widely for asthma care [9] and mental health care [10] and have recently been tested for pediatric physiatry [11] and treatment of attention-deficit/hyperactivity disorder [12].

- Remote patient monitoring, remote physiologic monitoring, or more simply, telemonitoring involves the monitoring of patient-generated data. These programs have been used in pediatrics primarily for management of type 1 diabetes [13,14] and asthma [15,16] and monitoring of congenital heart disease and cardiovascular implantable devices [13].

For the purposes of this review, the focus is on the most common use of telemedicine in pediatric care, virtual visits, and recently emerging evidence around this model of care.

LESSONS LEARNED

The accelerated uptake of telemedicine during the pandemic has resulted in valuable experience and evidence on the delivery of telemedicine for pediatric patients. Here the focus is on the lessons learned in 4 main areas: education and training, developing and adapting clinical workflows, patient assessment and treatment, and family-centered care.

Education and training

Education and training in telemedicine is important for improving pediatric providers' acceptance of and comfort with virtual visits [17]. Telemedicine-specific training may also improve the quality of the visits and increase the experience of the encounters for providers, patients, and families [3]. In addition to training focused on delivering care over video, site-specific training around telemedicine workflows and processes is necessary for ensuring comprehensive and compliant documentation.

Training tools for telemedicine, including toolkits, webinars, and learning modules, can be used to improve adoption and implementation of telemedicine. The development and use of online educational modules was one strategy adopted during the pandemic to rapidly train providers. These modules are mandatory in some clinics and/or health systems and train providers on how to interface with the electronic health record during telemedicine visits, how to optimize sound and lighting, and how to best engage patients, for example, by adjusting the computer to simulate eye contact [18]. Tutorials have also been used for onboarding new providers, including educational materials on navigating the telemedicine software, supporting documentation, and outlining compliance and billing requirements [2]. Such training modules have also been required by medical staff offices for physician privileging purposes. Tip sheets are another useful tool that can help providers maintain professional, consistent, high-quality care [3,19]. These sheets may include strategies for optimizing audio and visual quality, assessing patients over video, documenting the visit, and billing. Training resources for pediatric telehealth continue to be developed, including by the American Academy of Pediatrics [3].

The appointment of official telemedicine "champions" within a clinic is another strategy that has been used to improve both telemedicine adoption and training among providers [2]. It has been well documented that physician champions can help change attitudes among their peers, influencing the success of implementation and increasing the likelihood of sustainability. Champions can also act as peer educators, improving the skills and confidence of other providers, and have been used for one-on-one trainings to support other providers as practices transitioned to telemedicine during the pandemic [18]. Having a designated peer to answer questions and provide resources as needed can make providers feel supported. The presence of a provider telemedicine champion can also be an effective strategy for introducing new information on evidence-based practices, processes, and policies.

Medical education is an area in which high-quality telemedicine training is especially relevant. Incorporating telemedicine into the formal curriculum will improve the delivery of virtual visits and increase confidence. Despite the fact that trainees in all specialties are frequently seeing patients over telemedicine, fewer than 50% of pediatric training programs report having a formalized telemedicine curriculum and formal curricula that do exist are rated low in overall adequacy [20]. Recently, the American Association of Medical Colleges released a list of telehealth competencies relevant to medical education for physicians upon entry into residency or practice, and for experienced faculty physicians postresidency [21]. These competencies are organized across the following 6 domains:

- Patient safety and appropriate use of telehealth
- Access and equity in telehealth
- Communication via telehealth
- Data collection and assessment via telehealth
- Technology for telehealth
- Ethical practices and legal requirements for telehealth

Although these competencies add to emerging areas to help guide curricular and professional development, performance assessment, and cross-continuum collaborations, there remain opportunities to further develop curricula that incorporate evidence-based practices that add value to patients, providers, and payors. To this end, medical education, training programs, and ongoing continuing professional education should remain current and incorporate new clinical information on best practices as it becomes available.

Developing and adapting clinical workflows

The accelerated uptake of telemedicine during the pandemic also necessitated rapid adaptations to clinical workflows. Clinics and providers were forced to triage patients to determine whether an in-person visit was necessary or if a virtual visit would be appropriate. Oftentimes, this triage would occur over a virtual visit [18,22]. Some providers and clinic offices created specific, well-defined guidelines for determining whether a patient should receive an in-person or telemedicine visit [18,22]. Often, the determination as to whether the encounter/visit could be done by telemedicine depended on the provider specialty, the patient diagnosis, or the urgency of the referral or medical condition. Others also described approaches that considered personal preferences, such as at the request of the provider or the patient [23,24].

Scheduling telemedicine visits also required workflow changes for many clinics. Scheduling systems were updated to accommodate video visits and schedulers adopted additional roles as telemedicine coordinators or navigators, helping patients to schedule, test electronic access, and participate in virtual visits. For example, navigators were often tasked with obtaining consent for the encounter, explaining to each patient how to connect to the telemedicine platform and assessing their technological capacity to successfully conduct the visit, and describing the benefits and risks of virtual visits to patients [18]. These processes often caused confusion as some parents reported missed telemedicine visits because they forgot to schedule follow-up visits, which were previously scheduled by going to the front desk at the end of an in-person visit [23]. Thus, integrating scheduling and support into the telemedicine workflow can prevent delays in care caused by scheduling and technical issues.

Providing team-based care over telemedicine poses additional challenges and also requires thoughtful changes in operations and clinical workflows. To continue providing team-based care, many provider teams developed systems that would allow all members of the usual in-person team to be present during the video visit [25]. This included virtual "rooming" by the medical assistant or nurse, who would take the patient's history, review medications, and begin visit documentation. Despite the operational and technical challenges, telemedicine shows promise for improving care coordination for children, especially those with chronic disease [26]. By allowing more members of the patient's care team to be present, including family members or distant caregivers, virtual visit telemedicine encounters could help to improve the shared decision-making process. Such encounters could include team members who may not typically join a patient's visit with a physician, such as pharmacists, physical or occupational therapists, and providers, such as a primary care provider [27,28]. Practicing virtual visits with all members of the caregiver team may help to improve the quality of these visits [25].

Assessment and treatment

The inability to conduct a comprehensive physical examination has been frequently cited by both providers and caregivers as another disadvantage of virtual visits. Despite this, during the pandemic, providers found new ways to assess patients over video, many of which have been published [18,29]. For primary care and nonurgent conditions, a review of pediatric musculoskeletal teleassessments found that minimizing background noise and distractions, gathering items the child can use to demonstrate fine motor skills, ensuring the child is dressed in comfortable clothing, and preparing children for what to expect can help to facilitate an effective examination [30]. Other published studies found virtual examinations to be effective for diagnosing and treating common musculoskeletal conditions [29]. Eye examinations have also been conducted virtually during the pandemic for children, relying on parents to position their child's eye in the camera [22]. Training caregivers to conduct physical examinations may improve the quality of examinations; tools such as dolls, cards, and checklists could help to facilitate effective and efficient virtual visits [25,29,31].

In addition to providing routine, scheduled visits to children with chronic health conditions, virtual visits have been increasingly used during the pandemic for the diagnosis and treatment of acute conditions such as upper and lower respiratory tract infections [8,32]. One large study of 47 primary care practices found high concordance with antibiotic-prescribing guidelines for children with acute respiratory tract infections assessed over telemedicine when encounters occurred within the medical home [32]. However, there is evidence that when third-party clinical services are used outside the medical home, guideline-concordant antibiotic management for respiratory infections is lower compared with in-person visits with children's primary care provider [33]. Other studies also found acceptable concordance with guideline-based care for the assessment and treatment of children with behavior health and externalizing disorders, including attention and disruptive behavior problems [34]. Importantly, telemedicine can also be used to facilitate COVID-19 screening, diagnosis, and monitoring from home [35].

Patient-generated data for the purposes of remote physiologic monitoring can also help to support virtual visits by providing information that is typically collected in person. For example, home spirometry and peak flow meters can help to provide an idea of a patient's lung function between in-office spirometry measurements for patients with asthma [36,37]. Patients with diabetes mellitus commonly use devices such as insulin pumps, smart pens, and continuous glucose monitors, which provide data directly to providers that can be discussed during a virtual visit [38,39]. However, some research has shown that increased home monitoring may not result in improved outcomes and may even increase health care utilization given the closer monitoring and more convenient access to care [40]. In addition, although patient-generated measurements have the potential to increase the provider confidence and support a shift to alternating or supplementing in-person and telemedicine visits, parents may have low self-efficacy with regard to home measurements [23,31]. Thus, appropriate training of caregivers and better evidence are necessary to ensure successful use of home monitoring devices and a positive caregiver experience.

Family-centered care

It is increasingly recognized that telemedicine can be used to promote family-centered care [41], defined as a partnership approach to decision making between the family and the provider [42]. [43]. For children with complex medical needs, telemedicine has been shown to reduce care days outside of the home, serious illness, and health care costs [44], as well as improve a family's sense of security [45,46]. The use of telemedicine for postsurgical and palliative care is also promising, resulting in lower anxiety for parents and enhanced communication between providers and families [43,47].

During the pandemic, telemedicine was leveraged to provide family-centered care for hospitalized children [41,48]. When restrictions on physical presence were in place, family-centered rounds using telemedicine in the neonatal intensive care unit (NICU), pediatric intensive care unit (PICU), and inpatient ward allowed families and caregivers to be actively engaged in their child's care [29,49,50]. In the settings of both inpatient and outpatient care, telemedicine allows both parents (and other caregivers and family members) to be present. This can result in improved parent/caregiver experience [23] and may have larger implications for the child's care long term.

The accelerated move to video visits has also given providers an opportunity to see pediatric patients in their home environments, which may lead to a deeper understanding of the social and environmental factors that may be affecting the child. This unique and personal experience can help to provide more personalized care. However, providers should be cognizant of any potential negative impacts. For example, some adolescents may feel uneasy discussing sensitive topics while at home, which could lead to limited or inaccurate responses [4,51,52]. Future research should explore how this aspect of virtual visits can bring value to pediatric care while ensuring confidentiality when needed.

OPPORTUNITIES

The rapid adoption of telemedicine during the pandemic has highlighted the limitations of current technologies, workflows, and knowledge related to the delivery of telemedicine for pediatric patients. Key opportunities for growth exist in the areas of engaging pediatric patients, improving and measuring access to care, addressing health equity, and expanding the evidence base.

Improving engagement with pediatric patients

Research has consistently found that adult patients are generally satisfied with physicians' ability to develop rapport and communicate effectively over telemedicine [53,54]. However, engaging with pediatric patients over video may be more challenging, particularly for children who are introverted or who lack communication skills [23]. This challenge may be exacerbated by a virtual encounter with a new provider who has never met the child in person [23]. Strategies and resources that aid providers in developing therapeutic alliance with patients could enhance virtual visits by increasing trust, improving patient and parent experience, and encouraging better communication by pediatric patients.

Improving and measuring access to care

Telemedicine has long been recognized as a potential strategy to improve access to care, particularly for rural populations; this is especially true for children requiring pediatric subspecialty care because pediatric subspecialists are often scarce and concentrated at urban academic medical centers. Although it is widely accepted that telemedicine can reduce burdens on families related to travel and missed school and work days [26], the magnitude of this impact has not been quantified. In fact, during this pandemic, large-scale analyses on administrative data show that rural populations are less likely to use telemedicine with their provider [55]. It is likely that there are subgroups of patients for whom the availability of telemedicine could significantly impact health care utilization and ultimately, patient outcomes. Identifying these subgroups could help to target specific patients who could benefit most from telemedicine services.

Addressing health equity

There is concern that a shift to telemedicine use could lead to widening health disparities by improving access to care for those who already experience relatively lower burdens and better outcomes [56–58]. It is increasingly recognized that unless there is a specific focus on equity, interventions are likely to be implemented in a way that benefits those who already have relative advantages [59]. Identifying specific practices that promote equity within the delivery of telemedicine is important for developing evidence-based recommendations for best practices. Interventions that target patients less likely to access telemedicine could significantly contribute to health equity.

Expanding the evidence base for pediatric telemedicine

Telemedicine has often been tested as a single component (eg, telemedicine vs in-person care) despite the fact that it is a complex intervention comprising a set of processes. Examining specific practices within the delivery of telemedicine for each condition is necessary for developing a set of best practices. Understanding the essential "core components" of pediatric virtual care for a specific condition can help to create standards of care that could be thoughtfully and intentionally adapted for different local contexts. Dissemination and implementation science approaches are particularly relevant to telemedicine interventions but have been underutilized. Rigorous studies on the implementation of telemedicine, including how programs can be adapted to meet the needs of patients in different local contexts, are necessary for advancing the field.

SUMMARY

Despite an abundance of recent studies describing increased telemedicine use, there remain important gaps in the field. Opportunities exist to better understand telemedicine's role in education and training; how to best optimize clinical workflows, where telemedicine can improve patient assessment and treatment, and how telemedicine can be best used to support family-centered care. Educational resources that incorporate the most recent evidence on pediatric telemedicine care are needed. The availability of these resources can promote consistency across providers in addition to improving provider confidence and quality of care. Special care should be taken to ensure that these resources can be updated as evidence changes in this rapidly growing field. Patient-generated data, including remote physiologic monitoring, could improve the quality of virtual visits, but issues with measurement quality and parent self-efficacy must be addressed. Rigorous studies examining specific practices within telemedicine delivery and use are needed to develop evidence-based guidelines around virtual care for pediatric conditions. Implementation science methods and frameworks could be applied to identify and test these practices. Finally, a focus on equity is essential for ensuring that telemedicine interventions do not widen health disparities.

Disclosure

The authors have nothing to disclose.

References

[1] Bosworth A, Ruther J, Smason L, et al. Medicare beneficiary use of telehealth visits: early data from the start of the COVID-19 pandemic. Washington, DC: Office of the assistant secretary for planning and evaluation, US Department of Health and Human Services; 2020.
[2] Howie F, Kreofsky BL, Ravi A, et al. Rapid rise of pediatric telehealth during COVID-19 in a large multispecialty health system. Telemed J E Health 2022;28(1):3–10.
[3] Curfman A, McSwain SD, Chuo J, et al. Pediatric Telehealth in the COVID-19 Pandemic Era and Beyond. Pediatrics 2021;148(3):e2020047795.
[4] North S. Telemedicine in the time of COVID and beyond. J Adolesc Health 2020;67(2): 145.
[5] Olson CA, McSwain SD, Curfman AL, et al. The current pediatric telehealth landscape. Pediatrics 2018;141(3):e20172334.
[6] França UL, McManus ML. Availability of definitive hospital care for children. JAMA Pediatr 2017;171(9):e171096.
[7] França UL, McManus ML. Trends in regionalization of hospital care for common pediatric conditions. Pediatrics 2018;141(1):e20171940.
[8] Tomines A. Pediatric telehealth: Approaches by specialty and implications for general pediatric care. Adv Pediatr 2019;66:55–85.
[9] Kim CH, Lieng MK, Rylee TL, et al. School-based telemedicine interventions for asthma: a systematic review. Acad Pediatr 2020;20(7):893–901.
[10] Love H, Panchal N, Schlitt J, et al. The use of telehealth in school-based health centers. Glob Pediatr Health 2019;6:2333794X19884194.
[11] Davidson L, Haynes SC, Favila-Meza A, et al. Parent Experience and Cost Savings Associated with a Novel Tele-physiatry Program for Children Living in Rural and Underserved Communities. Arch Phys Med Rehabil 2021;103(1):8–13.
[12] Wenderlich AM, Li R, Baldwin CD, et al. A Quality Improvement Initiative to Improve ADHD Follow-up rates Using School-based Telemedicine. Acad Pediatr 2021;21(7):1253–61.
[13] Sasangohar F, Davis E, Kash BA, et al. Remote patient monitoring and telemedicine in neonatal and pediatric settings: Scoping literature review. J Med Internet Res 2018;20(12):e295.
[14] Kompala T, Neinstein AB. Telehealth in type 1 diabetes. Curr Opin Endocrinol Diabetes Obes 2021;28(1):21–9.
[15] MacGeorge, C.A., Andrews, A.L., King, K.L. (2021). Telehealth for Pediatric Asthma. In: Ford, D.W., Valenta, S.R. (eds) Telemedicine. Respiratory Medicine. Humana, Cham. https://doi.org/10.1007/978-3-030-64050-7_8.
[16] Davies B, Kenia P, Nagakumar P, et al. Paediatric and adolescent asthma: a narrative review of telemedicine and emerging technologies for the post-COVID-19 era. Clin Exp Allergy 2021;51(3):393–401.
[17] Costich M, Robbins-Milne L, Bracho-Sanchez E, et al. Design and implementation of an interactive, competency-based pilot pediatric telemedicine curriculum. Med Education Online 2021;26(1):1911019.
[18] Yang L, Brown-Johnson CG, Miller-Kuhlmann R, et al. Accelerated launch of video visits in ambulatory neurology during COVID-19: Key lessons from the Stanford experience. Neurology 2020;95(7):305–11.

[19] Contreras CM, Metzger GA, Beane JD, et al. Telemedicine: patient-provider clinical engagement during the COVID-19 pandemic and beyond. J Gastrointest Surg 2020;24(7):1692–7.
[20] Fitzgerald M, Bhatt A, Thompson LA, et al. Telemedicine in pediatric training: a national needs assessment of the current state of telemedicine education in pediatric training. Acad Pediatr 2021.
[21] Association of American Medical Colleges. Telehealth competencies. 2021. Available at: https://www.aamc.org/data-reports/report/telehealth-competencies. Accessed November 24, 2021.
[22] Kapoor S, Eldib A, Hiasat J, et al. Developing a pediatric ophthalmology telemedicine program in the COVID-19 crisis. J Am Assoc Pediatr Ophthalmol Strabismus 2020;24(4): 204–208 e202.
[23] Haynes SC, Kamerman-Kretzmer RJ, Khan SS, et al. Telemedicine use for pediatric asthma care: a mixed methods study. J Asthma 2022.
[24] Haynes SC, Kompala T, Tancredi DJ, et al. Factors associated with discontinuation of subspecialty diabetes care during the COVID-19 pandemic: a multi-site retrospective cohort study. Diabetes Care 2022;45(2):e34–6.
[25] Sinsky CA, Jerzak JT, Hopkins KD. Telemedicine and Team-Based Care: The Perils and the Promise. Mayo Clinic Proceedings. 96:2 (2021): 429-437.
[26] Fiks AG, Jenssen BP, Ray KN. A defining moment for pediatric primary care telehealth. JAMA Pediatr 2021;175(1):9–10.
[27] Griffith ML, Siminerio L, Payne T, et al. A shared decision-making approach to telemedicine: engaging rural patients in glycemic management. J Clin Med 2016;5(11):103.
[28] Murry LT, Kennelty K. Opportunity for pharmacists in telehealth, team-based care: clinical inertia. Telemed J E-Health 2020;26(10):1199–201.
[29] Tanaka MJ, Oh LS, Martin SD, et al. Telemedicine in the era of COVID-19: the virtual orthopaedic examination. J Bone Joint Surg Am 2020.
[30] Noutsios CD, Boisvert-Plante V, Laberge E, et al. The telemedicine-based pediatric examination of the back and lower limbs: a narrative review. J Pain Res 2021;14:2959.
[31] Belcher RH, Phillips J, Virgin F, et al. Pediatric otolaryngology telehealth in response to COVID-19 pandemic: lessons learned and impact on the future management of pediatric patients. Ann Otol Rhinol Laryngol 2021;130(7):788–95.
[32] Ray KN, Martin JM, Wolfson D, et al. Antibiotic prescribing for acute respiratory tract infections during telemedicine visits within a pediatric primary care network. Acad Pediatr 2021;21(7):1239–43.
[33] Ray KN, Shi Z, Gidengil CA, et al. Antibiotic prescribing during pediatric direct-to-consumer telemedicine visits. Pediatrics 2019;143(5):e20182491.
[34] Ros-DeMarize R, ChungMD P, StewartPhD R. Pediatric behavioral telehealth in the age of COVID-19: Brief evidence review and practice considerations. Curr Probl Pediatr Adolesc Health Care 2021;51(1):100949.
[35] Lukas H, Xu C, Yu Y, et al. Emerging telemedicine tools for remote COVID-19 diagnosis, monitoring, and management. ACS Nano 2020;14(12):16180–93.
[36] Van Der Kamp MR, Tabak M, de Rooij SE, et al. COVID-19: technology-supported remote assessment of pediatric asthma at home. Front Pediatr 2020;8:529.
[37] Barreto M, Evangelisti M, Montesano M, et al. Pulmonary function testing in asthmatic children. Tests to assess outpatients during the Covid-19 pandemic. Front Pediatr 2020;8: 571112.
[38] Crossen S, Raymond J, Neinstein A. Top 10 tips for successfully implementing a diabetes telehealth program. Diabetes Technol Ther 2020;22(12):920–8.
[39] Crossen SS, Romero CC, Loomba LA, et al. Patient Perspectives on Use of Video Telemedicine for Type 1 Diabetes Care in the United States during the COVID-19 Pandemic. Endocrines 2021;2(4):449–56.

[40] Medoff Cooper B, Marino BS, Fleck DA, et al. Telehealth Home Monitoring and Postcardiac Surgery for Congenital Heart Disease. Pediatrics 2020;146(3).
[41] Hart JL, Turnbull AE, Oppenheim IM, et al. Family-centered care during the COVID-19 era. J Pain Symptom Manage 2020;60(2):e93–7.
[42] Neff JM, Eichner JM, Hardy DR, et al. Family-centered care and the pediatrician's role. Pediatrics 2003;112(3):691.
[43] Morgan GJ, Craig B, Grant B, et al. Home videoconferencing for patients with severe congenital heart disease following discharge. Congenit Heart Dis 2008;3(5):317–24.
[44] Mosquera RA, Avritscher EBC, Pedroza C, et al. Telemedicine for children with medical complexity: a randomized clinical trial. Pediatrics 2021;148(3):e2021050400.
[45] Young NL, Bennie J, Barden W, et al. An examination of quality of life of children and parents during their Tele-Homecare experience. Telemed J E-Health 2006;12(6):663–71.
[46] Young NL, Barden W, McKeever P, et al. Taking the call-bell home: a qualitative evaluation of Tele-HomeCare for children. Health Soc Care Community 2006;14(3):231–41.
[47] Bradford N, Armfield NR, Young J, et al. The case for home based telehealth in pediatric palliative care: a systematic review. BMC Palliat Care 2013;12(1):1–13.
[48] Rosenthal JL, Sauers-Ford HS, Williams J, et al. Virtual family-centered rounds in the neonatal intensive care unit: a randomized controlled pilot trial. Acad Pediat 2021;21(7):1244–52.
[49] Umoren RA, Gray MM, Handley S, et al. In-hospital telehealth supports care for neonatal patients in strict isolation. Am J Perinatol 2020;37(08):857–60.
[50] Yager PH. Remote parent participation in intensive care unit rounds. Pediatr Clin 2020;67(4):655–9.
[51] Sequeira GM, Kidd KM, Rankine J, et al. Gender-diverse youth's experiences and satisfaction with telemedicine for gender-affirming care during the COVID-19 pandemic. Transgender Health 2021.
[52] Barney A, Buckelew S, Mesheriakova V, et al. The COVID-19 pandemic and rapid implementation of adolescent and young adult telemedicine: challenges and opportunities for innovation. J Adolesc Health 2020;67(2):164–71.
[53] Agha Z, Schapira RM, Laud PW, et al. Patient satisfaction with physician–patient communication during telemedicine. Telemed J E-Health 2009;15(9):830–9.
[54] Donelan K, Barreto EA, Sossong S, et al. Patient and clinician experiences with telehealth for patient follow-up care. Am J Manag Care 2019;25(1):40–4.
[55] FAIR Health. Monthly telehealth regional tracker. 2021. Available at: https://www.fairhealth.org/states-by-the-numbers/telehealth. Accessed November 24, 2021.
[56] Eberly LA, Kallan MJ, Julien HM, et al. Patient characteristics associated with telemedicine access for primary and specialty ambulatory care during the COVID-19 pandemic. JAMA Netw open 2020;3(12):e2031640.
[57] Nouri S, Khoong EC, Lyles CR, et al. Addressing equity in telemedicine for chronic disease management during the Covid-19 pandemic. NEJM Catalyst Innov Care Deliv 2020;1(3).
[58] Bakhtiar M, Elbuluk N, Lipoff JB. The digital divide: how Covid-19's telemedicine expansion could exacerbate disparities. J Am Acad Dermatol 2020;83(5):e345–6.
[59] Brownson RC, Kumanyika SK, Kreuter MW, et al. Implementation science should give higher priority to health equity. Implementation Sci 2021;16(1):28.

Advances in Pediatrics 69 (2022) 13–21

ADVANCES IN PEDIATRICS

Helping Our Toddlers, Developing Our Children's Skills

Innovative Behavioral Management Training for Pediatric Residents

Heather Agazzi, PhD[a,*], Sarah Dickinson, PhD[a], Rebecca M. Plant, MD[b]

[a]Department of Pediatrics, University of South Florida, 13101 North Bruce B Downs Boulevard, CMS 2078, Tampa, FL 33612, USA; [b]University of South Florida, Department of Neurology, 2 Tampa General Circle, 5007 Tampa, FL 33606, USA

Keywords

• Development • Behavior • Childhood • Pediatrics • Resident

Key points

- Behavioral health concerns are commonly reported among caregivers in primary care pediatric visits.
- Most children have a pediatrician, making the primary care visits an ideal time to counsel caregivers on effective parenting strategies.
- Providing behavioral management training for resident pediatricians is critical to preventing long-term behavioral issues.
- Behavioral management training can be incorporated with success into pediatric residency without significant time burdens.

INTRODUCTION

Behavioral health concerns are common among young children in the United States and can be very challenging for their caregivers to manage [1,2]. Approximately 1 in 6 children aged 2 to 8 years are reported to have an emotional, behavioral, or developmental condition but only about half of them receive adequate mental health support [3]. Additionally, young children aged younger than 7 years with challenging behavior are at increased risk for maltreatment compared with older children [4]. Children with developmental disabilities

*Corresponding author. *E-mail address:* hcurtis@usf.edu

https://doi.org/10.1016/j.yapd.2022.03.007

are 1.5 to 3.5 times more likely to be maltreated than their typically developing peers [4]; often times, this is due to developmental behaviors that parents find overwhelming. Unaddressed behavioral health disorders early in childhood increase the risk for long-term poor outcomes including school failure, substance abuse, delinquency, chronic health problems, and suicide [5]. The negative outcomes associated with untreated challenging behaviors of early childhood reflect an important need for early prevention and intervention services.

Supporting caregivers is key to prevention and early intervention for child behavioral health concerns. Caregiver support for childhood mental health conditions also promotes maternal mental health and reduces the risk for maternal depression. There are many evidence-based programs with demonstrated success at improving child behavior problems, parenting stress, and parenting skills, but access to these behavioral health services is limited for many families [6]. Thus, embedding behavioral health resources into primary care settings is crucial to prevention, early detection, and treatment of mental, emotional, and behavioral disorders among children and adolescents. Optimal integrated health care involves screening children for developmental and behavioral concerns, coordinating appropriate care for children, and providing in-the-moment behavioral management training for caregivers.

More than 90% of children in the United States receive routine care in outpatient primary care settings. This setting offers an accessible and safe resource for families who have concerns about their child's behavior or development. Indeed, more than half of pediatric primary care visits include emotional, behavioral, psychological, or educational concerns [7]. Receiving mental health services in the primary care setting is particularly helpful for families who are economically disadvantaged and have limited access and/or utilization of mental health care. However, primary care providers have varying degrees of training in providing brief, evidence-based behavioral interventions and parenting strategies, and thus, may not feel confident in their abilities to manage these concerns [6].

The American Academy of Pediatrics developed a policy statement in 2009 on mental health competencies for pediatric primary care physicians [8]. Additionally, the American Board of Pediatrics published "Entrustable Professional Activities (EPA) 9," which describes the assessment and management of patients with common behavioral or mental health problems that graduating pediatric residents should be prepared to manage [9]. Specifically, EPA-9 notes pediatricians should be able to manage common social-emotional concerns in young children, including the coordination of community referrals and resources. Despite these policy statements, Rosenberg and colleagues (2011) surveyed graduates 5 years postgraduation and found that behavioral and developmental issues were among the top 3 weakest aspects of training for primary care pediatrics [10]. Since 2011, there have been improvements in the recognition and treatment of behavioral and mental health competencies during pediatric training but there is still much work to be done before most programs can reach general competency [11]. Providing behavioral management

Fig. 1. HOT DOCS information Web page.

training for resident pediatricians is key to this endeavor. McCormick et al. (2014) evaluated the effect of Primary Care Positive Parenting Program (Triple P) on pediatric resident practices and on parent self-efficacy, use of positive discipline strategies, and on child disruptive behaviors. Results suggested that training residents had a positive impact on their consultation skills and on parent disciplinary practices. This study adds strength to the call for increased resident training in behavior and development.

We describe an innovative training method that promotes resident knowledge of child development and behavioral management of common early childhood disruptive behaviors. Specifically, we adapted a 12-hour curriculum typically delivered during 6 consecutive weeks with caregivers of children into 2 condensed formats, in-person and virtual, for pediatric residents and combined medicine-pediatric residents at a large academic medical center in the southeast United States. We describe the development of this training experience and present data regarding changes in resident knowledge of child development and behavioral management techniques.

GENERAL CONTENT

Program development

Helping Our Toddlers, Developing Our Children's Skills (HOT DOCS; [12]) is a behavioral parent-training program for caregivers of children with disruptive behaviors and professionals who deliver behavioral health services to children aged from birth to 5 years (Fig. 1 for quick response (QR) code link to HOT DOCS web page). HOT DOCS is a group intervention that occurs during 6 weekly 2-hour sessions and is offered in-person in community settings as well as virtually [13]. After participation in HOT DOCS, caregiver participants have reported decreases in parenting stress and child disruptive behaviors, increases in knowledge of effective strategies, and high satisfaction with the program [13–15]. Community allied health professionals (eg, nurses, physicians, speech-language pathologists, social workers, and so forth) who have completed HOT DOCS reported satisfaction with the program and gains in knowledge of early childhood disruptive behaviors and effective behavior management strategies [16]. As such, we adapted the traditional delivery of HOT DOCS to a condensed training for pediatric residents delivered in a 3-hour training focused on practical information and resources for physicians to share with caregivers during primary care visits. This condensed training is offered to residents annually, and most residents attended at least one of these sessions during their busy training years. These trainings are typically offered in the evening at a local restaurant or a faculty member's home and include a meal. Alternatively, the condensed training can easily be taught during protected educational time such as academic half day or noon conferences. The condensed training focuses on high-frequency behavioral and social-emotional concerns presenting in primary care such as managing noncompliance, temper tantrums, addressing feeding and sleeping routines, and transitioning between daytime and nighttime routines (eg, stopping play to take a bath). The trainings include a didactic lecture, group activities including a case study problem-solving activity, and a HOT DOCS Trainer Manual with associated caregiver materials and handouts.

When COVID-19 disrupted in-person group meetings, the HOT DOCS program was swiftly adapted to 6 webinar recordings that residents completed on their month-long rotation in development and behavior. The recordings include a review of the didactic content that is used in the group-delivered program by a HOT DOCS Professional Trainer. In-person, group-based activities are modified for webinars such that the trainer walks through a scenario of a child engaging in challenging behavior and then prompts participants with probing questions (eg, "How did the caregiver react to the child when the child ran away from the dinner table?") to teach the steps to problem-solve the scenario. This model supported a swift transition to virtual learning with the onset of the global pandemic and ensured continued learning experiences via asynchronous webinars relevant to the development and behavior rotation while protecting resident health.

Research

We conducted 2 studies to measure the value of delivering the HOT DOCS program to pediatric residents using 2 different modalities: in-person and virtual. Both studies were approved by the University of South Florida Institutional Review Board for the Protection of Human Subjects. In both studies, we collected pretest and posttest data of knowledge, and collected follow-up data on the clinical utility of the programs as described below.

Modality 1

Description of modality 1. Residents received the content of the HOT DOCS program in person as a 3-hour lecture as described above. Residents were taught several fundamental characteristics of social learning and behavior theory associated with behavior change. Residents first learned how to problem-solve behaviors to determine the function, or motivation, of the behavior (to "get something" or "get out of something"). Residents then learned how to respond to behaviors in a functionally appropriate way by developing preventions, teaching children new skills, and identifying new caregiver responses to problem behaviors. Some examples of preventions included the following:

- Helping children make choices
- Teaching caregivers to deliver effective commands
- Engaging in special play time daily
- Making a "busy bag" to occupy a child during outings where disruptive behaviors are expected.

Residents also learned how to teach children new skills, which involved the following:

1. Breaking down the steps of a desired behavior
2. Teaching the behavior explicitly
3. Modeling how to engage in the behavior
4. Reinforcing successive approximations toward the desired skill.

Finally, residents were taught how to use appropriate responses to challenging behaviors such as:

- Planned ignoring
- Redirection
- Hand-over-hand follow through, a technique that promotes compliance with direct commands by offering physical assistance to the child.

Participants and method. Twenty-four residents in various stages of training in pediatrics and medicine-pediatrics attended a 3-hour workshop hosted in a local restaurant (7 residents in first year; 5 in second year; and 9 in third and fourth years). The program was offered to all pediatric (36) and combined Medicine-Pediatric (20) trainees; participation was voluntary. Each resident completed the HOT DOCS Knowledge Test [17] before the workshop and again at the conclusion of the workshop. The HOT DOCS Knowledge Test is a 15-item test that assesses knowledge of behavioral theory, effective behavior management techniques, and general knowledge of child development milestones.

The HOT DOCS Knowledge Test has demonstrated adequate reliability with Cronbach's alpha = .78. Pretest to posttest changes in knowledge were analyzed using a paired samples *t*-test. In addition, residents were contacted at 1-year follow-up to complete a brief survey about the utility of HOT DOCS to their clinical practice. The 1-year follow-up survey was analyzed using descriptive statistics.

Results. Average scores on the HOT DOCS Knowledge Test at pretest were 80.9% (SD = 9.4), whereas average scores at posttest were 95%, revealing significant improvement in knowledge (SD = 6.2; $P < .001$). Further, 88% of residents' scores improved from pretest to posttest (scores for the remaining 12% did not change).

A total of 12 residents completed the 1-year follow-up survey and 100% of residents reported they regularly use skills taught in the HOT DOCS course in their day-to-day pediatric primary care practices. Most residents agreed or strongly agreed that their behavioral counseling skills improved after they participated in the training program, and they regularly use HOT DOCS skills in their day-to-day practice in pediatric primary care. Residents overall reported increased use of evidence-based behavior management techniques following participation in HOT DOCS.

MODALITY 2

Description of modality 2. Residents received the full content of the HOT DOCS program via 6 webinar recordings of the traditional group-delivered model. Similar to modality 1, residents were taught fundamental characteristics of social learning and behavior theory and how to determine the function of behavior (to "get something" or "get out of something"). Residents then learned how to respond to behaviors in a functionally appropriate way by developing preventions, teaching new skills, and identifying new responses to problem behaviors. These recordings did not involve live interactions with a HOT DOCS Professional Trainer.

At the start of their rotation, residents received a schedule with the HOT DOCS webinars embedded across 2 half-day sessions. The webinars required about 6 hours to complete, and residents were asked to take the same Knowledge Test described above via Qualtrics link before starting the webinars and on completion. This model requires 1 day to finish and can be completed virtually from the resident's home because the webinars are housed on a Panopto platform through the university server. All links to the webinars and the pretest are assigned to the residents on their monthly schedule, and on completion of the final webinar, residents contact internal staff to receive a link to the posttest.

Participants and method. Twenty-two residents in pediatrics and medicine-pediatrics enrolled in the webinar series during their Developmental Rotation in their first or second year of training, 21 of whom completed all videos and answered the HOT DOCS posttest (12 residents in first year; 9 in second year). Each resident completed the HOT DOCS Knowledge Test [17] before viewing the lectures, and they were contacted 6-months to 1-year later to complete a brief survey about the value of HOT DOCS to their clinical practice. Pretest to posttest changes in knowledge (ie, HOT DOCS Knowledge Test) were analyzed using a paired samples *t*-test for the 21 completers. The follow-up survey was analyzed using descriptive statistics.

Results. Average scores on the HOT DOCS Knowledge Test at pretest were 84.2% (SD = 8.6), whereas average scores at posttest were 97.3%, revealing significant improvement in knowledge (SD = 4.8; $P < .001$). Further, 85.7% of residents' scores improved from pretest to posttest (the remaining 14.3% showed unchanging scores).

Of the 8 residents who completed the follow-up survey, 88% reported they regularly use skills taught in the HOT DOCS course in their day-to-day practice in pediatric primary care.

All residents agreed or strongly agreed that their behavioral counseling skills improved after they participated in the training program.

Discussion. HOT DOCS is a well-established evidence-based behavioral management course for caregivers of young children [13,18]. This innovative and engaging course increased the pediatric resident's skill set for managing difficult childhood behaviors in primary care through in-person training or virtual formats adapted for residents due to the COVID-19 pandemic. Both training methods resulted in statistically significant improvements in residents' knowledge of appropriate behavioral management skills for young children. The in-person voluntary trainings consisted of a mixture of first through fourth-year residents; the virtual format is now a required part of the Developmental Rotation during the first or second year of residency. This very practical information is useful in their daily practice within continuity clinic to further solidify their newly learned skills while under the supervision of an academic pediatrician. As a required rotation early during their residency, the trainees have more time to practice these skills in an observed format.

The HOT DOCS curriculum can provide practical training within pediatric residency without imposing significant time burdens. The 2 formats described in this article are easily scheduled within the individual resident's rotation schedule (required development rotations, continuity clinic curriculum, pediatric psychology and/or psychiatry electives, and so forth) or within resident didactic time such as noon conferences and/or academic half days. Anecdotally, our residents enjoyed time outside of typical work hours to enjoy a meal and learn together in a more relaxed environment and have requested continuation of the in-person option. The virtual format has been especially critical during the COVID-19 pandemic whereas our residents have converted many of their didactic sessions to virtual-only. The virtual option also allows for dissemination to other institutions and broader collaboration across locations and specialties. Additionally, qualitative posttraining surveys have shown that participants use the materials presented during the course frequently in their pediatric practice (both during and after the completion of training). Most residents who participated in HOT DOCS have reported using the information regularly in their practice, which supports our key objective of increasing our residents' knowledge and skills regarding effective behavioral management techniques for common referrals in pediatric primary care.

Another advantage of the residents participating in a condensed version of the same course that caretakers participate in is a shared language to discuss behavioral management. The trainees are taught the same techniques as the caregivers during the course, providing a shared understanding of strategies such as special play, hand-over-hand follow through, and planned ignoring. By the parent and pediatrician using similar language and having a similar background in behavioral management strategies, communication and management may be more effective and efficient.

These results are limited by the following:

- Two small samples of resident trainees at one institution in southwest Florida.
- Self-selection bias within the in-person trainings because they were voluntary.
- Differences in length of training and therefore previous medical knowledge within each modality; the in-person format had a mixture of first through fourth-year trainees versus the virtual format is nearly exclusively first-year trainees.
- Pretest and posttest methodology.
- Self-report of the value of skills learned.

Future studies should include the following:

- Demographic variables.
- Increased sample sizes within residency training programs and survey additional residency training program to allow for more comparisons among groups.
- Objective assessments of residents' use of techniques within the primary care setting.
- Caregivers' perspectives on the treating provider's ability to share helpful techniques.

SUMMARY

Behavioral management training is critical during pediatric residency education given the high prevalence of childhood disruptive behaviors and the ideal position of pediatricians to support caregivers in managing these behaviors. Addressing most behavioral referrals in primary care decreases the likelihood that child behavior problems go unnoticed, untreated, and escalate to more serious future mental health problems. This is especially important given that most children with behavioral health problems never receive intervention. The HOT DOCS program is one behavioral management training that can be effectively integrated within the pediatric residency through several training formats. HOT DOCS increased resident knowledge in effective behavior management strategies and resulted in application of that knowledge within their clinical practice.

Disclosure

HOT DOCS is funded by the Children's Board of Hillsborough County; the authors have no other commercial/financial interests to disclose.

References

[1] Ellingson KD, Briggs-Gowan MJ, Carter AS, et al. Parent identification of early emerging child behavior problems: predictors of sharing parental concern with health providers. Arch Pediatr Adolesc Med 2004;158(8):766–72.

[2] Neece CL, Green SA, Baker BL. Parenting stress and child behavior problems: A transactional relationship across time. Am J Intellect Dev disabilities 2012;117(1):48–66.
[3] Cree R, Bitsko R, Robinson L, et al. Health care, family, and ocmmunity factors associated with mental, behavioral, and developmental disorders and poverty among children aged 2-8 years – United States, 2016. MMWR Morbidity Mortality Weekly Rep 2018;67: 1377–83.
[4] Child Welfare Information Gateway. The risk and prevention of maltreatment of children with disabilities. Washington, DC: U.S. Department of Health and Human Services, Children's Bureau.; 2018.
[5] Webster-Stratton C, Taylor T. Nipping early risk factors in the bud: Preventing substance abuse, delinquency, and violence in adolescence through interventions targeted at young children (0–8 years). Prev Sci 2001;2(3):165–92.
[6] McCormick E, Kerns SEU, McPhillips H, et al. Training Pediatric Residents to Provide Parent Education: A Randomized Controlled Trial. Acad Pediatr 2014;14(4):353–60.
[7] Cooper S, Valleley RJ, Polaha J, et al. Running out of time: Physician management of behavioral health concerns in rural pediatric primary care. Pediatrics 2006;118(1):e132–8.
[8] American Academy of Pediatrics. Policy statement–The future of pediatrics: mental health competencies for pediatric primary care. Pediatrics 2009;124(1):410–21.
[9] Kenya McNeal-Trice MA, Burke Ann, Barone Michael, et al. Entrustable professional Actvities 9: assess and manage patients with common behavior/mental health problems. online: American Board of Pediatrics; 2013.
[10] Rosenberg AA, Kamin C, Glicken AD, et al. Training gaps for pediatric residents planning a career in primary care: a qualitative and quantitative study. J graduate Med Educ 2011;3(3):309–14.
[11] Poynter SE, McNeal-Trice K, Gonzalez del Rey J. Addressing the Behavioral and Mental Health Educational Gap in Pediatric Residency Training. Pediatrics 2020;146(1):e20200805.
[12] Agazzi H, Childres J, Armstrong K. Helping our Toddlers, developing our Children's skills (HOT DOCS). 4th edition. Tampa, FL: University of South Florida, Department of Pediatrics; 2020.
[13] Agazzi H, Hayford H, Thomas N, et al. A nonrandomized trial of a behavioral parent training intervention for parents with children with challenging behaviors: In-person versus internet-HOT DOCS. Clin Child Psychol Psychiatry 2021;26(4).
[14] Agazzi H, Salinas A, Williams J, et al. Adaptation of a behavioral parent-training curriculum for Hispanic caregivers: HOT DOCS Español. Infant Ment Health J 2010;31(2): 182–200.
[15] Childres J, Agazzi H, Armstrong K. Evaluating outcomes of a behavioral parent training program for caregivers of young children: Waitlist-control vs. immediate treatment. J Early Child Infant Psychol 2011;7:25–44.
[16] Williams J, Salinas A. Mixed Methods Evaluation of the HOT DOCS Parent Training Program. In: USF health Research Day. Tampa, FL: Child Development Division, Department of Pediatrics, University of South Florida.; 2007.
[17] Agazzi H, Williams J. An instrument to assess caregiver knowledge of behavioral principles as applied to young children. University of South Florida; 2010.
[18] Dunlop S, Kimonis E, Agazzi H. Adapting and Implementing the "Helping Our Toddlers, Developing Our Children's Skills (HOT DOCS)" Parent Training Program in an Australian Context: A Feasibility Study. Evidence-based Pract Child Adolesc Ment Health 2021;6(1):28–46.

Advances in Pediatrics 69 (2022) 23–39

ADVANCES IN PEDIATRICS

Childhood Hearing Health and Early Language Exposure

A Culturally Sensitive Approach

Parul Bhatia, MD[a,*], Julie Rems-Smario, EdD[b], Katrin Jaradeh, BS[c], Dylan K. Chan, MD, PhD[d]

[a]Department of Pediatrics, Keck School of Medicine USC, Children's Hospital Los Angeles, 4650 Sunset Boulevard, #76, Los Angeles, CA 90027, USA; [b]California School for the Deaf, California Department of Education, CORE, 39350 Gallaudet Drive, Fremont, CA 94538, USA; [c]School of Medicine, University of California, San Francisco, 533 Parnassus Avenue, San Francisco, CA 94143, USA; [d]Department of Otolaryngology-Head & Neck Surgery, University of California, San Francisco, 2233 Post Street Box 1225, San Francisco, CA 94115, USA

Keywords

• Deaf • Hearing • Screen • Culture • Language • Child • EHDI

Key points

- Use positive terminology when discussing hearing health and language opportunities with patients and families.
- Advocate for deaf or hard of hearing children to have the earliest possible exposure to rich language, whether spoken, signed, or a combination, with the goal of developing age-appropriate language milestones.
- Understand the short critical window for auditory pathway development in early childhood, therefore necessitating timely and adequate access to sound for patients who choose spoken communication. This typically necessitates a hearing aid or cochlear implant early in life.
- Pay careful attention to thoughtful delivery of culturally sensitive care when working with families from ethnic/linguistic minorities.
- Recognize risk factors for progressive or late onset hearing levels and rescreen in the appropriate time frame, typically within 3 to 9 months from occurrence.

In discussing hearing health and early language exposure in children, the authors seek to present information in an inclusive manner for persons of

*Corresponding author. *E-mail address:* pbhatia@chla.usc.edu

https://doi.org/10.1016/j.yapd.2022.04.003

different cultural backgrounds. Additionally, and equally important, we strive to approach children with different physical traits using descriptive terms rather than terms that suggest inferiority. Regarding the diverse group of individuals who are deaf or hard of hearing (DHH), we would like to bring awareness to terms often used in the medical literature that create a sense of otherness. The authors come from different professions in the health care and education fields, including General Pediatrics, Otolaryngology Head and Neck Surgery (OHNS), and the state Department of Education and use different languages, including spoken and American Sign Language (ASL). The authors understand that the strength of our society is in our diversity, and the incredible value of this diversity surfaced in the preparation of this article.

TERMINOLOGY

The medical literature often uses terms like "hearing loss," "hearing impairment," or "hearing deficit" when describing an individual who is DHH. These terms, while accurate when using a medical construct, marginalize those who identify as part of the Deaf culture and may create bias in hearing families of children who are DHH. For the Deaf community, deafness is a neutral or positive trait to be embraced. Fortunately, the literature is rich with descriptive language that can be substituted for traditional medical terms without taking away from the health care narrative. For this article, the authors use the term *hearing level* (HL) when describing the hearing of individuals who are DHH.

In addition, it is important to be aware of the nomenclature deaf versus Deaf. The term deaf, with a lowercase "d," refers to the individual's hearing status. It reflects the physical trait. This contrasts with Deaf with a capital "D," which reflects an identity, culture, or community [1]. According to the literature, at the center of Deaf culture is the commonality of signed language, which in the United States is ASL [2]. Other characteristics that bond members of the Deaf culture include a shared history, customs, technology, art, humor, and set of values[3]. For this article, the authors are using *deaf* to describe individuals who have HL and *Deaf* to describe individuals or communities who identify with the Deaf culture.

It is important to understand that the terms deaf and Deaf do not always apply to the same individual. For example, an individual can be fully hearing, such as a fully hearing child of Deaf adults, who uses both spoken and signed language. This individual is not deaf, as the hearing pathways are present, but may identify as a member of the Deaf community [4]. In another example, an individual may be deaf and exclusively use spoken communication. This person may identify solely with the hearing community and not the Deaf community. It behooves us to remember that identity is a very personal choice, can change over time, and is up to the individual to decide what is best for them. The earliest recipients of the universal newborn hearing screening (NBHS) programs are just now entering late adolescence and young adulthood, and as this developmental age is characterized by self-identity exploration, much is to be learned from their lived experiences.

Finally, in medicine, there is a move toward person-first language, acknowledging the person first and any related attributes or features second to not define that individual by the feature or attribute. For many in the Deaf community, this is counter intuitive as being Deaf is an important, positive attribute, and an integral part of their identity. As described above, there are wide variations in how people of all ages who are DHH identify. For this reason, to be consistent with guidelines published by the Joint Commission on Infant Hearing (JCIH) and endorsed by the American Academy of Pediatrics [5], people-first language will be used by the authors unless referring specifically to individuals or communities who identify as part of the Deaf culture.

BACKGROUND

With the implementation of universal NBHS, children born DHH are now identified earlier than ever before. The first states to adopt universal NBHS were Hawaii and Rhode Island in the early 1990s, and by the mid-2000s, NBHS became the standard of practice across the United States and in many countries worldwide. In the United States, an average of 1.7/1000 children are reported to be born DHH [6], making it the most common birth condition for which we screen during the newborn period. This rises to 2.83/1000 in school-aged children and 3.5/1000 in adolescents due to late onset HL [5,7]. Of patients born DHH, 50% are born without recognizable risk factors, and 90% are born to parents who are hearing [8].

EARLY HEARING DETECTION AND INTERVENTION GOALS

Early hearing detection and intervention (EHDI) programs at the national and state level continuously assess data and update protocols to best advocate for children who are identified as DHH. The primary goal of EHDI is to promote early identification with immediate language exposure so that infants and young children who are DHH can appropriately meet their developmental language milestones. Consequences of late identification and late language exposure are well-documented and occur over several developmental domains including social-emotional, communication, speech, literacy, and academic achievement. In fact, success in meeting age-appropriate language milestones more closely correlates with early age of identification and language exposure compared with the degree of HL [9].

To avoid delays, the nationally accepted EHDI benchmarks for early infancy are to screen all newborns before 1 month of age, establish hearing thresholds for those who require further assessment before 3 months of age, and initiate early language services, also known as early intervention, before 6 months of age. Hearing coordination centers are an integral part of the state EHDI system and are responsible for tracking all newborns through this process to help decrease the frequency with which patients are lost to follow-up. Additionally, for families who choose to include spoken language for their

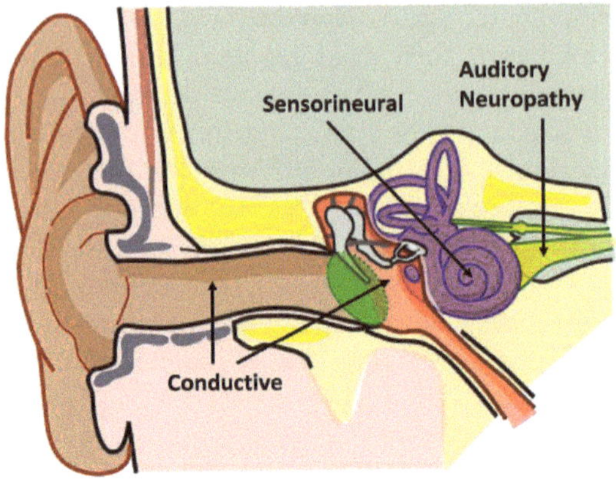

Fig. 1. Description of hearing changes based on location. (*Adapted from* Chittka L, Brockmann A. Perception space–the final frontier. PLoS Biol. Apr 2005;3(4):e137. https://doi.org/10.1371/journal.pbio.0030137.)

child, hearing aids (HAs) should be fit as soon as hearing thresholds are established due to the critical window for the development of hearing pathways. Even newborns can receive HAs. States that meet this "1-3-6 month" benchmark are challenged to move toward a "1-2-3 month" timeline to give infants the earliest possible exposure to language [5].

HEARING SCREENING AND AUDIOMETRY

Audiologists describe the hearing health of an individual based on several characteristics of the sound pathways.

- *Laterality*: unilateral versus bilateral
- *Location*: (Fig. 1):
- *Thresholds*: defined as the softest sound perceptible in the respective ear [10].
  - Mild (20–40 db)
  - Moderate (41–70 db)
  - Severe (71–90 db)
  - Profound (>90 db)

In this article, mild, moderate, severe, or profound HL refers to hearing thresholds in the respective ranges. Typically, *hard of hearing* refers to HL in the mild-to-severe range, and *deaf* refers to HL in the profound range with minimal to no sound perception.

- *Frequency*: ranges from 500 to 8000 Hz
- *Timing*:
  - Congenital—HL present at birth
  - Late onset—full hearing at birth; HL develop in childhood
- Stability
  - Progressive—HL may be present at birth and continue to progress with time
  - Stable—HL remains constant

NBHS typically uses one of two devices: automated otoacoustic emissions or OAE and automated auditory brainstem response or ABR. For automated OAE, a sound in various frequencies is introduced to the ear canal via a probe. If hearing is intact, the device detects naturally occurring sounds created by the cochlear hair cells in response to the original sound. Detection of the OAE takes seconds and indicates a healthy pathway to the level of the cochlea. The screen can be completed in less than a minute in a quiet or sleeping infant. Automated ABR is similarly an easy-to-use point of care tool, but it relies on sounds detected at the level of the brainstem, and thus it is inclusive of the peripheral auditory nerve. For the newborn screenings, the results are preset to display in a binary fashion (pass/refer), making interpretation straightforward. Either tool can be used in healthy newborns, but EHDI protocols recommend ABR for babies who are in the neonatal intensive care unit due to the inherent increased risk for auditory neuropathy.

Infants who do not pass the NBHS are referred to audiology for diagnostic testing with the diagnostic ABR and a battery of other tests to check the auditory pathways. Older infants and children respond to sound more reliably and thus can participate in age and developmentally appropriate behavioral audiometry (Table 1).

LANGUAGE OPPORTUNITIES

According to the Individuals with Disabilities Education Act Part C, once an infant is identified as DHH, a referral must be placed for early intervention services within 7 days of diagnosis [11]. State and local programs should present families with resources that expose them to languages in a respectful and nonjudgmental manner. As an example, the California SB210 Committee for Children who are Deaf or Hard of Hearing: Birth to Five Years created a parent-friendly guide, *Language Development Milestones*, to help monitor children in meeting their goals in spoken and signed languages [12] (Table 2).

Spoken language with or without visual tools such as cued speech and signed exact English, signed language such as ASL, and bilingual (signed plus spoken) language, are all excellent opportunities for patients; which modalities a child experiences depend on numerous factors, including parental identity, resources, and available support. Early exposure to language is perhaps the most important factor determining successful communication for all children, regardless of hearing status. Because of the short critical period of initial auditory and language development in the first 3 years of life, this exposure to language for children who are DHH means:

1. Early access to rich spoken language *plus* timely and adequate access to sound, usually necessitating early placement of an HA or cochlear implant (CI)
2. Early access to rich signed language *plus* timely and adequate access to Deaf mentors, community, and education programs
3. Both of the above

Table 1
Behavioral audiometry in children

Behavioral screen	Age of child	Description
Behavioral observation audiometry	6 mo	The child turns their head or makes movement in response to sounds. This is not a conditioned response, and independently is not considered a valid hearing test.
Visual reinforced audiometry	6–24 mo	With the use of visual reinforcers, such a puppets that light up, the child is conditioned to respond to sounds, allowing the audiologist to determine hearing thresholds.
Conditioned play audiometry	24+ mo	With the assistance of toys, the child engages in an interactive game of listening for sounds, allowing the audiologist to determine hearing thresholds.
Conventional audiometry	>3–4 y	The child follows instructions to indicate when they hear the sound, typically by raising a hand.

Table 2
Parent guide for Universal Language Acquisition Milestones for spoken language and signed language: Sample of milestones

Age	Signed and/or spoken language milestone
Birth to 1 y Old	Your baby smiles when they see you. Your baby looks around and is attentive to people's faces. Your baby shows awareness of the environment. By 12 mo, your baby has 1–3 signs or words.
1–2 y Old	Your baby recognizes their own name when it is signed or spoken. Your baby uses signed or spoken names to refer to self and others. Your baby takes 1–2 turns in a conversation and uses exclamatory expressions.
2–3 y Old	By 2½ years of age, your child answers questions with yes or no. Your child uses intelligible signs or words about 80% of the time. Your child vocalizes or signs for all needs.
3–4 y Old	Your child answers questions logically. Your child starts to understand different perspectives. Your child communicates fluently, clearly, and is easily understood by family and familiar adults.
4–5 y Old	Your child uses 2,500 + words and/or signs. Your child begins to ask the meanings of words or signs. Your child puts sequencing concepts together. At this stage, your child is Kindergarten-ready for literacy.

Adapted from Senate Bill 210 (Galgiani) Committee. SB 210 Language Development Milestones. California Department of Education. Updated July 3, 2020. Accessed November 15, 2021. https://www.cde.ca.gov/sp/ss/dh/sb210langmilestones.asp.

This approach provides the greatest access to language and culture; however, the ability of families, particularly those with limited resources, to take on these multiple paths can be daunting.

Most children born deaf have parents who are hearing, and typically the child is the first meaningful interaction the family has with an individual who is deaf. In response, the Health Resources and Services Administration introduced grant funding for the Deaf Mentor program, with the goal of "increasing the number of families enrolled in DHH adult-to-family support services by no later than 9 months of age" [13]. The Deaf Mentor program entails "mentoring by a variety of DHH adults including those who use ASL, cued speech, spoken language, and combinations of modalities. Trained DHH adults are uniquely qualified to provide families with a positive and hopeful perspective from their day-to-day, real-life experiences as a DHH person living in a hearing world." [14].

In the following sections, we will provide an overview of cultural considerations in the care of children who are DHH and their families. Achieving an understanding of a family's perspective will help to develop a culturally congruent care plan to support the growth and well-being of all children.

DEAF COMMUNITY

Deaf individuals often struggle with low-quality interpretation services and systemic barriers that reflect the audism in our society. One framework applied in communities of color to overcome the obstacles that prevent social mobility and that create differentials in power is the community cultural wealth capital framework [15]. This framework focuses on the strengths within marginalized communities, which are nurtured by families and communities, through various forms of capital. Here, we are using the Deaf community cultural wealth capital framework to describe the skills, abilities, and knowledge Deaf adults utilize to overcome the systemic barriers they face in their day-to-day lives [16].

- *Navigational Capital:* Navigational capital includes the skills of maneuvering through social institutions, namely the ability to maneuver through spaces not designed for individuals who are DHH [16]. It includes the ways people who are DHH access society. Examples include adapted technology such as clocks that vibrate or flashing doorbells, video relay services for phone calls, and video conference calls.
- *Aspirational Capital:* Aspirational capital includes the ability to maintain hopes and dreams for the future. It is an important source of motivation and inspiration for the DHH community, especially children, to aim high despite the challenges and stereotypes that exist regarding deafness [16]. Many Deaf role models in politics and pop culture media have successfully broken the glass ceiling and serve as reminders that individuals who are DHH experience the same successes and achievements as hearing individuals when given equal opportunities.
- *Social Capital:* Social capital includes the networks of people and community resources that provide instrumental and emotional support to navigate society's

institutions [16]. Social capital for families of children who are DHH may include a network of Deaf mentors from the Deaf community.
- *Linguistic Capital:* Linguistic capital refers to intellectual and social skills attained through a variety of language experiences [16]. Healthy language acquisition supports the well-being of children who are DHH in many areas of their life, including the social-emotional, medical, and academic arenas.

NON-AUDIOLOGIC EVALUATION

Once a child is identified as DHH by an audiologist, medical workup can be initiated to learn the underlying biology of the child's hearing. Understanding the biological cause can be impactful in several ways because it can provide (1) prognostic information regarding likelihood of future changes in the child's hearing status; (2) early identification of important syndromic associations which may affect medical, educational, and audiological choices; (3) genetic information for family counseling; (4) specific knowledge to drive interventions such as cochlear implantation; and (5) for some families, knowledge that can support acceptance of their child's hearing. Exact choice and sequence of etiologic tests depend on a number of factors, including the child's age, HL, laterality, clinical history, and family goals.

Although universal NBHS has changed the landscape of early identification of infants who are DHH, it is not without its limitations. For example, the NBHS may miss mild HL due to the design of the screening tools [5], and by definition cannot identify late onset HL since it is not present at birth. Fortunately, some of the risk factors for the later onset HL are known. Infants with these risk factors should be rescreened in the first year of life despite having passed the NBHS, even in the absence of hearing related symptoms. A sample of risk factors for late onset HL is listed in Table 3.

Although history and physical examination can occasionally reveal a clear etiology relating to birth history, family history, intrauterine or postnatal exposures, or syndromic associations (Table 4), most children who are DHH present with no obvious biological explanation. For these children, three principal evaluations are considered, each accounting for the three major causes of congenital or childhood-onset permanent sensorineural HL.

Genetic

Genetic etiologies account for more than 50% of all causes of congenital deafness, and 70% of these are non-syndromic and otherwise invisible on examination [17]. The most commonly affected of these is GJB2, a gene that codes for the cochlear gap junction protein, connexin 26 [18,19]. GJB2 is inherited in an autosomal recessive pattern, and variants in this gene lead to permanent damage of the cochlear hair cells. It accounts for 20% of all children who are born deaf, making it the single most common known etiology for congenital deafness. However, variants in GJB2 are often found in individuals of European or Asian ancestry, and rarely in those of African or indigenous American descent [20]. The genetics of hearing in these traditionally underrepresented minority groups, including Latinx in the United States, is poorly understood [21–24]. This disparity should be addressed, especially because identifying a genetic etiology can provide valuable prognostic knowledge and lead to early identification of critical associations. Genetic etiologies are best identified with deafness gene panel testing, which assesses for causative variants in 150 to 200 genes known to be related to hearing [25]. In recent years, deafness gene panels have become much more widely available to the primary care provider.

Infectious

In the United States, one in every 200 babies is born with congenital cytomegalovirus (cCMV) [26]. Congenital CMV is the second most common etiology for permanent HL in early childhood [27] and is diagnosed by performing viral culture or polymerase chain reaction from the urine, saliva, or blood in infants under 3 weeks of age. Testing to confirm whether a baby has cCMV cannot take place after the first 3 weeks of life due to the possibility of postnatal horizontal transfer of the virus. Thus, the detection of cCMV requires either early screening or use of archival testing of dried blood spots [28,29].

CMV is ubiquitous in our society, with 1 in every 3 children already infected by age 5 years [30]. These children shed the virus in the urine, saliva, and other bodily fluids, easily transmitting it to others. Currently, the best prevention measure for cCMV is good public education about the importance of handwashing during pregnancy, especially after changing diapers, and not sharing utensils or drinks with young children [30]. Despite this, according to a 2005 HealthStyles survey by the CDC, only 14% of female respondents had heard of CMV [31].

Because cCMV-associated deafness is frequently progressive or late-onset, early consideration of CMV testing in the newborn period can be highly impactful [32–34]. Research is still ongoing regarding the best approach to cCMV screening as it relates to hearing, and therefore, individual states and hospitals vary tremendously in their cCMV protocols [35]. There are generally three approaches to cCMV testing in the newborn period:

1. Symptom-based: Screen only if non-hearing CMV-related symptoms are present
2. Targeted: Perform symptom-based cCMV screening as above *plus* screen newborns who do not pass the NBHS
3. Universal: Screen all newborns for cCMV

Imaging

Imaging with MRI or computed tomography (CT) can reveal anatomic etiologies for HL and is also necessary for determination of candidacy for cochlear implantation. Studies show that imaging is more likely to reveal an etiology, such as isolated structural changes in the temporal bone, in patients who are unilaterally DHH as opposed to bilateral [36].

In summary, the following approach can be applied to the medical evaluation of children with permanent sensorineural HL [5,25,37].

Table 3
A sample of risk factors for early childhood hearing loss: Guidelines for infants who pass the newborn hearing screening

Risk factor classification	Recommended diagnostic follow up
Caregiver concern regarding hearing, speech, language developmental delay	Immediate referral
Family History of childhood hearing loss	By 9 mo
Neonatal intensive care unit admission for >5 d	By 9 mo
Hyperbilirubinemia requiring exchange transfusion	By 9 mo
Aminoglycoside administration for >5 d	By 9 mo
Asphyxia or hypoxic ischemic encephalopathy	By 9 mo
Extracorporeal membrane oxygenation	By 3 mo after occurrence
In utero infections such as herpes, rubella, syphilis, and toxoplasmosis	By 9 mo
In utero infections with CMV	By 3 mo after birth
Craniofacial features that may affect hearing	By 9 mo
Phenotypic or genetic features that suggest syndromes associated with hearing changes	By 9 mo
Meningitis, encephalitis, of other infection known to affect hearing	By 3 mo after occurrence
Significant head trauma, especially basal skull or temporal bone fracture	By 3 mo after occurrence

Refer to the Joint Commission on Infant Hearing 2019 Position Statement for a more complete list.
Data from the Joint Committee on Infant Hearing. Year 2019 Position Statement: Principles and Guidelines for Early Hearing Detection and Intervention Programs. J Early Hear Detect Interv. 2019;4(2):1-44.

- Obtain a thorough history and physical examination, with special attention to family history and birth history
- Assess for known perinatal or acquired causes
- Evaluate for syndromic features
- Consider cCMV testing if patient less than 3 weeks of age, or cCMV dried blood spot testing if available, for patients greater than 3 weeks of age.
- Consider genetic testing, including deafness gene panel testing, targeted panels for syndromic causes, or single-gene testing for GJB2 (Connexin 26), depending on clinical picture and testing availability
- Consider imaging, including MRI and CT [25,36,37]
- Consider EKG to evaluate for prolonged QT [5].

Finally, referrals should be initiated soon after identification and ongoing care supported, with the following specialists. These include [5]:

- Language specialists through the child's educational service provider(s)
- Audiology
- OHNS
- Ophthalmology
- Genetics

Table 4
Examples of syndromes associated with deafness or hard of hearing

Syndrome	Non-auditory clinical characteristics
Pendred	Enlarged vestibular aqueduct; thyroid goiter
Usher	Retinitis pigmentosa
Branchio-oto-renal	Branchial cysts or fistula; external and middle ear changes; renal abnormalities
Jervell and Lange-Nielsen	Cardiac arrhythmia (prolonged QT interval)
Waardenburg	Pigmentary changes of skin, hair, iris
Stickler	Joint laxity or arthritis; myopia; vitreoretinal degeneration; Pierre Robin sequence; cleft palate
Treacher Collins	Underdevelopment of facial bones and tissues; cleft palate; eyelid coloboma; external and middle ear changes
Alport	Glomerular kidney disease; eye changes

INTERVENTION FOR ACCESS TO SOUND

According to a national survey conducted in 2018 by the National Center for Hearing Assessment and Management, almost 50% of families of children who are DHH use spoken language alone for their child's communication modality, and an additional 17% use mostly spoken language supplemented by sign language, cued speech, or other [8]. Early access to sound during the critical period of auditory system development in the first few years of life provides the basis for development of hearing, listening skills, speech, and spoken language. Access to sound with HAs or CIs by 6 months of age is strongly associated with improved spoken language outcomes [9,38], with age-appropriate spoken language outcomes able to be achieved with timely access [38]. Children identified as DHH have many different opportunities for obtaining access to sound. For children with sensorineural deafness, meaningful access to sound requires the use of a hearing device. For children of all HL, mild to profound, strong evidence from multiple prospective, longitudinal studies demonstrate that earlier access to sound through appropriate fitting and subsequent utilization of hearing devices is associated with improved spoken language outcomes.

There are three classes of devices used to improve access to sound in children with sensorineural HL: (1) air-conduction HAs, (2) bone-conduction hearing devices (BCHDs), and (3) CIs. HAs are nonsurgical and typically involve a behind-the-ear component together with an earmold that fits into the auditory meatus. BCHDs, which are often used for conductive HL and microtia/aural atresia, are also used in single-sided sensorineural deafness to send sound from the affected ear to the contralateral, typical hearing ear. The BCHDs are available as either a nonsurgical, removable device, such as a soft headband or an adhesive sticker behind the ear, or as a surgical implant, involving a small

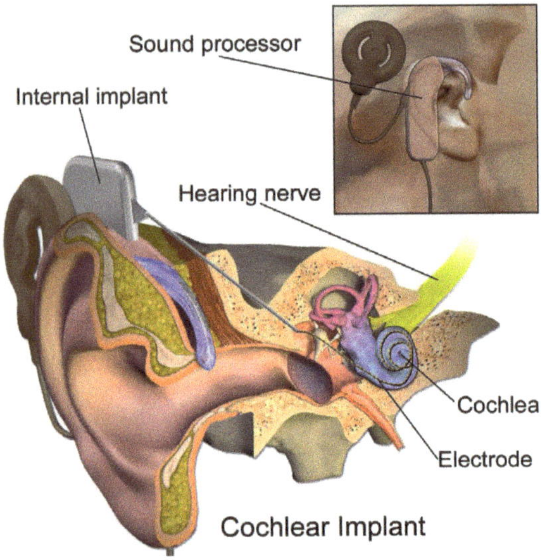

Fig. 2. Cochlear implant. (*Adapted from* Blausen M. Medical gallery of blausen medical 2014. WikiJournal of Medicine. 2014;1(2):1-79. https://doi.org/10.15347/wjm/2014.010.)

implant into the temporal bone behind the ear with an external removable processor. Finally, CIs involve a device surgically implanted within the temporal bone and attached to an electrode array that coils through the cochlea to directly stimulate the auditory nerve. The external, removable segment sits on the scalp over the device via a simple magnet. This external component is required to process sound and transmit signals to the internal implant. When the child removes this external portion, the internal component is nonfunctional and the child does not have access to sound (Fig. 2).

Hearing devices are principally managed by audiologists, who are responsible for decision-making surrounding hearing device candidacy, choice of hearing device, and subsequent management of fitting, adjustment, and monitoring. In general, HAs and nonsurgical BCHDs can be fit at any age, even in newborns. Surgical BCHDs and CIs vary in their minimum age depending on exact device and indication; generally, surgical BCHDs are considered beginning around age 5 years, and CIs beginning around age 6 months. Infants with acquired deafness due to meningitis are at specific risk for progressive cochlear fibrosis and ossification that worsen CI outcomes; for these children, cochlear implantation is considered an emergency and can be done as young as 2 to 3 months of age [39].

Hearing aid fitting requires medical clearance from an OHNS, which will also evaluate all medical and surgical options as well as contraindications for hearing device use. The OHNS also performs surgical placement of BCHDs and CIs, typically as outpatient procedures. The most significant surgical risk of cochlear implantation is meningitis. Because of the associated increased lifetime risk of meningitis, CI recipients should receive the PPSV23 pneumococcal vaccines at age 2 years, in addition to the standard PCV-13 series [40].

Choice of hearing devices takes into account hearing threshold and sidedness. Mild-to-moderate sensorineural HL generally responds well to HAs regardless of sidedness. Bilateral sensorineural HL with thresholds of greater than 70 dB HL can benefit from CI. Unilateral sensorineural HL of greater than 70 dB can be managed with any of the three device options, although emerging evidence from high-quality prospective studies has demonstrated that CI for single-sided deafness provides improved hearing in noise, sound localization, and development of spoken language [41,42]. This is important to consider as children with unilateral permanent sensorineural HL comprise a significant number of those identified through the NBHS, making up almost 40% of cases [6]. As with all clinical management strategies, assessment of parental concerns and goals with subsequent shared decision-making between family and clinical providers is paramount.

CULTURAL INTERSECTIONALITY

The United States is a very diverse multicultural and ethnic country with 44.9 million foreign-born individuals and 17.8 million children under 18 having one foreign-born parent as of 2020 [43]. Nationwide, approximately 67.8 million people speak a language other than English in the home [44]. Given this great diversity, careful attention to thoughtful delivery of culturally sensitive care is important when working with families from ethnic and linguistic minorities. Furthermore, it is imperative that health care providers and educators acknowledge the intersectionalities of an individual's various identities and treat each individual as their own rather than as part of a monolith.

As mentioned previously in this article, NBHS became the standard practice across the United States by the mid-2000s. However, to this day, many countries still do not perform NBHS, and some children are often first identified as DHH after they migrate to the United States [45]. For some parents who are hearing, it can be disruptive and sometimes a traumatic experience when they are told for the first time that their child is deaf. The subsequent path these parents take with regards to their child's health care, education, and developmental needs is often an investment of time and finances that can leave some families overwhelmed when making decisions regarding their child's next steps.

It has been previously documented that families often face stressors, including the pressure related to deadlines and difficulties with decision-making, when raising a child who is DHH [46,47]. Health care providers and educators must be aware of these stressors and meet families where they are when discussing opportunities for their child's language development. This stress is amplified in families from ethnic minority groups or immigrant families who use languages other than English or ASL [48]. Typically, immigrant families will often require resources once they migrate to the United

States; this is even more so when navigating the complexities of the health care and educational systems. Members of an immigrant family typically face stress, depression, and anxiety themselves, which is compounded when facing the cultural stigma of having a family member with a "disability" [49,50]. Recognizing that a personalized approach to patient care in the clinic is imperative, a trauma-informed approach may be a useful framework within the clinical encounter when working with families with various lived experiences [51]. Of importance, people from various cultures may approach deafness differently, and as health care providers and educators, it is our duty to be aware of these differences and approach conversations in a culturally informed manner.

Deaf individuals whose language is ASL regard themselves as a linguistic minority, similar to people from ethnic minority groups whose first language is not English [52]. Immigrant children who are DHH living in the United States possess "dual minority" membership; they may simultaneously seek acculturation into the American and Deaf cultures [53]. Health care providers should pay close attention to the cultural intersectionalities of our patients and approach each individual with compassion and respect.

THE MEDICAL HOME

The pediatrician plays a unique role in the care of the youngest members of the DHH communities. In the medical home model, the pediatrician is empowered to provide comprehensive, patient-centered, culturally sensitive care with compassion and respect for all individuals. The following recommendations may help in providing this care for children who are DHH:

- Remember to review all language opportunities with patient and family
- Use ASL interpreters when this is the preferred language
- Recognize the limitations of the NBHS and repeat hearing screens in a timely manner based on the JCIH risk factors for late onset or progressive HL
- For children using spoken language, early and timely access to sound is critical and can often be achieved with the assistance of hearing devices, even in the newborn period
- Make timely referrals and complete etiologic work up in a shared decision-making model with the family
- Recognize cultural intersectionality and support families using a trauma-informed care framework
- Become familiar with local and national resources for people who are DHH

SUMMARY

With the implementation of universal NBHS, opportunities for early language exposure for children who are DHH are more robust than ever before. From improvements in hearing devices to expansion of deafness gene panel testing, our understanding of the medical and technological advances in hearing health is expanding. Equally as important is the growing strength and diversity of the culturally Deaf community. Children born DHH today have improved opportunities to explore languages and cultures from multiple perspectives. Each child and family's journey, from initial hearing screening to the development of robust language and all the steps in between, is unique. Celebrating this diversity and providing compassionate support will only improve the well-being of our patients and their families.

Acknowledgments

The authors would like to acknowledge Lynn Kysh, MLIS, MPP for her invaluable support in preparation of this article.

Disclosure

The authors have nothing to disclose.

References

[1] Simms L, Thumann H. In search of a new, linguistically and culturally sensitive paradigm in deaf education. Am Ann Deaf 2007;152(3):302–11.
[2] Pendergrass KM, Newman SD, Jones E, et al. Deaf: a concept analysis from a cultural perspective using the wilson method of concept analysis development. Clin Nurs Res 2019;28(1):79–93.
[3] Maxwell-McCaw D, Zea MC. The deaf acculturation scale (DAS): development and validation of a 58-item measure. J Deaf Stud Deaf Educ 2011;16(3):325–42.
[4] Kusters A, De Meulder M. Understanding Deafhood: in search of its meanings. Am Ann Deaf 2013;157(5):428–38.
[5] The Joint Committee on Infant Hearing. Year 2019 position statement: principles and guidelines for early hearing detection and intervention programs. J Early Hear Detect Interv 2019;4(2):1–44.
[6] National Center on Birth Defects and Developmental Disabilities. Type and severity summary of identified cases of hearing loss. Atlanta, GA: Centers for Disease Control and Prevention; 2019. Available at: https://www.cdc.gov/ncbddd/hearingloss/2019-data/12-type-and-severity.html. Accessed November 15, 2021.
[7] Korver AM, Smith RJ, Van Camp G, et al. Congenital hearing loss. Nat Rev Dis Primers 2017;3:16094.
[8] White KR. Demographic considerations in serving children who are hard of hearing or deaf. J Early Hear Detect Interv 2018;3(2):14–7.
[9] Yoshinaga-Itano C, Sedey AL, Coulter DK, et al. Language of early- and later-identified children with hearing loss. Pediatrics 1998;102(5):1161–71.
[10] American Speech-Language Hearing Association.. Audiology information series: type, degree, and configuartion of hearing loss. 2015. Available at: https://www.asha.org/siteassets/ais/ais-hearing-loss-types-degree-configuration.pdf. Access date: May 2, 2022.
[11] Early intervention program for infants and toddlers with disabilities. Final regulations. Fed Regist 2011;76(188):60140–309.
[12] Senate Bill 210 (Galgiani) Committee. SB 210 Language Development Milestones. California Department of Education. Available at: https://www.cde.ca.gov/sp/ss/dh/sb210langmilestones.asp. Accessed November 15, 2021.
[13] Maternal and Child Health Bureau. HRSA-20-047 frequently asked questions. Rockville, MD: Health Resources and Servicecs Administration; 2019. Available at: https://mchb.hrsa.gov/funding-opportunities/faqs-hrsa-20-047. Accessed November 19, 2021.
[14] Hands & voices family leadership in language & learning (FL3). DHH guidelines: guidelines for deaf and hard of hearing mentor/guide/role model programs. 2013. Available at: https://handsandvoices.org/fl3/fl3-docs/DHH-Guidelines.pdf. Access date: May 2, 2022.

[15] Yosso TJ. Whose culture has capital? A critical race theory discussion of community cultural wealth. Race Ethn Educ 2005;8(1):69–91.
[16] Fleischer F, Garrow W, Narr R. Chapter 18: developing deaf education. In: Murawski WW, Scott KL, editors. What really works in secondary education. Sage Publications; 2015.
[17] National Center on Birth Defects and Developmental Disabilities. Genetics of hearing loss. Atlanta, GA: Centers for Disease Control and Prevention; 2020. Available at;. https://www.cdc.gov/ncbddd/hearingloss/genetics.html. Accessed November 19, 2021.
[18] Chari DA, Chan DK. Diagnosis and treatment of congenital sensorineural hearing loss. Curr Otorhinolaryngol Rep 2017;5(4):251–8.
[19] Chan DK, Chang KW. GJB2-associated hearing loss: systematic review of worldwide prevalence, genotype, and auditory phenotype. Laryngoscope 2014;124(2):E34–53.
[20] Shan J, Chobot-Rodd J, Castellanos R, et al. GJB2 mutation spectrum in 209 hearing impaired individuals of predominantly Caribbean Hispanic and African descent. Int J Pediatr Otorhinolaryngol 2010;74(6):611–8.
[21] Sloan-Heggen CM, Bierer AO, Shearer AE, et al. Comprehensive genetic testing in the clinical evaluation of 1119 patients with hearing loss. Hum Genet 2016;135(4):441–50.
[22] Yan D, Tekin D, Bademci G, et al. Spectrum of DNA variants for non-syndromic deafness in a large cohort from multiple continents. Hum Genet 2016;135(8):953–61.
[23] Florentine MM, Rouse SL, Stephans J, et al. Racial and ethnic disparities in diagnostic efficacy of comprehensive genetic testing for sensorineural hearing loss. Hum Genet 2021; https://doi.org/10.1007/s00439-021-02338-4.
[24] Rouse SL, Florentine MM, Taketa E, et al. Racial and ethnic disparities in genetic testing for hearing loss: a systematic review and synthesis. Hum Genet 2021; https://doi.org/10.1007/s00439-021-02335-7.
[25] Liming BJ, Carter J, Cheng A, et al. International pediatric otolaryngology group (IPOG) consensus recommendations: Hearing loss in the pediatric patient. Int J Pediatr Otorhinolaryngol 2016;90:251–8.
[26] Stagno S, Britt W. Chapter 23 - Cytomegalovirus infections. In: Remington JS, Klein JO, Wilson CB, et al, editors. Infectious diseases of the fetus and newborn infant. 6th edition. W.B. Saunders; 2006. p. 739–81.
[27] Stehel EK, Shoup AG, Owen KE, et al. Newborn hearing screening and detection of congenital cytomegalovirus infection. Pediatrics 2008;121(5):970–5.
[28] Boppana SB, Ross SA, Novak Z, et al. Dried blood spot real-time polymerase chain reaction assays to screen newborns for congenital cytomegalovirus infection. JAMA 2010;303(14):1375–82.
[29] Kenneson A, Cannon MJ. Review and meta-analysis of the epidemiology of congenital cytomegalovirus (CMV) infection. Rev Med Virol 2007;17(4):253–76.
[30] Centers for Disease Control and Prevention. Pregnancy: preventing infections. Available at: https://www.cdc.gov/pregnancy/infections.html. Accessed November 24, 2021.
[31] Ross DS, Victor M, Sumartojo E, et al. Women's knowledge of congenital cytomegalovirus: results from the 2005 HealthStyles survey. J Womens Health (Larchmt) 2008;17(5):849–58.
[32] Lanzieri TM, Chung W, Flores M, et al. Hearing loss in children with asymptomatic congenital cytomegalovirus infection. Pediatrics 2017;139(3):e20162610.
[33] Diener ML, Zick CD, McVicar SB, et al. Outcomes from a hearing-targeted cytomegalovirus screening program. Pediatrics 2017;139(2); https://doi.org/10.1542/peds.2016-0789.
[34] Lee ER, Chan DK. Implications of dried blood spot testing for congenital CMV on management of children with hearing loss: A preliminary report. Int J Pediatr Otorhinolaryngol 2019;119:10–4.
[35] Advocacy in Action. National CMV Foundation. Available at: https://www.nationalcmv.org/about-us/advocacy. Accessed November 19, 2021.

[36] van Beeck Calkoen EA, Engel MSD, van de Kamp JM, et al. The etiological evaluation of sensorineural hearing loss in children. Eur J Pediatr 2019;178(8):1195–205.
[37] Lin PH, Hsu CJ, Lin YH, et al. Etiologic and audiologic characteristics of patients with pediatric-onset unilateral and asymmetric sensorineural hearing loss. JAMA Otolaryngol Head Neck Surg 2017;143(9):912–9.
[38] TYC Ching, Dillon H, Button L, et al. Age at intervention for permanent hearing loss and 5-year language outcomes. Pediatrics 2017;140(3):e20164274.
[39] Singhal K, Singhal J, Muzaffar J, et al. Outcomes of cochlear implantation in patients with post-meningitis deafness: a systematic review and narrative synthesis. J Int Adv Otol 2020;16(3):395–410.
[40] National Center for Immunization and Respiratory Diseases. Cochlear impants and vaccination recommendations. Centers for Disease Control and Prevention; 2019. Available at: https://www.cdc.gov/vaccines/vpd/mening/public/dis-cochlear-faq-gen.html. Accessed November 16, 2021.
[41] Benchetrit L, Ronner EA, Anne S, et al. Cochlear Implantation in Children With Single-Sided Deafness: A Systematic Review and Meta-analysis. JAMA Otolaryngol Head Neck Surg 2021;147(1):58–69.
[42] Arras T, Boudewyns A, Dhooge I, et al. Assessment of Receptive and Expressive Language Skills Among Young Children With Prelingual Single-Sided Deafness Managed With Early Cochlear Implantation. JAMA Netw Open 2021;4(8):e2122591.
[43] Migration Policy Institute. United States: Demographics & Social. Available at: https://www.migrationpolicy.org/data/state-profiles/state/demographics/US. Accessed November 16, 2021.
[44] Migration Policy Institute. United States: Language & Education. Available at: https://www.migrationpolicy.org/data/state-profiles/state/language/US. Accessed November 16, 2021.
[45] Neumann K, Euler HA, Chadha S, et al. A survey on the global status of newborn and infant hearing screening. J Early Hear Detect Interv 2020;5(2):63–84.
[46] Quittner AL, Barker DH, Cruz I, et al. Parenting stress among parents of deaf and hearing children: associations with language delays and behavior problems. Parent Sci Pract 2010;10(2):136–55.
[47] Spahn C, Burger T, Löschmann C, et al. Quality of life and psychological distress in parents of children with a cochlear implant. Cochlear Implants Int 2004;5(1):13–27.
[48] Ding H, Hargraves L. Stress-associated poor health among adult immigrants with a language barrier in the United States. J Immigr Minor Health 2009;11(6):446–52.
[49] Othman EH, Ong LZ, Omar IA, et al. Experiences of muslim mothers of children with disabilities: a qualitative study. J Disabil Religion 2021;1–25; https://doi.org/10.1080/23312521.2021.1911734.
[50] Su C, Khanlou N, Mustafa N. Chinese Immigrant Mothers of Children with Developmental Disabilities: Stressors and Social Support. Int J Ment Health Addict 2021;19(1):1–18; https://doi.org/10.1007/s11469-018-9882-z.
[51] Substance Abuse and mental health services (SAMHSA) trauma and justice strategic initiative. SAMHSA's concept of trauma and guidance for a trauma-informed approach. U.S. Department of Health and Human Services. 2014. Available at: https://ncsacw.samhsa.gov/userfiles/files/SAMHSA_Trauma.pdf. Access date: May 2, 2022.
[52] Charrow VR, Wilbur RB. The deaf child as a linguistic minority. Theor Into Pract 1975;14(5):353–9.
[53] Cohen OP, Fischgrund JE, Redding R. Deaf children from ethnic, linguistic and racial minority backgrounds: an overview. Am Ann Deaf 1990;135(2):67–73.

Advances in Pediatrics 69 (2022) 41–58

ADVANCES IN PEDIATRICS

A Pediatrician's Guide to Working with Children on the Autism Spectrum in Coronavirus Disease 2019 and Beyond: Retrospect and Prospect

Thusa Sabapathy, MD, FAAP[a,*], Megan Goss, MD[b], Jessica L. Borelli, PhD[c], Robin Steinberg-Epstein, MD, FAAP[d]

[a]University of California, Irvine School of Medicine, The Center for Autism & Neurodevelopmental Disorders, 2500 Red Hill Avenue, Suite 100, Santa Ana, CA 92705, USA; [b]UC Irvine/CHOC Children's Hospital of Orange County, 505 S. Main Street, Suite 525, Orange, CA 92868, USA; [c]Department of Psychological Science, University of California, Irvine, 4201 Social & Behavioral Sciences Gateway, Irvine, CA 92697, USA; [d]University of California, Irvine School of Medicine, The Center for Autism and Neurodevelopmental Disorders, 2500 Red Hill Avenue, Suite 100, Santa Ana, CA 92705, USA

Keywords

• Autism • COVID-19 • Pandemic • Health • Services • Vulnerable • Adapt • Resilience

Key points

- The COVID-19 pandemic is an unprecedented event with observable consequences and devastating effects on autistic children and families, highlighting and broadening disparities in the care.
- Abrupt reduction in services and access to care during the pandemic compromised physical and mental health and led to missed intervention opportunities at critical times.
- However, many autistic children and providers demonstrated resilience in adapting to these challenges.

INTRODUCTION

The coronavirus disease 2019 (COVID-19) pandemic is an unprecedented event with observable consequences and devastating effects on children and families.

*Corresponding author. *E-mail address:* tsabapat@hs.uci.edu

https://doi.org/10.1016/j.yapd.2022.04.001

This global occurrence highlighted and broadened gaps and disparities in the care of children with developmental disabilities, while simultaneously catalyzing innovation. Initially not seen as direct victims of the disease, children are inherently vulnerable to the impacts of COVID-19, resulting in increased stress, anxiety, isolation, and health challenges. The impact is further amplified in autistic children and children with other neurodevelopmental considerations. These children are uniquely vulnerable due to communication impairments, comorbid medical disorders, poor adaptability, and reliance on therapeutic interventions. Abrupt reduction in services and access to care during the pandemic led to compromised physical and mental health and missed opportunities for intervention at critical times, which may have profound consequences further down the road [1]. There are, however, bright spots in this story, because many autistic children demonstrated resilience in their abilities to adapt to these challenges. It is important to examine the effects that the pandemic triggered, address deficiencies, and recognize new opportunities to improve systems of care to prepare for unforeseen futures. This review outlines the impacts of the first year and a half of the pandemic on autistic children and provides tools for professionals, recognizing the ever-evolving nature of the situation (Fig. 1).

CAVEATS ABOUT THE STATE OF THE SCIENCE

This article reviews findings from the available published scientific literature, combined with clinical experience from the trenches during the first year and a half of the COVID-19 pandemic to generate comprehensive recommendations for practitioners serving autistic individuals and their families during

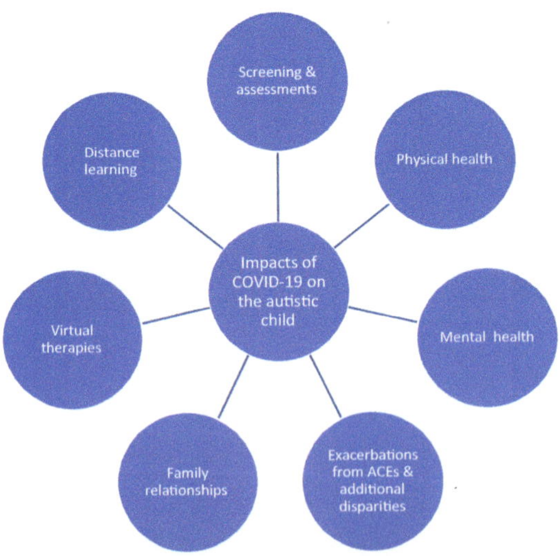
Screening &
assessments
Distance
learning
Physical health
Impacts of
COVID-19 on
the autistic
child
Virtual
therapies
Mental health
Family
relationships
Exacerbations
from ACEs &
additional
disparities

Fig. 1. The multidimensional impact of COVID-19 on autistic children. ACE, adverse childhood event.

times of crisis. It is important to note that the research literature at this time is incomplete, evolving, and has significant gaps in key areas. Generating ways of examining these groups through creative and nontraditional means is an important public health priority within this field, and as a result, many of the available studies oftentimes involved smaller and narrower sample sizes. Clinical experience as medical and mental health providers at a university-based medical institution supplemented the available literature to provide a thorough summary and meaningful recommendations on this topic.

MEDICAL CARE

Early in the pandemic, most children did not seem to become severely ill from COVID-19 compared with adults [2], although the COVID-19 landscape is ever-changing with the emergence of new variants. However, analysis during the pandemic found that autistic children without comorbidities were hospitalized at much higher rates than other children, and even more so if they had autism with comorbid intellectual disability [3]. Comparatively, autistic children were hospitalized at higher rates than children with other medical problems including obesity and heart failure [3]. Hospitalizations of autistic children with COVID-19 were also longer than their neurotypical peers with increased risk of mortality [3,4].

These higher risks in the autistic population are likely multifactorial, including decreased ability to wear masks and convey symptoms and communication barriers limiting the ability to follow safety directions [4]. More severely impaired autistic individuals often live in group homes, placing them at greater risk for rapid viral spread [5]. Before the pandemic, autistic children were found to have poor cooperation and noncompliance in inpatient settings [6]. The use of insensitive techniques in pediatrics can inadvertently increase behavioral outbursts and complicate the ability to provide life-saving treatments, necessitating the use of chemical or physical restraints, which can further exacerbate aggressive behaviors [7]. Although some health care workers are receiving formal training on aggression and challenging behavior management, this is not yet standard of care and more research working with the pediatric autistic population, specifically, is needed [7–9]. Given these multi-tiered risk factors, autistic children must be recognized as a high-risk population for COVID-19.

During the initial part of the pandemic, the autistic community voiced fears of "health care rationing," an example of which is prioritizing a neurotypical patient over a patient with a neurodevelopmental disorder should only one ventilator be available [10]. Many US states and several European countries issued crisis care guidelines at the pandemic's peak, raising community concerns for exclusion of care in specific adult populations, such as individuals with disabilities and the elderly [11,12]. Such policies must receive critical evaluation, especially given the aforementioned heightened risk for hospitalization and death of the autistic population so that autistic patients are treated fairly and ethically.

Owing to scientific innovation and collaboration, at the time of this article, the US Food and Drug Administration (FDA) authorized 3 vaccines against COVID-19 [13]. Before the pandemic, autistic children were vaccinated at lower rates than neurotypical children [14]. Studies published after the pandemic's onset found that reasons for vaccine hesitancy in parents of autistic children included beliefs that vaccines led to autism and developmental plateaus [15,16].

However, a large study of autistic adults found higher rates of COVID-19 vaccination compared with age-matched controls, while acknowledging varying vaccine practices across countries and populations [17]. This higher rate could be due to many factors including parental oversight of autistic individuals and concern for more severe COVID-19 illness. A small study found no increased COVID-19 vaccine side effects, such as fever or fatigue, in autistic patients compared with nonautistic patients [18]. These data support favorable trends in combating the pandemic in autistic individuals, and providers should continue to refer to FDA recommendations regarding updates on vaccination age cutoffs and booster doses to best protect autistic patients.

Autistic children should be considered a high-risk population for medical complications of COVID-19, due to factors predisposing them to infections and difficulties with inpatient hospitalizations. Given these risks, standardized interventions to address behaviors complicating hospital stays should be investigated and implemented even beyond the pandemic. Policies in times of crises must be critically evaluated for ethical care of a neurodiverse population. Although vaccination has historically been a contentious subject in the autistic community, efforts to prioritize *COVID-19 vaccination in autistic patients should be encouraged.*

TELEHEALTH

Owing to physical distancing measures and parental fears, a steep drop in pediatric well-child and sick visits was observed during the pandemic and telehealth quickly became an important mode of patient interaction [19]; this required providers to overcome technological barriers to access, insurance repayment logistics, and concerns regarding HIPAA compliance. Sometimes providers enjoyed this method of interaction, as telehealth offered a window into patients' home environments, offering unique insight into care previously unavailable [20].

Some families even preferred telehealth appointments, with parents not wanting to miss time from work and minimizing transportation barriers [21].

However, there were drawbacks to this modality of patient care with technology utilization challenges and loss of personal perspectives with telemedicine [22]. Providers experienced discomfort with diagnostic reliability, due to lack of in-person physical examinations, lack of play observations, and difficulties in screening for mental health disorders over telehealth calls. Despite increased use of telemedicine, a developmental-behavioral study of preschoolers found that most medication initiations and changes still took place in the in-person setting [23]. These findings suggest ongoing telehealth should continue to remain an option, but that a hybrid model is the best compromise between convenience and comprehensive care.

The COVID-19 pandemic forced a dramatic shift toward telehealth models. Both providers and families found satisfaction and even benefit from telehealth appointments; however, in-person visits are still important for medication changes, severe behavioral concerns, families with technology limitations, and to verify certain therapeutic modalities.

AUTISM SCREENING AND DIAGNOSIS

With the drop in in-person pediatric visits during the early days of the pandemic, opportunities were missed for timely developmental screenings. It is accepted that for some children, autism can be reliably diagnosed by experienced clinicians by 14 months of age or earlier, and that children younger than 5 years show tremendous benefit from earlier intervention [24]. The early US data on autism identification during the pandemic highlights a multitiered challenge: decreased referral rates, increased wait times for evaluation, and decreased number of children receiving early intervention (EI) services, although there were notable gaps in the data available at this time [25,26].

Given these challenges, several groups developed new and modified existing approaches in autism screening and assessments. Typically, broadband level 1 screening tests, like the Modified Checklist for Autism in Toddlers, Revised, with Follow-Up (M-CHAT-R/F), are first line in identifying toddlers at risk for autism by screening all patients in primary care, compared with level 2 tools that rely on trained clinician's observations using a structured, play-based model and are typically given when a toddler is identified as at risk [27,28].

Although the specificity and sensitivity of level 1 screening tests are high in low-risk settings, a study before the pandemic found that combining level 1 screeners and level 2 screeners, such as the STAT (Screening Tool for Autism in Toddlers and Young Children), improved specificity and could streamline referrals and decrease wait times for diagnostic evaluations [29]. Research to validate these tools are ongoing, but preliminary data are very positive [30].

Furthermore, virtual validated tools could potentially be used to identify high-risk children for EI, enabling them to begin services in a timelier manner. Limited data currently exist to support this approach. However, if data from the pandemic can demonstrate strong psychometric properties and these methods are accepted by insurers, the COVID-19 pandemic may serve as a catalyst to use alternate virtual assessment tools, such as the SORF (Systematic Observation of Red Flags of Autism Spectrum Disorder) [31], TELE-ASD-PEDS [32], or the BOSA (Brief Observation of Symptoms of Autism) [33], which are opening the door for further diagnostic access. Use of these tools would afford earlier access to care and service to underresourced and rural communities, improving patient outcomes and health equity.

During the COVID pandemic, screening for and referrals for formal assessment of autism decreased. There has been limited access to evaluations and EI in some parts of the country; this created opportunities for using innovative multitiered screeners for earlier autism identification and developing new virtual assessment tools that are hoped to improve patient outcomes and lessen health disparities.

SERVICES

COVID-19 pandemic restrictions greatly reduced the delivery of critical therapeutic interventions needed by the autistic community [34]. Autistic children often receive various treatment interventions, which can include applied behavior analysis (ABA), speech therapy, occupational therapy, physical therapy, and cognitive behavioral therapy (CBT) [35]. These therapies are typically delivered in one-to-one in-person settings, either in the home or in clinics. These children can also receive interventions through their school districts, as outlined in their Individualized Education Programs (IEPs). Therapists work closely with families to address tailored goals, which can include building social, adaptive, and communication skills and coping with sensory and behavioral challenges. Families rely on their therapy teams to help them navigate challenges and set their children up for successful outcomes.

When the pandemic struck, delivery of many vital therapy services came to an immediate halt and families lost their support networks. Concurrently, therapists faced unprecedented practice regulations, restrictions, and closures [36], and one survey of ABA therapists reported decreased productivity and job insecurity [37]. Restructuring efforts to provide virtual services were deployed. Providing therapies via telehealth is not a new concept, as the World Federation of Occupational Therapists and Confederation for Physical Therapy has encouraged their providers for many years to offer telehealth programs [38,39]. During the pandemic's peak, therapy providers implemented nuanced decision-making models that considered the risks and benefits of restarting in-person therapies versus transitioning to teletherapies [40]. During this time of mass transition, many challenges with the virtual modality of therapy delivery arose including Internet connection issues, Web literacy gaps, and difficulties following therapists' instructions remotely [41]. In one study from the SPARK/Simmons Foundation community dataset of more than 97,000 autistic individuals, the benefits of teletherapy were perceived to be low and impacted by the lack of interactive play, peer-to-peer interactions, and reinforcers, which are hard to deliver remotely [42]. For many families, there was appropriate fear that the disruption in services would lead to a regression in skills and ultimately impact prognosis.

Despite these challenges, the rise of teletherapies in many settings is exciting given its potential to make therapies more accessible by decreasing time and costs related to travel. In one intervention model, in which virtual parental support and rehabilitation was provided, parents reported increased child growth and development and increased feelings of self-relevance, engagement, perceived support, and recognition [43]. Helpful parenting tips have emerged, including scheduling regular online consultations with therapy providers, maintaining online therapy, creating structured daily schedules and reinforcement systems, and scheduling daily child-appropriate activities [43].

As service providers explored optimal best practices when offering telehealth options, several virtual tools emerged. The acronym "VIRTUAL" was developed to highlight important domains needed to deliver effective teletherapy: Visual, Information, Relationships, Technology, Unique, Access, and Legal [44]. Innovative parent coaching programs that include counseling and support have also emerged. One program focused on teaching parents to implement simple token reward systems that were positively reinforcing for all [45]. Within CBT models, therapists adopted creative solutions to several challenges posed by the virtual session format, including expanding their virtual rapport-building activities, implementing virtual visual aids/handouts, and navigating distractions [46]. Noted advantages to virtual CBT sessions included some children engaging more from the comfort of their home, sharing aspects of their physical environment, and more flexibility in scheduling sessions [46]. The COVID-19 pandemic prompted both families and service providers to become creative in the ways autistic children receive services when in-person options are not possible.

Vital therapy services for autistic children came to an immediate halt due to the COVID-19 pandemic, leaving families isolated and fearful. Virtual therapies were implemented, but not all patients were able to participate. Although virtual programs were expanded, special consideration was made to continue one-to-one therapies for some autistic children where virtual therapies were unrealistic. The COVID-19 crisis opened the door for opportunities to increase accessibility to services through virtual options that can be used even beyond the pandemic.

EDUCATION

To reduce the spread of COVID-19, schools closed globally in early 2020. Every US state closed its schools in mid-March 2020, and a US study found significant decreases in incidence of and mortality from COVID-19 in states where in-person schools remained closed [47]. Stay-at-home orders, which included school and nonessential business closures, were associated with decreased incidence of COVID-19 infections [48]. However, a study of schools that resumed in-person classes in fall 2020 found that the vast majority of students and staff members who contracted COVID-19 during the school year acquired their infections from exposures outside of school [49]. This finding suggests that interventions that fall short of school closures, such as canceling large gatherings, physical distancing, and masking, may have more effectively prevented COVID-19 spread than school closures. Although school closure focused on preventing deaths and avoiding overwhelming hospitals due to COVID-19 cases, models have demonstrated that the mass school closures will lead to higher years of life lost due to downstream impacts of educational losses than the estimated years of life saved from COVID-19 infections [50,51]. With the rise of new COVID-19 variants and lack of approved COVID-19 vaccines for younger children at this time, the risk of these factors must be weighed.

As the lockdown phase of the pandemic progressed, the US Department of Education released statements regarding providing special education and evaluations during times of physical distancing [52]. Meanwhile, it became clear that distance learning jeopardized the upholding of the Individuals with Disabilities Education Act (IDEA) and providing Free and Appropriate Public Education (FAPE). Around the world, children's special education was discontinued during the pandemic [53]. As most schools transitioned online, the impact of distance learning on autistic children was varied and complex. A study exploring the core pandemic experiences of parents of autistic children found that families lacked tools to provide education at home, feared downstream implications of distance learning, and lamented the loss of attention that their children previously received in-person [54]. Behaviors such as noncompliance, inflexibility, and tantrums worsened with distance learning [55]. The Core Experiences Study demonstrated higher educational losses in students learning in virtual environments compared with peers learning in person [56], and more isolation and decreased physical activity [57]. Contrasted with these findings, some children benefited from the distance learning environment, became more relaxed while learning at home, developed independence, and built better relationships with their parents [58–60]. Although some parents reported preference for virtual learning, this type of education likely failed to meet children's socialization needs. Clinical experience found that in some cases, distance learning was so preferred that there was real fear and anxiety about returning to in-person learning. However, the options for home-charter schools and medical home programs would not adequately support the needs of children with higher support needs because neither program typically offers sufficient special education support.

These findings prompt many questions regarding the future of education for autistic children. If some parents have preference for and data support that students fare better with distance learning during the pandemic, is IDEA obligated to continue facilitating this option? What emerging lessons can be harnessed to provide the best education to autistic children? How will the education system catch up on the backlogs of IEPs? How will students be provided the opportunity to make up for what they lost, especially those in special education and those attending underserved schools? Although early studies are only beginning to highlight the educational impact of COVID-19 on students, time and future studies are needed to fully grasp the impact of the pandemic on education, especially the education of autistic children.

In the autistic population, many children struggled with virtual learning during the pandemic, with limited or completely halted education and worsening of behaviors at home, whereas some benefited in many ways from distance learning at home. Further studies are needed to assess the full degree of impact on autistic children. Many more studies so far have been conducted of the neurotypical population, showing greater negative impacts of distance learning related to social determinants of health, and models showing higher years of life lost due to school closures than years of life saved by halting in-person education. The experience thus far has frankly led to more questions than answers about what is best educationally for autistic children moving forward, questions that should guide innovative thinking for education system structuring so that it can most benefit autistic children.

MENTAL HEALTH

Autistic children are at greater risk to psychological challenges during the COVID-19 pandemic than their neurotypical peers due to the nature of autism, which demands consistency and is highly associated with comorbid anxiety, depression, and attention-deficit/hyperactivity disorder. One study found increased aggression, behavioral outbursts, and regression more in the autistic population than in other children with neurodevelopmental considerations during the restrictions [55]. Anxiety and depression were highest among those with prepandemic psychiatric conditions, those who were younger, and those with fewer emotional contacts [55,61]. These effects were worse earlier in the pandemic and compounded by limited access to educational services [53,55]. When compared with neurotypical groups, there was a clear pattern that disrupted schedules and services were more problematic for autistic children compared with neurotypical subjects [61]. However, there were benefits found in some studies, wherein autistic adults reported enjoying isolation with reduced sensory and social overload [61].

Examining the utilization of the mental health emergency care system during the pandemic demonstrated an increase in mental health acuity, including increased suicide attempts [62,63]. Immediately after stay-at-home orders were enacted, the number of pediatric emergency department (ED) visits dropped, but over the next several months, whereas ED visits remained low, the proportion of ED visits for mental health crises increased dramatically, most notably in patients older than 12 years [63,64]. Patients with mental health conditions presented more severely during the COVID-19 pandemic and more frequently required admission to the hospital [65]. Unfortunately, in clinical experience, children were boarded in the ED for hours to days because inpatient psychiatric facilities were overwhelmed with patients due to the increase in acute mental health needs from COVID-19 [66].

With the reality of increased mental health needs during the pandemic, it is important to understand factors that aid in resilience. Having strong family function prepandemic and contact with the school system even indirectly were found to be protective [55,67]. In autistic adults' telehealth check-ins, telehealth with a therapist, journaling, maintaining a schedule, walking/exercise, and keeping in touch with family via phone/chat were critically important in coping during times of physical distancing [68]. Families reported that social stories, providing breaks, telehealth, hobbies, cooking, and virtual connections were helpful as well. These findings underscore the importance of targeting emotional regulation, continued services, social connection, and creating routine among the chaos. Understanding factors that support resilience are critical in offering tools moving forward.

The growing literature suggests that the mental health of children declined during the COVID-19 pandemic, more significantly so in autistic children and those with pre-COVID-19 behavioral concerns. However, autistic individuals without service disruptions, with schedules, and with ongoing social support fared better. As this population reintegrates and the state of normalcy returns, providers should also watch for a spike in behaviors, because this will create another change in routines, new social demands, and sensory inputs.

FAMILY RELATIONSHIPS

The COVID-19 pandemic presented many challenges to the families of autistic children. Schools are an important influence in children's lives because many autistic children receive services in the school setting, thrive in a structured and organized classroom, and benefit from the opportunities in school to socialize with peers [69,70]. The loss of in-person education significantly disrupted the lives of autistic children, and in many cases placed more pressure and stress on families to make up for these losses. More time spent in restricted spaces at home with fewer resources, such as being limited to the same toys, can exacerbate children's restricted interests, thus worsening autism symptoms and challenging family dynamics. Parents had difficulties setting limits on play and screen time, leading to more conflict in parent-child relationships [71]. Parents of autistic children are already at heightened risk for mental health problems such as stress, depression, and anxiety, which was likely exacerbated during the pandemic, due to decreased access to respite care and increased demands in the home environment [72]. Emerging data during the pandemic found that children were at increased risk for abuse in the home in the setting of parental job loss [73]. The mental health of parents and children were linked during COVID-19, so when parents struggled, children were more likely to struggle, and vice versa [74].

Despite these challenges, some families saw benefits in certain domains for their children that improved family dynamics. For example, some children experienced less stress due to the decreased social demands and decreased academic pressures of distance learning [60,75]. However, this was less likely to be the case for families in which their child had behavioral or learning difficulties. Half of the parents in one small study reported their children being happier and calmer during quarantine [76]. Not having to endure battles over homework completion, for instance, during the first 6 months of homeschooling, reduced parent and child stress levels and conflict. During the pandemic and the period of remote learning, children were allowed to honor their rhythms of sleep/wake cycles, eating, and physical activity in a way that was more individually beneficial rather than having to meet the needs of an entire student body, which could reduce overall stress load in the home.

Disrupted routines and changes presented opportunities for innovation in families with autistic children during the pandemic. Families that were able to implement routines in the home environment, adequately limit children's exposure to screens or restricted interests, continue to expose their children to social environments, and reduce challenges that children face in the in-person school environment, such as teasing, bullying, and academic stressors, may have created an optimal home life for autistic children.

CONSIDERATION OF FURTHER EXACERBATIONS FROM DISPARITIES AND ADVERSE CHILDHOOD EVENTS

It is important to consider how the disparities that many autistic children experience may have exacerbated the negative impacts the pandemic had on them. Before the COVID-19 crisis, families of autistic children and children with developmental disabilities were at higher risk for food insecurity [77]. One study reported worsening of behaviors during the pandemic in autistic children from lower-income families and families who were food insecure [78]. During the pandemic, minority populations were found to have increased rates of food insecurity compared with nonminorities [79,80]. Consideration of these multiple factors is important because the pandemic likely created a situation of potentially compounding effects and multiple vulnerabilities for autistic children and their families.

The educational crisis during the COVID-19 pandemic exacerbated already present disparities in learning opportunities for children. Less participation in virtual learning activities was found in students in poverty [81] and students in rural communities [82]. Families with monetary means were able to provide innovative solutions to educate their children during times of school closures, such as paying out of pocket for educated adults to lead "pods" of students in a neighborhood [83]. Meanwhile a digital divide and worsening achievement gaps became apparent for students from low-income families who experienced limited access to digital equipment and Internet [84]. The implications of these findings for autistic children must be considered, especially given the additional challenges they faced with distance learning as mentioned previously.

These considerations are important due to the strong relationship between autism diagnosis and a higher number of adverse childhood events (ACEs) [85]. ACEs are a set of 10 potentially traumatic events occurring in childhood that have been linked to health problems in adulthood [86]; this is likely due to the families of autistic children being particularly vulnerable to financial difficulties, parental divorce/separation, and household mental illness/substance abuse. In addition to delayed diagnosis, the average age of entry into autism services was delayed in patients with higher ACE scores [87]. Given these baseline statistics, the COVID-19 pandemic has likely compounded these disparities further and has placed autistic children at higher risk for negative outcomes, although no study on this has been published at this time.

Families of autistic children have faced compounding vulnerabilities during the pandemic. The challenges of distance learning led parents to unique and discriminatory ways of coping, often serving only those with greater economic means and exacerbating already present educational disparities. It will be important for health care professionals to offer support and resources to families and to screen for ACEs and for further research to be conducted regarding these topics.

THE PEDIATRICIAN'S TOOLBOX FOR AUTISM CARE IN CORONAVIRUS DISEASE 2019 AND BEYOND

For the general pediatrician, it is important to understand the complex impact of the COVID-19 pandemic on autistic patients and their families, recognizing that every family experienced challenges and possibly even found some pleasant surprises along the way. During office visits physically or virtually, families should be asked open endedly about their experiences and check-in on their well-being. In addition, families should be helped to navigate challenges faced with their child's education and service interventions. The expansion of the use of telemedicine brings new opportunities for innovative ways to screen and diagnose patients and decrease wait times.

Advocacy for children and challenging of potentially unethical policies will be needed to lessen disparities and provide care with equity.

During the pandemic, several online services were augmented or created to provide information about autism and tips for care. Many intervention programs were adapted and are now available as caregiver-delivered programs, increasing caregivers' abilities to support their children over the long-term. Webinars and resources were created to help parents encourage prosocial behaviors at home, including Baby Navigator, Autism Speaks, Triad Family First, and Help is in Your Hands (Fig. 2). These services are hoped to outlive COVID-19 pandemic as useful educational tools for parents and a bridge to services.

When autistic children and their families are exposed to unforeseen circumstances, such as the COVID-19 pandemic, pediatricians can help in many ways as a primary point of contact for these families during difficult times. Fig. 2 is the Pediatrician's Toolbox for care of the autistic child based on the early findings and needs that have come to light during the COVID-19 crisis. Through all the darkness of this pandemic there is hope and possibility for improvement in care for autistic patients.

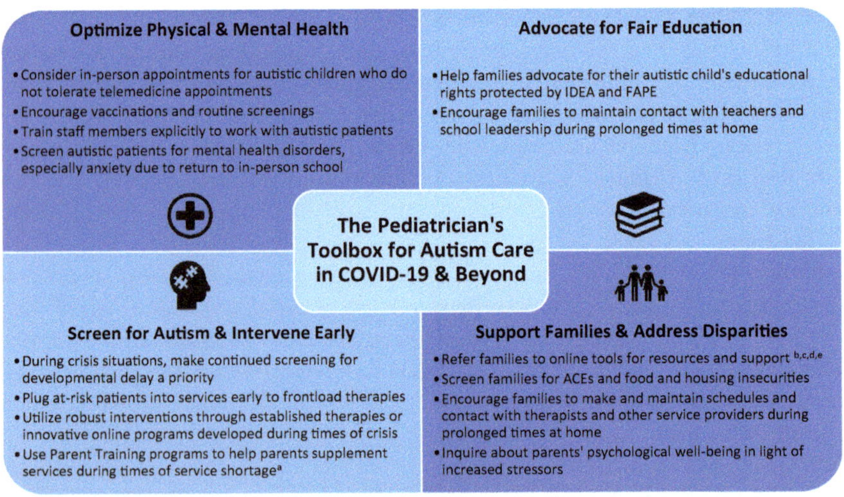

Fig. 2. A pediatrician's toolbox for autism care in coronavirus disease 2019 and beyond. Web tools: [a]*Autism Speaks Parent Training*: https://www.autismspeaks.org/covid-19-information-and-resources-families#ParentTraining; [b]*Baby Navigator:* babynavigator.com; [c]*Autism Speaks:* autismspeaks.org; [d]*TRIAD Families First Program:* vkc.vumc.org/vkc/triad/fam/; [e]*The AAP Parenting Website:* https://www.healthychildren.org/English/Pages/default.aspx.

DISCLOSURE

The authors have nothing to disclose.

CLINICS CARE POINTS

- This paper reviewed the available literature up until the time of submission, which was incomplete and developing, and notably most available studies involved small sample sizes
- Autistic children with COVID-19 were hospitalized more frequently and for longer periods than their neurotypical peers
- COVID-19 vaccination in autistic patients should be encouraged given their higher risk for more severe illness
- The pandemic forced a dramatic shift toward telehealth models, and while both providers and families found benefit in telehealth appointments, in-person visits are still important for medication changes, severe behavioral concerns and families with technology limitation
- The COVID-19 pandemic led to a fall in screening for and referrals for formal assessment of autism, simultaneously creating opportunities for utilizing multi-tiered screeners for earlier autism identification and the development of virtual assessment tools
- Therapy services for autistic children came to a halt due to the COVID-19 pandemic, and while virtual therapies were implemented, not all patients were able to participate
- In the autistic population, while many children struggled with virtual learning during the pandemic, with limited or completely halted education and worsening of behaviors at home, some benefited in many ways from distance learning at home; further studies are needed to assess the full degree of impact of virtual learning on autistic children
- The challenges of distance learning led parents to unique ways of coping, often serving only those with greater economic means and exacerbating already present disparities
- Utilization of routines and reduction of challenges that autistic children face in the in-person school environment, such as bullying and social stressors, may have created an optimal home life for autistic children during the pandemic
- When autistic children and their families are exposed to unforeseen circumstances, such as the COVID-19 pandemic, pediatricians can help as the primary point of contact for these families during difficult times, including pointing them to online resources and engaging in advocacy

Acknowledgments

The authors wish to thank Dr Peter Chung, Dr Geeta Grover, and Dr Marc Lerner for their advice regarding the content of this article, as well as Jenny Zanger for assisting with reference organization.

References

[1] White LC, Law JK, Daniels AM, et al. Brief Report: Impact of COVID-19 on individuals with ASD and their caregivers: A perspective from the SPARK cohort. J Autism Dev Disord 2021;51(10):3766–73.

[2] CDC. COVID data tracker: demographic trends of COVID-19 cases and deaths in the US reported to CDC. Atlanta (GA): US Department of Health and Human Services, CDC; 2021. Available at: https://covid.cdc.gov/covid-data-tracker/#demographics.
[3] Karpur A, Vasudevan V, Shih A, et al. Brief report: Impact of COVID-19 in individuals with autism spectrum disorders: Analysis of a national private claims insurance database. J Autism Dev Dis 2021; https://doi.org/10.1007/s10803-021-05100-x.
[4] Oakley B, Tillmann J, Ruigrok A, et al. COVID-19 health and social care access for autistic people: European policy review. BMJ Open 2021;11(6):e045341.
[5] Landes SD, Turk MA, Formica MK, McDonald KE, Stevens JD. COVID-19 outcomes among people with intellectual and developmental disability living in residential group homes in New York State. Disabil Health J 2020;13(4):100969.
[6] Johnson NL, Rodriguez D. Children with autism spectrum disorder at a pediatric hospital: a systematic review of the literature. Pediatr Nurs 2013;39(3):131–41. Available at: https://pubmed.ncbi.nlm.nih.gov/23926752/.
[7] Dalton EM, Herndon AC, Cundiff A, et al. Decreasing the use of restraints on children admitted for behavioral health conditions. Pediatrics 2021;148(1):e2020003939.
[8] Matuska G, Gallagher A. The needs of people with intellectual disabilities and autism during the pandemic: Making the invisible visible. Nurs Ethics 2020;27(7):1487–9.
[9] Mitchell MJ, Newall FH, Sokol J, et al. Simulation-based education for staff managing aggression and externalizing behaviors in children with autism spectrum disorder in the hospital setting: pilot and feasibility study protocol for a cluster randomized controlled trial. JMIR Res Protoc 2020;9(6):e18105.
[10] den Houting J. Stepping out of isolation: Autistic people and COVID-19. Autism Adulthood 2020;2(2):103–5.
[11] Scully JL. Disability, disablism, and COVID-19 pandemic triage. J Bioeth Inq 2020;17(4):601–5.
[12] Epstein S, Campanile J, Cerilli C, et al. New obstacles and widening gaps: A qualitative study of the effects of the COVID-19 pandemic on U.S. adults with disabilities. Disabil Health J 2021;14(3):101103.
[13] COVID-19 Vaccines. US Food and Drug Administration. 2021. Available at: https://www.fda.gov/emergency-preparedness-and-response/coronavirus-disease-2019- covid-19/covid-19-vaccines. Accessed October 30, 2021.
[14] Zerbo O, Modaressi S, Goddard K, et al. Vaccination patterns in children after autism spectrum disorder diagnosis and in their younger siblings. JAMA Pediatr 2018;172(5):469–75.
[15] Goin-Kochel RP, Fombonne E, Mire SS, et al. Beliefs about causes of autism and vaccine hesitancy among parents of children with autism spectrum disorder. Vaccine 2020;38(40):6327–33.
[16] Bonsu NEM, Mire SS, Sahni LC, et al. Understanding vaccine hesitancy among parents of children with autism spectrum disorder and parents of children with non-autism developmental delays. J Child Neurol 2021;36(10):911–8.
[17] Weinstein O, Krieger I, Cohen AD, et al. COVID-19 vaccination among individuals with autism spectrum disorder: A population-based study. Res Autism Spectr Disord 2021;89.
[18] Brondino N, Bertoglio F, Forneris F, et al. A pilot study on covid and autism: Prevalence, clinical presentation and vaccine side effects. Brain Sci 2021;11(7):860.
[19] Crawley E, Loades M, Feder G, et al. Wider collateral damage to children in the UK because of the social distancing measures designed to reduce the impact of COVID-19 in adults. BMJ Paediatr Open 2020;4(1):e000701.
[20] Knutsen J, Wolfe A, Burke BL, et al. A systematic review of telemedicine in autism spectrum disorders. Rev J Autism Dev Disord 2016;3:330–44.
[21] Burke BL Jr, Hall RW, Section on Telehealth Care. Telemedicine: Pediatric applications. Pediatrics 2015;136(1):e293–308.

[22] Simacek J, Elmquist M, Dimian AF, et al. Current trends in telehealth applications to deliver social communication interventions for young children with or at risk for autism spectrum disorder [published online ahead of print, 2020 Oct 12]. Curr Dev Disord Rep 2020;1–9.
[23] Harstad E, Shults J, Barbaresi W, et al. Preschool attention-deficit/hyperactivity disorder and telephone medication management at developmental-behavioral pediatric network sites. J Dev Behav Pediatr 2021;42(6):481–4.
[24] Landa RJ, Gross AL, Stuart EA, et al. Developmental trajectories in children with and without autism spectrum disorders: The first 3 years. Child Dev 2013;84(2):429–42.
[25] Delayed Interventions: Early Indicators of the Pandemic's Impact on Infants and Toddlers. Advocates for children of New York. 2021. Available at: https://www.advocatesforchildren.org/custom_search?amp=. Accessed October 31, 2021.
[26] The Impact of COVID-19 on Early Intervention: How States can Support our Youngest Learners. The Education Trust. 2021. Available at: https://edtrust.org/wp-content/uploads/2014/09/The- Impact-of-COVID-19-on-Early-Intervention-How-States-Can-Support-Our-Youngest- Learners-May-2021.pdf. Accessed October 31, 2021.
[27] Robins DL, Casagrande K, Barton M, et al. Validation of the modified checklist for Autism in toddlers, revised with follow-up (M-CHAT-R/F). Pediatrics 2014;133(1):37–45.
[28] Brewer N, Young RL, Lucas CA. Autism screening in early childhood: Discriminating autism from other developmental concerns. Front Neurol 2020;11:594381.
[29] Khowaja M, Robins DL, Adamson LB. Utilizing two-tiered screening for early detection of autism spectrum disorder. Autism 2018;22(7):881–90.
[30] Berger NI, Wainer AL, Kuhn J, et al. Characterizing available tools for synchronous virtual assessment of toddlers with suspected autism spectrum disorder: A brief report. J Autism Dev Disord 2021; https://doi.org/10.1007/s10803-021-04911-2.
[31] Dow D, Day TN, Kutta TJ, et al. Screening for autism spectrum disorder in a naturalistic home setting using the systematic observation of red flags (SORF) at 18-24 months. Autism Res 2020;13(1):122–33.
[32] Corona L, Hine J, Nicholson A, et al. TELE-ASD-PEDS: a telemedicine-based ASD evaluation tool for toddlers and Young children. Vanderbilt University Medical Center; 2020. Available at: https://vkc.vumc.org/vkc/triad/tele-asd-peds.
[33] Lord C, Dow D, Holbrook A, et al. Brief observation of symptoms of autism (BOSA). Western Psychological Services; 2020.
[34] Masi A, Mendoza Diaz A, Tully L, et al. Impact of the COVID-19 pandemic on the well- being of children with neurodevelopmental disabilities and their parents. J Paediatr Child Health 2021;57(5):631–6.
[35] Lord C, Elsabbagh M, Baird G, et al. Autism spectrum disorder. Lancet 2018;392(10146): 508–20.
[36] Litke N, Daniel T, Wallacher S, et al. Einfluss der COVID-19 Pandemie auf die ambulante physiotherapie [Impact of the COVID-19 pandemic on outpatient physical therapy in Germany]. Z Evid Fortbild Qual Gesundhwes 2021;165:58–67.
[37] Jimenez-Gomez C, Sawhney G, Albert KM. Impact of COVID-19 on the applied behavior analysis workforce: Comparison across remote and nonremote workers. Behav Anal Pract 2021;1–10; https://doi.org/10.1007/s40617-021-00625-0.
[38] Jacobs K, Cason J, McCullough A. The process for the formulation of the international telehealth position statement for occupational therapy. Int J Telerehabilitation 2015;7(1): 21–32.
[39] Report of the WCPT/INPTRA Digital Physical Therapy Practice Task Force. World Physiotherapy. 2020. Available at: https://world.physio/sites/default/files/2020-06/WCPT-INPTRA-Digital- Physical-Therapy-Practice-Task-force-March2020.pdf. Accessed August 11, 2021..
[40] degli Espinosa F, Metko A, Raimondi M, et al. A model of support for families of children with autism living in the COVID-19 lockdown: Lessons from Italy. Behav Anal Pract 2020;13(3): 550–8.

[41] Camden C, Silva M. Pediatric teleheath: Opportunities created by the COVID-19 and suggestions to sustain its use to support families of children with disabilities. Phys Occup Ther Pediatr 2021;41(1):1–17.
[42] Shorey S, Tiang Lau LS, Tan JX, et al. Families with children with neurodevelopmental disorders during COVID-19: A scoping review. J Pediatr Psychol 2021;46(5):514–25.
[43] Provenzi L, Grumi S, Gardani A, et al. Italian parents welcomed a telehealth family-centered rehabilitation programme for children with disability during COVID-19 lockdown. Acta Paediatr 2020;110(1):194–6.
[44] Colombo RA, Wallace M, Taylor R. An essential service decision model for ABA providers during crisis. Behav Anal Pract 2020;13:306–11.
[45] LeBlanc LA, Lazo-Pearson JF, Pollard JS, et al. The role of compassion and ethics in decision making regarding access to applied behavior analysis services during the COVID-19 crisis: A response to Cox, Plavnick, and Brodhead. Behav Anal Pract 2020;13(3):604–8.
[46] Kalvin CB, Jordan RP, Rowley SN, et al. Conducting CBT for anxiety in children with autism spectrum disorder during COVID-19 pandemic. J Autism Dev Disord 2020; https://doi.org/10.1007/s10803-020-04845-1.
[47] Auger KA, Shah SS, Richardson T, et al. Association between statewide school closure and COVID-19 incidence and mortality in the US. JAMA 2020;324(9):859–70.
[48] Lyu W, Wehby GL. Comparison of estimated rates of coronavirus disease 2019 (COVID-19) in border counties in Iowa without a stay-at-home order and border counties in Illinois with a stay-at-home order. JAMA Netw Open 2020;3(5):e2011102.
[49] Zimmerman KO, Akinboyo IC, Brookhart MA, et al. Incidence and secondary transmission of SARS-COV-2 infections in schools. Pediatrics 2021;147(4):e2020048090.
[50] Christakis DA, Van Cleve W, Zimmerman FJ. Estimation of US children's educational attainment and years of life lost associated with primary school closures during the coronavirus disease 2019 pandemic. JAMA Netw Open 2020;3(11); https://doi.org/10.1001/jamanetworkopen.2020.28786.
[51] Zimmerman FJ, Anderson NW. Association of the timing of school closings and behavioral changes with the evolution of the coronavirus disease 2019 pandemic in the US. JAMA Pediatr 2021;175(5):501–9; https://doi.org/10.1001/jamapediatrics.2020.6371.
[52] Office for Civil Rights & Office of Special Education and Rehabilitative Services. Addressing the risk of COVID-19 in preschool, elementary and Secondary Schools while serving children with disabilities. US Dept of Education; 2020.
[53] Mutluer T, Doenyas C, Aslan Genc H. Behavioral implications of the COVID-19 process for autism spectrum disorder, and individuals' comprehension of and reactions to the pandemic conditions. Front Psychiatry 2020;11:561882.
[54] Tokatly Latzer I, Leitner Y, Karnieli-Miller O. Core experiences of parents of children with autism during the COVID-19 pandemic lockdown. Autism 2021;25(4):1047–59.
[55] Colizzi M, Sironi E, Antonini F, et al. Psychosocial and behavioral impact of COVID-19 in autism spectrum disorder: an online parent survey. Brain Sci 2020;10(6):341.
[56] Verlenden JV, Pampati S, Rasberry CN, et al. Association of children's mode of school instruction with child and parent experiences and well-being during the COVID-19 pandemic — COVID experiences surveyUnited States, October 8 pandemic — COVID experiences survey, United States, October 8–November 13, 2020. MMWR 2021;70(11):369–76.
[57] Takaku R, Yokoyama I. What the COVID-19 school closure left in its wake: Evidence from a regression discontinuity analysis in Japan. J Public Econ 2021;195:104364.
[58] Pesch MH, Julian MM, Munzer TG. Reflections on children with developmental and behavioral challenges who are thriving while sheltering in place. J Dev Behav Pediatr 2020;41(7): 506–7.
[59] Meral BF. Parental views of families of children with autism spectrum disorder and developmental disorders during the COVID-19 pandemic. J Autism Dev Disord 2021; https://doi.org/10.1007/s10803-021-05070-0.

[60] Mumbardó-Adam C, Barnet-López S, Balboni G. How have youth with Autism Spectrum Disorder managed quarantine derived from COVID-19 pandemic? An approach to families perspectives. Res Dev Disabil 2021;110:103860.
[61] Oomen D, Nijhof AD, Wiersema JR. The psychological impact of the COVID-19 pandemic on adults with autism: a survey study across three countries. Mol Autism 2021;12; https://doi.org/10.1186/s13229-021-00424-y.
[62] Hill RM, Rufino K, Kurian S, et al. Suicide ideation and attempts in a pediatric emergency department before and during COVID-19. Pediatrics 2021;147(3); https://doi.org/10.1542/peds.2020-029280.
[63] Leeb RT, Bitsko RH, Radhakrishnan L, et al. Mental health– related emergency department visits among children aged <18 years during the COVID- 19 pandemic — United States, January 1–October 17, 2020. MMWR 2020;69(45):1675–80.
[64] Gill PJ, Mahant S, Hall M, et al. Reasons for admissions to US children's hospitals during the COVID-19 pandemic. JAMA 2021;325(16):1676–9.
[65] Krass P, Dalton E, Doupnik SK, Esposito J. US pediatric emergency department visits for mental health conditions during the COVID-19 pandemic. JAMA Netw Open 2021;4(4): e218533.
[66] Hoffmann JA, Duffy SJ. Supporting youth mental health during the COVID-19 pandemic. Acad Emerg Med 2021; https://doi.org/10.1111/acem.14398.
[67] Penner F, Hernandez Ortiz J, Sharp C. Change in youth mental health during the COVID- 19 pandemic in a majority Hispanic/Latinx US Sample. J Am Acad Child Adolesc Psychiatry 2021;60(4):513–23.
[68] Ameis SH, Lai MC, Mulsant BH, et al. Coping, fostering resilience, and driving care innovation for autistic people and their families during the COVID-19 pandemic and beyond. Mol Autism 2020;11; https://doi.org/10.1186/s13229-020-00365-y.
[69] Golberstein E, Wen H, Miller BF. Coronavirus disease 2019 (COVID-19) and mental health for children and adolescents. JAMA Pediatr 2020;174(9):819–20.
[70] Shattuck PT, Orsmond GI, Wagner M, Cooper BP. Participation in social activities among adolescents with an autism spectrum disorder. PLoS One 2011;6(11); https://doi.org/10.1371/journal.pone.0027176.
[71] Fitzpatrick SE, Srivorakiat L, Wink LK, Pedapati EV, Erickson CA. Aggression in autism spectrum disorder: Presentation and treatment options. Neuropsychiatr Dis Treat 2016;12: 1525–38.
[72] Keenan BM, Newman LK, Gray KM, et al. Parents of children with ASD experience more psychological distress, parenting stress, and attachment-related anxiety. J Autism Developmental Disord 2016;46(9):2979–91.
[73] Lawson M, Piel MH, Simon M. Child maltreatment during the COVID-19 pandemic: Consequences of parental job loss on psychological and physical abuse towards children. Child Abuse Negl 2020;110(Pt 2):104709.
[74] Bate J, Pham PT, Borelli JL. Be my safe haven: Parent–child relationships and emotional health during COVID-19. J Pediatr Psychol 2021;46(6):624–34.
[75] Liu G, Wang S, Liao J, et al. The efficacy of WeChat-based parenting training on the psychological well-being of mothers with children with autism during the COVID-19 pandemic: Quasi-experimental study. JMIR Ment Health 2021;8(2); https://doi.org/10.2196/23917.
[76] Forrest DL, Kroeger RA, Stroope S. Autism spectrum disorder symptoms and bullying victimization among children with autism in the United States. J Autism Dev Disord 2020;50: 560–71.
[77] Karpur A, Vasudevan V, Lello A, et al. Food insecurity in the households of children with autism spectrum disorders and intellectual disabilities in the United States: Analysis of the National Survey of Children's Health Data 2016–2018. Autism 2021; https://doi.org/10.1177/13623613211019159.

[78] Panjwani AA, Bailey RL, Kelleher BL. COVID-19 and behaviors in children with autism spectrum disorder: disparities by income and food security status. Res Dev Disabil 2021;115: 104002.
[79] Fitzpatrick KM, Harris C, Drawve G, Willis DE. Assessing food insecurity among US adults during the COVID-19 pandemic. J Hunger Environ Nutr 2020;16(1):1–18.
[80] Dubowitz T, Dastidar MG, Troxel WM, et al. Food Insecurity in a Low-Income, Predominantly African American Cohort Following the COVID-19 Pandemic. Am J Public Health 2021;111(3):494–7.
[81] Hash PM. Remote learning in school bands during the COVID-19 shutdown. J Res Music Educ 2020;68(4):381–97.
[82] Onyema EM, Eucheria NC, Obafemi FA, et al. Impact of coronavirus pandemic on education. J Educ Pract 2020;11(No. 13); https://doi.org/10.7176/jep/11-13-12.
[83] Carpenter D, Dunn J. We're all teachers now: Remote learning during COVID-19. J Sch Choice 2020;14(4):567–94.
[84] Goudeau S, Sanrey C, Stanczak A, et al. Why lockdown and distance learning during the COVID-19 pandemic are likely to increase the social class achievement gap. Nat Hum Behav 2021;5(10):1273–81.
[85] Rigles B. The relationship between adverse childhood events, resiliency and health among children with autism. J Autism Dev Disord 2017;47(1):187–202.
[86] Felitti VJ, Anda RF, Nordenberg D, et al. Relationship of childhood abuse and household dysfunction to many of the leading causes of death in adults. The Adverse Childhood Experiences (ACE) Study. Am J Prev Med 1998;14(4):245–58.
[87] Berg KL, Acharya K, Shiu CS, et al. Delayed diagnosis and treatment among children with autism who experience adversity. J Autism Dev Disord 2018;48(1):45–54.

Advances in Pediatrics 69 (2022) 59–74

ADVANCES IN PEDIATRICS

Brain Surgery for Medically Intractable Epilepsy

Vincent Joris, MD[a], Alexander G. Weil, MD, FRCSC[b], Aria Fallah, MD, MSc, FRCSC[c,*]

[a]Fellow, Department of Neurosurgery, Sainte-Justine University Hospital Centre, 3175 Chemin de la Côte-Sainte-Catherine, Montreal, Quebec H3T 1C5, Canada; [b]Associate Professor, Department of Neurosurgery, Sainte-Justine University Hospital Centre, 3175 Chemin de la Côte-Sainte-Catherine, Montreal, Quebec H3T 1C5, Canada; [c]Associate Professor, Department of Neurosurgery, David Geffen School of Medicine at University of California, Los Angeles, 300 Stein Plaza, Suite 525, Los Angeles, CA 90095, USA

Keywords

• Epilepsy surgery • Outcomes • Medically intractable epilepsy • Surgical selection • Resection

Key points

- Children suffering from drug-resistant epilepsy must be quickly referred to a comprehensive pediatric epilepsy center for a thorough presurgical evaluation.
- Early referral allows for early treatment, which reduces the risk of secondary epileptic focus and increases the possibility of greater functional neuroplasticity following resective surgery.
- Hemispheric, lobar, or lesional epilepsies are often amenable to complete resection, which increases chances of seizure freedom after surgery.
- Bihemispheric and generalized epilepsies can benefit from palliative surgeries or from neuromodulation.
- Neuromodulation techniques infrequently allow for seizure freedom but can significantly reduce seizure burden and increase quality of life.

INTRODUCTION

In North America, an estimated 100/100,000 children are diagnosed each year with epilepsy [1], which is defined as recurrent seizures, and affects between 0.5% and 1% of the population. Of those patients, 50% will be controlled by

*Corresponding author. *E-mail address:* afallah@mednet.ucla.edu

https://doi.org/10.1016/j.yapd.2022.03.014
0065-3101/22/

a first antiepileptic drug (AED) and 15% will be controlled by a second AED [2]. After 2 AED, the chance of seizure control drops significatively, meaning that 15% to 30% of children [3] will be pharmaco-resistant [4] and suffer from intractable epilepsy.

Patients suffering from intractable epilepsy are more at risk of injury [5], low self-esteem [6], and even death [7] (sudden unexpected death in epilepsy or SUDEP). Since the first randomized clinical trial (RCT) [8] in adults demonstrating that temporal lobectomy could allow better seizure control than AED in certain cases, tremendous progress has been made to better define patient and surgical procedures that could help achieve seizure freedom. In a recent RCT by Dwivedi and colleagues [9], surgical management of various epilepsy disorders in children led to 77% seizure freedom at 12 months compared with 7% with medical treatment.

The most important steps are patient selection and procedure definition. This is achieved through the presurgical workup, which will classify, roughly, the patient between focal epilepsy (temporal lobe epilepsy [TLE] or extratemporal lobe epilepsy [ETLE]) versus generalized epilepsy as well as lesional versus nonlesional epilepsy. Once the epilepsy type has been well described, surgical procedures can be tailored to the patient and the epileptic region.

The authors divided the article as follows:

- Presurgical workup
  - Noninvasive investigations
  - Invasive investigations
  - Timing of surgery
- TLE
- ETLE
- Multifocal and generalized epilepsy
  - Palliative procedures
  - Neuromodulation

PRESURGICAL WORKUP

Noninvasive investigations

Once epilepsy has been diagnosed and failure of 2 AED has been noted, the diagnosis of *intractable epilepsy* is given [4]. At that point, patients should be referred to a comprehensive epilepsy center. The first step will be to confirm drug resistance. Indeed, the 2 AED given to the patient might have been inadequate for the epilepsy type [10].

Once drug resistance is confirmed, a complete workup is undergone to best define the epileptic zone based on anatomicoelectroclinical findings.

- Since the development of *electroencephalography* (EEG) in 1950, seizure diagnosis has always relied on it. This test can detect interictal or ictal epileptiform activity but can be negative in up to 50% [11] of cases because of its short duration. With improvement of technology and data-storage capacities,

video-EEG was developed, which allows recordings of EEG activities and clinical manifestations simultaneously over several days. Those recordings allow better electroclinical correlation and determination of the epilepsy type based on semiology and electric origin.
- As opposed to the video-EEG, which has good temporal accuracy but poor spatial accuracy, the field of intractable epilepsy has also significantly benefited from the progress in *MRI*. This diagnosis tool is the gold standard for epilepsy assessment that facilitates identification of an epileptogenic lesion, such as focal cortical dysplasia (FCD), glioneuronal tumors, or mesiotemporal sclerosis. The evolution to the 3-T magnet has increased spatial resolution and increased lesional diagnosis to 65% [12]. With the emergence of the 7-T magnet, one can expect even better spatial definition and increased diagnostic yield with as much as 43% more lesional cases identified [13].

Although these tests are sufficient for a subset of patients, others require more advanced technologies to help identify and delineate the epileptogenic focus.

- *PET-computed tomography* and *ictal*–single-photon emission computed tomography rely on abnormal brain metabolism secondary to the seizure focus during the interictal or ictal phase, respectively. This is usually used to confirm the affected lobe when MRI and EEG are incongruent, or when the lesion is subtle.
- *Magnetoencephalography (MEG)* detects magnetic dipole parallel to the brain surface. Its advantage compared with the EEG is the absence of artifacts generated by the skull and the scalp, but the depth resolution is poor. Unfortunately, very few centers have access to MEG. However, this technology is a good add on when EEG cannot well define the boundaries of epileptogenic cortex.
- *Functional MRI* and *tractography* are advanced MRI sequences that allow visualization of eloquent brain regions as well as main white matter tracts. Those sequences are useful when epileptic zones are near or in eloquent cortex.
- A more thorough *neuropsychological testing*, especially in TLE, might also prove useful to better localize cognitive dysfunction, such as memory and language deficits.
- *Biological and genetic testing* might help in refining the diagnosis and establishing a prognosis for the patient as well as a treatment strategy. These tests are improving each year, and more than 265 genes [14] have already been linked to various epilepsy syndromes.

Once the workup has been completed, a *multidisciplinary meeting* is organized involving epileptologists, neurosurgeons, neuroradiologists, neuropsychologists, and nursing staff. The purpose of this meeting is to answer 2 questions: (1) Can the epileptogenic zone be identified? and if so, (2) Is it safe to remove that region of the brain? In other words, does the deficit associated with removing that region of the brain result in an acceptable deficit to the patient? The best treatment plan is then defined in regard to all that information. Table 1 lists frequent diagnoses [15] and epilepsy type related to it.

Table 1
Common drug resistant epilepsy causes

Common causes	Epilepsy type
Focal cortical dysplasia	Lesional/lobar/multilobar
Hippocampal sclerosis	
Tumor: Ganglioglioma, DNET, glioma, hypothalamic hamartoma	
Tuberous sclerosis complex (hamartoma)	
Polymicrogyria	
Hemimegalencephaly	Hemispheric epilepsy
Hemispheric cortical dysplasia	
Sturge-Weber syndrome	
Rasmussen encephalitis	
Stroke	
Encephalopathic epilepsies: Lennox-Gastaut syndrome, West syndrome	Generalized epilepsy

DNET, Dysembryoplastic Neuroepithelial Tumor

If the noninvasive evaluation is inconclusive or not sufficiently congruent, a phase 2 investigation through invasive EEG evaluation can be performed to better define the seizure-onset zone and identify surrounding eloquent brain regions.

Invasive investigation
In some instances, the noninvasive assessment is insufficient to determine with precision the extent of the epileptogenic zone. This may often be the case in FCD or nonlesional epilepsy whereby MRI is usually not adequate to visualize the boundaries of the epileptogenic region or when the presumed epileptogenic region is adjacent or involving eloquent cortex. In these instances, representing up to 40% of surgical candidates, *invasive EEG* may help in understanding the epileptic network [16].

Invasive recordings can be performed in the following different ways:

- *Subdural grids* has long been the most frequent technique for invasive evaluation in North America. In this procedure, the EEG grids are placed on the surface of the brain through a craniotomy and a large dural opening. This allows the surgeon to place a large number of electrodes directly on the cortex under direct vision. When this procedure is performed, a potential resection procedure can be planned a few days after the recordings, making this a two-stage procedure. In those instances, subdural EEG grids can also be used during the surgery to guide resection.
- *Depth electrodes* have been the preferred approach over the past several decades in Europe, especially under the French and Italian school of epilepsy. The advantage compared with subdural grids is the possibility of depth analysis, accessing both sides of the brain and sampling over a wider area of the brain. In addition, these electrodes are placed in a percutaneous fashion obviating a craniotomy [17]. The main disadvantage is the inability to perform brain mapping, which allows identification of eloquent brain

regions. The appearance of *surgical robots* has facilitated its widespread use through North America more recently. Contrary to subdural grids, the depth electrodes can be removed through a very short operation, and the definitive surgical procedure is often delayed for about 6 weeks to minimize the risk of infection.

Timing of surgery

Persistence of seizures despite medical treatment is sometimes seen as trivial by the families and even caretakers, especially in the case of focal seizures or well-known stereotypical seizures. This might lead to a delay in referral to surgical epilepsy centers. This delay added to the time-consuming workup can lead to a significant delay before appropriate treatment can be initiated.

The importance of early surgical intervention is well documented. Children operated before 12 months of epilepsy history seem to have a better psychomotor prognosis [18]. With the absence of seizure control, a secondary epileptogenesis can develop leading to a propagation of seizure onset zones [19]. With time, new independent epileptic foci will appear and transform a curable epilepsy into an incurable epilepsy [20]. Furthermore, younger patients will benefit from neuroplasticity [21], and surgery around eloquent zones can be more aggressive with limited long-term impact (see later discussion).

Even though a definite timing for treatment has not yet been defined, a widespread consensus for treatment is "as soon as possible."

TEMPORAL LOBE EPILEPSY

TLE accounts for 15% to 20% of epilepsies in children [22]. Its prognosis compared with extratemporal epilepsy is usually better. As in all epilepsies, the presence of a lesion in relation to the epilepsy or abnormal MRI as well as the absence of generalized seizures usually indicates better prognosis of seizure freedom [23].

In contrast with adults whereby TLE is the most frequent cause of epilepsy, pediatric TLE is less frequent and usually involves more complex networks [24]. Indeed, adult TLE is frequently related to mesiotemporal sclerosis [25], whereas TLE in children is usually caused by FCD [26], glioneuronal tumors [27] or both, which involves more lateral cortex and sometimes other lobes.

A full workup is done to confirm the electroclinicoanatomic origin of the seizures. Involvement of surrounding regions, the frontal operculum and the insula, in particular, needs to be excluded. Neuropsychological workups are especially useful to rule out memory impairment before surgery and determine if memory function in the contralateral hippocampus is sufficient. Functional MRI is also useful to determine the dominant hemisphere and exclude language areas surrounding the epileptogenic foci.

- The typical surgery is the *anterior temporal lobectomy*, which consists of a resection of the anterior temporal lobe as well as the mesiotemporal structures comprising the amygdala, the hippocampus, and the parahippocampal gyrus, which have all been shown to be involved in mesial TLE. In the dominant

hemisphere, the superior temporal gyrus is usually spared to avoid language impairment.
- The resection can be tailored with the use of *electrocorticography* (ECoG), which consists of intraoperative recording of interictal activities with subdural grids. The strength of this approach is to better determine, intraoperatively, which regions should be resected and which regions should be spared. The weakness is the lack of ictal recordings as well as the limited duration of the recordings, which might lead to false negatives. The literature is still inconclusive on the added benefit of ECoG.
- Apart from the traditional tailored anterior temporal lobectomy, a newer procedure using *laser interstitial thermal therapy (LITT)* has emerged [28]. The main indication in temporal epilepsy is to target the mesiotemporal structures while minimizing collateral damage to the nearby optic radiations and language networks, which course in the lateral part of the temporal lobe. Selective approaches in pediatric neurosurgery are exceptional because the epileptic network usually involves the lateral cortex but might still be indicated in older children with networks closer to those of the adult population.
- In some cases, the neuropsychological assessment shows that most of the memory function is on the side of the temporal epilepsy. In those cases, hippocampus resection cannot be performed, and the multidisciplinary teams will need to resort to *neuromodulation techniques*, which is discussed later in the article.

Overall, prognosis after lobectomy is good in children, with 76% achieving seizure freedom [23], with a trend toward better results in cases of lesional epilepsy where total resection is possible.

EXTRATEMPORAL LOBE EPILEPSY

Most lobar epilepsies are extratemporal in children. They have been traditionally separated from temporal epilepsy because lobectomies are often partial owing to the presence of eloquent cortex (central region and visual cortex), which leads to less robust seizure control [29]. ETLE is further divided depending on the affected lobe, including the frontal, parietal, and occipital lobe in decreasing order of frequency.

The workup is especially important in those epilepsies to analyze the involvement of the eloquent cortex, which mostly limits resections. Functional MRI and tractography may be of special interest for this aspect. Second-phase investigation with intracranial recordings is often performed to completely rule out involvement in other regions, which has a direct impact on prognosis, as well as strictly defining the location and involvement of eloquent cortex. Intraoperative ECoG is often a useful adjunct to help tailor resections based on interictal EEG recordings.

Lesionectomy

More frequently than in temporal epilepsy, the resection might be tailored to a lesion when present and when the epilepsy assessment confirms that the seizure onset zone is limited to that lesion. Surgical technique is comparable to a tumorectomy and involves diverse techniques of microdissection, which is beyond the scope of this article. Prognosis for those lesional epilepsies is significantly better than nonlesional epilepsies.

- Specific lesions to consider are *FCDs*. FCDs have been classified into 3 groups [30]: type 1 is related to architectonic disorder only; type 2 includes architectonic disorder as well as dysmorphic neurons (balloon cells); and type 3 is the association of an FCD with another lesion (tumor or scar tissue). The diagnosis of FCD has significantly improved with the increase of spatial definition on MRI [31]. Typically, FCD is seen on the MRI as blurring of the gray-white junction of the neocortex. Other signs such as a transmantle sign can be seen but are not always present. The imaging abnormality can be extremely subtle so advanced MRI sequences such as voxel-based morphometry can be promising [32]. The main difficulty remains the delineation of the boundaries of the FCD, which will influence the extent of resection. Type 2 FCDs are usually more focal and better delineated than type 1 FCDs, which makes seizure control more likely [33]. Again, ECoG during surgery might help in determining resection boundaries, but results in the literature are not always consistent.
- Another special condition is *hypothalamic hamartoma*. This deep-seated lesion can cause a specific type of seizure called gelastic seizures, which are characterized by involuntary laughter. Those seizures are often intractable but respond well after resection [34]. Unfortunately, direct resection can cause harm to the hypothalamus, which in turn can lead to complications, such as obesity or diabetes insipidus. Because this lesion is benign from an oncologic standpoint, the risk-benefit balance is not always in favor of resection. Nowadays, LITT is the preferred approach to these lesions, allowing for maximal ablation while reducing the risks of approach-related morbidities [35].

Altogether, surgery for lesional ETLE achieves seizure freedom in about 66% of cases versus only 34% for nonlesional ETLE [36].

Frontal lobectomy

In medically intractable frontal lobe epilepsy without an identifiable lesion, a frontal lobectomy can be considered. The main determinant is hemisphere dominance, which will indicate the presence of language function. The functional limits are the primary motor cortex posteriorly and the language cortex inferiorly if present. The trend nowadays is to tailor the resection instead of doing standard lobectomy. For this purpose, these cases are commonly done with ECoG or preresection invasive EEG evaluations. Care must be taken to avoid injuring major veins and arteries, as morbidity often comes from those lesions. Transient neurologic impairment is frequent after such surgeries but resolves in the following weeks.

Posterior quadrant resections

A posterior quadrant resection consists of parieto-occipital resection that can be extended to the temporal lobe if needed. Although the posterior quadrant resection is an uncommon procedure, most children undergoing a large multilobal resection are less than the age of 2 years and have an identifiable lesion, commonly FCD, that spares the frontal lobe.

This resection spares the central area and, in the absence of a vascular lesion, should thus not lead to hemiparesis. On the contrary, a complete hemianopia is a rule but is often present before surgery owing to the underlying disease. In the well-selected patient, seizure freedom can reach 75% [37].

Insulectomy

The insula is a deep-seated and quite thin lobe, underneath the Sylvian fissure. Its access is difficult and puts the main vascular structures of the brain at risk. Nevertheless, the insula is at a junction between the frontal, temporal, and parietal lobe through their opercular regions. It is commonly involved in limbic system epilepsy.

Its general involvement is probably underrecognized, as its investigation is difficult. Surface EEG can rarely distinguish insular activity from the surrounding opercular region, and invasive EEG implantation is thus frequently needed [38]. Subdural grids are difficult to place owing to the narrow space, even in the case of a large Sylvian split. Depth electrodes are the preferred technique, but targeting, owing to the vessels, might be complicated [39]. All the technical difficulties make the insula an understudied and less understood lobe compared with the others.

Failures in TLE are thought to be related to more extended seizure onset zones commonly referred to as temporal lobe plus epilepsy. The involvement of the insula in this entity is thought to play an important role [40].

Technically demanding, the insulectomy can be limited to the anterior or posterior lobe. A large Sylvian fissure split is required to expose the lobe, and resection is performed between the Sylvian vessels, or part of an operculum (usually the frontal operculum) is resected. Nevertheless, favorable outcome is possible with up to 69% achieving seizure freedom [41]. In order to avoid the vascular risks, some groups have resorted to the use of radiofrequency ablation or LITT for a more minimally invasive approach [42], but definite proof of superiority is still lacking.

Multiple subpial transection

If the seizure focus is located in an eloquent brain region, resection may not be an option, especially if it will lead to an unacceptable neurologic deficit, such as hemiparesis or aphasia.

In these situations, multiple subpial transection (MST) has been described as a technique to isolate the epileptogenic cortex from surrounding cortex without compromising neurologic function [43]. Some variations to the technique have been described, but the concept remains the same: interrupt the horizontal connections in the cortex to limit propagation and recruitment of gray matter in seizure generation and spread. This technique maintains the longitudinal connections from the cortex, which allows conserving the functional activity of the pathologic cortex.

MSTs can be performed alone if the seizure-onset zone is strictly limited to the eloquent cortex, or in addition to a resective procedure such as a lesionectomy or a lobectomy if the seizure-onset zone extends to the eloquent cortex. Good outcomes (>95% reduction of seizure) are reported in up to 87% of patients if MST is performed in conjunction with resection and in up to 71% of patients if performed alone [44]. Some studies report 50% of seizure freedom at 5 years [45] after MST only in eloquent cortex.

Neuroplasticity

Even if resection of eloquent cortex is usually avoided, there are special nuances for infants, toddlers, and younger children with respect to neuroplasticity. Contrary to previous theories, studies have shown that language lateralization only starts around 4 years old and is usually finished by age 7 years with different timing depending on the region of the brain involved [46]. Hand dominance usually occurs by the age of 2. In children less than 2 years of age, resection can generally be considered regardless of the brain region involved, as almost all functions lost can be completely reacquired.

Furthermore, recovery from a craniotomy is generally quicker and more complete than in adults [47]. This ability to recover is most evident in patients undergoing hemispherectomy, which will be discussed later. Even though a complete hemisphere is disconnected, patients usually maintain walking capacity, gross motor arm function, and the ability to communicate.

It is important to consider that the brain of patients with drug-resistant epilepsy might be wired differently. This is especially the case in "catastrophic" or syndromic epilepsies with diffuse brain involvement whereby neuroplasticity might also be impaired [21].

MULTILOBAR AND GENERALIZED EPILEPSY

Palliative surgeries

When the epileptogenic zone involves homotopic regions in both hemispheres, or when the epilepsy is generalized from its onset, curative resections cannot be achieved. Nevertheless, targeting the most impairing seizure types can be useful. These surgeries are called "palliative" in that they are meant to lower the seizure burden but not necessarily provide seizure freedom.

Corpus callosotomy

In some epileptic syndromes, such as Lennox-Gastaut syndrome, the most debilitating seizures are drop attacks in which the patient suddenly loses tone of the lower limbs, resulting in a fall. These seizures can cause serious injuries and can significantly decrease quality of life. In those cases, a *corpus callosotomy* can be performed to stop the epileptic activity from spreading from one hemisphere to the other. This can be very effective in eliminating drop attacks.

- This technique is a *partial callosotomy*, as it involves transection of the anterior two-thirds of the corpus callosum. By doing so, motor fibers, at the origin of the atonic seizures, are interrupted, but other fibers connecting both hemispheres are maintained, decreasing the risks of disconnection syndromes [48]. The most serious concern with a disconnection syndrome is the loss of bihemispheric communication. If drop attacks or other serious seizures originating from the spread of the epileptic activity between hemisphere persist, the callosotomy can be completed in a second-look surgery.

- In more debilitated patients with severe mental delay and those that are nonverbal, a *complete corpus callosotomy* can be performed in a single step, as the chance of controlling seizures, usually more complex in those cases, outweighs the risk of disconnection syndromes, usually less clinically relevant in this population.
- In a systematic review [49], 88% of patients with a complete corpus callosotomy experienced worthwhile seizure reduction (Engel class III) versus 58% in anterior two-thirds partial corpus callosotomy, but with 18% of patients developing a disconnection syndrome in the case of complete corpus callosotomy versus 0% in case of partial corpus callosotomy.

Some teams [50] have suggested performing this procedure with an endoscope to reduce blood loss and incision length, but no clear superiority to open procedures exists. Some investigators have also performed a callosotomy with LITT [51] with, again, lack of clear advantage compared with the classic open technique.

Functional hemispherotomy

Some patients suffer from a diffuse, even hemispheric, but unilateral epilepsy. Usual causes are Rasmussen encephalitis, hemimegalencephaly, large perinatal hemispheric stroke, or Struge-Weber syndrome. In those cases, the affected brain is not fully functional, and a full hemisphere can be disconnected to eliminate clinical seizures with limited impact on neurologic function. Even though this procedure might seem aggressive, it allows development of the normal hemisphere, which usually leads to functional improvement. Nevertheless, this surgery is obviously reserved for select candidates. The authors' research group has recently developed a prognosis score [52] based on a multicenter experience, which demonstrated that older patients at the time of seizure onset (>3.5 years), those without generalized seizure semiology, those without previous resection or contralateral hypometabolism, and those with epilepsy originating from poststroke gliosis had the highest likelihood of seizure freedom.

Different approaches have been described and can be roughly divided into 2 groups: lateral perisylvian hemispherectomies (developed by Villemure) and vertical parasagittal hemispherectomies (developed by Delalande). Again, some investigators have developed endoscopic disconnection to reduce invasiveness, but this is still not used on a widespread basis. In a large multicenter review [53] performed on 672 patients, seizure freedom was reached in 88% of patients at 1 year but decreased to 62% at 10 years with more durable seizure freedom in those that underwent a vertical hemispherotomy.

Neuromodulation procedures

Apart from corpus callosotomies, neuromodulation procedures can still be considered for palliative reduction in seizures. To date, no epilepsy types nor epileptogenic syndromes are formal contraindication for those procedures, which makes them a useful tool for the epilepsy neurosurgeon.

Those techniques rely on the introduction of electric current in the neurologic system to modulate brain activities. Even though these technologies rarely bring complete seizure freedom, they usually improve epilepsy control, which in turn increases quality of life.

The main complexity of those procedures comes from the adjustment of settings (ie, the adaptation of the current) after the surgeries, which requires a trained specialist. Most of the time, this task is performed by the treating epileptologist.

Deep brain stimulation

Deep brain stimulation (DBS) has initially been developed for the treatment of movement disorders. The aim is to modulate brain circuiting by stimulation at particular nodes of the circuit. The type of stimulation used can drive or inhibit the circuit. Interest in treating other condition such as epilepsy has rapidly emerged.

Limbic epilepsy, which is very common in adult epilepsy syndromes, commonly involves the circuit of Papez. The most commonly used target in this circuit seems to be the *anterior thalamic nucleus (ATN)*. Other targets have been tried, such as the centromedian nucleus of the thalamus, the mamillary body, or the hippocampus.

This surgery needs careful planning and targeting, which is made possible using a stereotactic head frame. The use of the frame is challenging in children under 4 years of age because of the skull thickness. Once the frame is positioned, 2 electrodes are inserted to the target and then connected to a generator in the pectoral region. This generator can later be interrogated, and current settings can be adjusted in order to optimize epilepsy control usually over the course of several months.

The group SANTE has performed [54] the largest RCT in adults to date and shows 56% seizure reduction at 2 years with 54% of patients having more than 50% of seizure reduction and 12.7% being seizure free. These outcomes improve at 5 years [55] with 69% mean seizure reduction and 68% of patients with more than 50% of seizure reduction, and further at 7 years [56] with 75% mean seizure reduction. The main side effect of ATN targeting is the occurrence of subjective depression and memory impairment in some cases, which might require therapy. However, these symptoms are not found following formal neuropsychological assessment [57]. Comparable data for children are still lacking, but a recent systematic review [58] found 12.5% seizure freedom and 85% seizure reduction in patients.

Even though this technology has been available for a few years, its use is still limited probably because of its falsely perceived greater aggressiveness compared with vagus nerve stimulation (VNS) without major added value proven yet.

Vagus nerve stimulation

VNS consists of placing an electrode around the vagus nerve in the neck. The electrode is connected to a stimulator under the skin in the pectoral region. The exact mechanism is still unclear. When the stimulator activates, an antidromic discharge travels backwards along the nerve and is thought to release neurotransmitters inside the brainstem, mainly in the locus coeruleus. Those neurotransmitters in turn are thought to reduce cortical excitability that leads to epileptogenesis.

This intervention is quite simple and can be performed in same-day surgery, which has made it easily available even in patients with severe disability. The results are somewhat limited with 50% of patients achieving greater than 50% seizure reduction. Better outcomes can be achieved in those with later age of seizure onset and fewer AED tried before VNS, probably meaning less severe epilepsy [59]. Still, this technique is frequently considered given the ease of implantation and the severity of treated patients.

Future developments are related to seizure detection in the hopes of developing closed-loop systems. Presently, the system can detect tachycardia, often related to seizure onset. It can use this indirect biomarker of a seizure to send an additional stimulation to try to abort the forthcoming seizure. This seems to improve seizure control but is not yet a true closed-loop system.

Responsive neurostimulation

Responsive neural stimulation is a closed-loop system in which 1 or 2 electrodes, inserted close to or inside epileptogenic focus, are connected to a generator. These electrodes contain detecting contacts, and when an ictal pattern is detected, a stimulation is induced.

Indication is usually limited to 2 epileptogenic foci, which may limit patient selection, but results for this selected population are quite good.

Similar to DBS, most of the data are from the adult population, but the authors conducted a recent retrospective multicenter analysis [60] on its use in children and young adults with 35 patients, which showed that 60% of patients have at least greater than 50% of seizure improvement and 6% of patients achieve seizure freedom. Only 3 patients presented complications (2 infection and 1 hemorrhage), and 4 patients had concurrent resection.

SUMMARY

Intractable epilepsy is a frequent diagnosis in children. A comprehensive assessment is necessary, which is initiated after referral to a dedicated pediatric epilepsy surgery center. Multiple surgical procedures are available and need to be tailored to each patient to achieve the best possible outcome. Curative procedures usually consist of resection, whereas palliative procedures comprise neuromodulation and disconnection techniques.

CLINICS CARE POINTS

- There is an increasing number of children that can benefit from epilepsy surgery.
- A surgical resection or disconnection offers a chance to cure.
- There is a shift toward minimally invasive procedures and neuromodulation.
- Individualized treatments are required for each patient to achieve the best outcomes.

Disclosure

The authors have nothing to disclose.

References

[1] Kim H, Thurman DJ, Durgin T, et al. Estimating Epilepsy Incidence and Prevalence in the US Pediatric Population Using Nationwide Health Insurance Claims Data. J Child Neurol 2016;31(6):743–9.
[2] Kwan P, Brodie MJ. Early identification of refractory epilepsy. N Engl J Med 2000;342(5): 314–9.
[3] Kalilani L, Sun X, Pelgrims B, et al. The epidemiology of drug-resistant epilepsy: A systematic review and meta-analysis. Epilepsia 2018;59(12):2179–93.
[4] Kwan P, Arzimanoglou A, Berg AT, et al. Definition of drug resistant epilepsy: consensus proposal by the ad hoc Task Force of the ILAE Commission on Therapeutic Strategies. Epilepsia 2010;51(6):1069–77.
[5] Rao S, Stino A, Seraji-Bozorgzad N, et al. Seizure-related injury and postictal aggression in refractory epilepsy patients. Epilepsy Res 2020;160:106281; https://doi.org/10.1016/j.eplepsyres.2020.106281.
[6] Deleo F, Quintas R, Pastori C, et al. Quality of life, psychiatric symptoms, and stigma perception in three groups of persons with epilepsy. Epilepsy Behav 2020;110:107170; https://doi.org/10.1016/j.yebeh.2020.107170.
[7] Harden C, Tomson T, Gloss D, et al. Practice Guideline Summary: Sudden Unexpected Death in Epilepsy Incidence Rates and Risk Factors: Report of the Guideline Development, Dissemination, and Implementation Subcommittee of the American Academy of Neurology and the American Epilepsy Society. Epilepsy Curr 2017;17(3):180–7.
[8] Wiebe S, Blume WT, Girvin JP, et al. Effectiveness, Efficiency of Surgery for Temporal Lobe Epilepsy Study G. A randomized, controlled trial of surgery for temporal-lobe epilepsy. N Engl J Med 2001;345(5):311–8.
[9] Dwivedi R, Ramanujam B, Chandra PS, et al. Surgery for Drug-Resistant Epilepsy in Children. N Engl J Med 2017;377(17):1639–47.
[10] Park KM, Kim SE, Lee BI. Antiepileptic Drug Therapy in Patients with Drug-Resistant Epilepsy. J Epilepsy Res 2019;9(1):14–26.
[11] Krumholz A, Wiebe S, Gronseth G, et al. Practice Parameter: evaluating an apparent unprovoked first seizure in adults (an evidence-based review): report of the Quality Standards Subcommittee of the American Academy of Neurology and the American Epilepsy Society. Neurology 2007;69(21):1996–2007.
[12] Knake S, Triantafyllou C, Wald LL, et al. 3T phased array MRI improves the presurgical evaluation in focal epilepsies: a prospective study. Neurology 2005;65(7):1026–31.
[13] Wang I, Oh S, Blumcke I, et al. Value of 7T MRI and post-processing in patients with nonlesional 3T MRI undergoing epilepsy presurgical evaluation. Epilepsia 2020;61(11): 2509–20.

[14] Gursoy S, Ercal D. Diagnostic Approach to Genetic Causes of Early-Onset Epileptic Encephalopathy. J Child Neurol 2016;31(4):523–32.
[15] Shorvon SD. The etiologic classification of epilepsy. Epilepsia 2011;52(6):1052–7.
[16] Kovac S, Vakharia VN, Scott C, et al. Invasive epilepsy surgery evaluation. Seizure 2017;44:125–36; https://doi.org/10.1016/j.seizure.2016.10.016.
[17] Isnard J, Taussig D, Bartolomei F, et al. French guidelines on stereoelectroencephalography (SEEG). Neurophysiol Clin 2018;48(1):5–13; https://doi.org/10.1016/j.neucli.2017.11.005.
[18] Sugano H, Arai H. Epilepsy surgery for pediatric epilepsy: optimal timing of surgical intervention. Neurol Med Chir (Tokyo) 2015;55(5):399–406.
[19] Morrell F. Varieties of human secondary epileptogenesis. J Clin Neurophysiol 1989;6(3):227–75.
[20] Holthausen H, Pieper T, Kudernatsch M. Towards early diagnosis and treatment to save children from catastrophic epilepsy – focus on epilepsy surgery. *Brain Dev* Sep 2013;35(8):730–41.
[21] Ismail FY, Fatemi A, Johnston MV. Cerebral plasticity: Windows of opportunity in the developing brain. Eur J Paediatr Neurol 2017;21(1):23–48.
[22] Benifla M, Otsubo H, Ochi A, et al. Temporal lobe surgery for intractable epilepsy in children: an analysis of outcomes in 126 children. Neurosurgery 2006;59(6):1203–13, discussion 1213-4.
[23] Englot DJ, Rolston JD, Wang DD, et al. Seizure outcomes after temporal lobectomy in pediatric patients. J Neurosurg Pediatr 2013;12(2):134–41.
[24] Bourgeois M, Sainte-Rose C, Lellouch-Tubiana A, et al. Surgery of epilepsy associated with focal lesions in childhood. J Neurosurg 1999;90(5):833–42.
[25] Barba C, Cossu M, Guerrini R, et al. Temporal lobe epilepsy surgery in children and adults: A multicenter study. Epilepsia 2021;62(1):128–42.
[26] Arya R, Mangano FT, Horn PS, et al. Long-term seizure outcomes after pediatric temporal lobectomy: does brain MRI lesion matter? J Neurosurg Pediatr 2019;24(2):200–8.
[27] Sinclair DB, Wheatley M, Aronyk K, et al. Pathology and neuroimaging in pediatric temporal lobectomy for intractable epilepsy. Pediatr Neurosurg 2001;35(5):239–46.
[28] Wu C, Jermakowicz WJ, Chakravorti S, et al. Effects of surgical targeting in laser interstitial thermal therapy for mesial temporal lobe epilepsy: A multicenter study of 234 patients. Epilepsia 2019;60(6):1171–83.
[29] Ansari SF, Maher CO, Tubbs RS, et al. Surgery for extratemporal nonlesional epilepsy in children: a meta-analysis. Childs Nerv Syst 2010;26(7):945–51.
[30] Najm IM, Sarnat HB, Blumcke I. Review: The international consensus classification of Focal Cortical Dysplasia - a critical update 2018. Neuropathol Appl Neurobiol 2018;44(1):18–31.
[31] Mellerio C, Labeyrie MA, Chassoux F, et al. 3T MRI improves the detection of transmantle sign in type 2 focal cortical dysplasia. Epilepsia 2014;55(1):117–22.
[32] Jin B, Krishnan B, Adler S, et al. Automated detection of focal cortical dysplasia type II with surface-based magnetic resonance imaging postprocessing and machine learning. Epilepsia 2018;59(5):982–92.
[33] Rowland NC, Englot DJ, Cage TA, et al. A meta-analysis of predictors of seizure freedom in the surgical management of focal cortical dysplasia. J Neurosurg 2012;116(5):1035–41.
[34] Scholly J, Staack AM, Kahane P, et al. Hypothalamic hamartoma: Epileptogenesis beyond the lesion? Epilepsia 2017;58(Suppl 2):32–40.
[35] Bourdillon P, Ferrand-Sorbet S, Apra C, et al. Surgical treatment of hypothalamic hamartomas. Neurosurg Rev 2021;44(2):753–62.
[36] Tellez-Zenteno JF, Hernandez Ronquillo L, Moien-Afshari F, et al. Surgical outcomes in lesional and non-lesional epilepsy: a systematic review and meta-analysis. Epilepsy Res 2010;89(2–3):310–8.

[37] Markosian C, Dodson V, Zhang HJ, et al. Total and partial posterior quadrant disconnection for medically refractory epilepsy: A systematic review. Seizure 2021;91:66–71; https://doi.org/10.1016/j.seizure.2021.05.018.
[38] Desai A, Bekelis K, Darcey TM, et al. Surgical techniques for investigating the role of the insula in epilepsy: a review. Neurosurg Focus 2012;32(3):E6; https://doi.org/10.3171/2012.1.FOCUS11325.
[39] Kappen P, Eltze C, Tisdall M, et al. Stereo-EEG exploration in the insula/operculum in paediatric patients with refractory epilepsy. Seizure 2020;78:63–70; https://doi.org/10.1016/j.seizure.2020.02.011.
[40] Barba C, Minotti L, Job AS, et al. The Insula in Temporal Plus Epilepsy. J Clin Neurophysiol 2017;34(4):324–7.
[41] Weil AG, Le NM, Jayakar P, et al. Medically resistant pediatric insular-opercular/perisylvian epilepsy. Part 2: outcome following resective surgery. J Neurosurg Pediatr 2016;18(5):523–35.
[42] Gireesh ED, Lee K, Skinner H, et al. Intracranial EEG and laser interstitial thermal therapy in MRI-negative insular and/or cingulate epilepsy: case series. J Neurosurg 2020;1–9; https://doi.org/10.3171/2020.7.JNS201912.
[43] Morrell F, Whisler WW, Bleck TP. Multiple subpial transection: a new approach to the surgical treatment of focal epilepsy. J Neurosurg 1989;70(2):231–9.
[44] Spencer SS, Schramm J, Wyler A, et al. Multiple subpial transection for intractable partial epilepsy: an international meta-analysis. Epilepsia 2002;43(2):141–5.
[45] Finet P, Santos LP, El Tahry R, et al. Clinical Outcome of Radiating Multiple Subpial Transections Alone for Drug Resistant Epilepsy After More Than 5 Years Follow-Up. World Neurosurg 2019;126:e1155–9; https://doi.org/10.1016/j.wneu.2019.02.218.
[46] Berl MM, Mayo J, Parks EN, et al. Regional differences in the developmental trajectory of lateralization of the language network. Hum Brain Mapp 2014;35(1):270–84.
[47] Anderson V, Spencer-Smith M, Wood A. Do children really recover better? Neurobehavioural plasticity after early brain insult. Brain 2011;134(Pt 8):2197–221.
[48] Jea A, Vachhrajani S, Widjaja E, et al. Corpus callosotomy in children and the disconnection syndromes: a review. Childs Nerv Syst 2008;24(6):685–92.
[49] Graham D, Tisdall MM, Gill D. Corpus callosotomy outcomes in pediatric patients: A systematic review. Epilepsia 2016;57(7):1053–68.
[50] Smyth MD, Vellimana AK, Asano E, et al. Corpus callosotomy-Open and endoscopic surgical techniques. Epilepsia 2017;58(Suppl 1):73–9.
[51] Roland JL, Akbari SHA, Salehi A, et al. Corpus callosotomy performed with laser interstitial thermal therapy. J Neurosurg 2019;1–9; https://doi.org/10.3171/2019.9.JNS191769.
[52] Weil AG, Lewis EC, Ibrahim GM, et al. Hemispherectomy Outcome Prediction Scale: Development and validation of a seizure freedom prediction tool. Epilepsia 2021;62(5):1064–73.
[53] Fallah A, Lewis E, Ibrahim GM, et al. Comparison of the real-world effectiveness of vertical versus lateral functional hemispherotomy techniques for pediatric drug-resistant epilepsy: A post hoc analysis of the HOPS study. Epilepsia 2021;62(11):2707–18.
[54] Fisher R, Salanova V, Witt T, et al. Electrical stimulation of the anterior nucleus of thalamus for treatment of refractory epilepsy. Epilepsia 2010;51(5):899–908.
[55] Salanova V, Witt T, Worth R, et al. Long-term efficacy and safety of thalamic stimulation for drug-resistant partial epilepsy. Neurology 2015;84(10):1017–25.
[56] Salanova V, Sperling MR, Gross RE, et al. The SANTE study at 10 years of follow-up: Effectiveness, safety, and sudden unexpected death in epilepsy. Epilepsia 2021;62(6):1306–17.
[57] Troster AI, Meador KJ, Irwin CP, et al. Memory and mood outcomes after anterior thalamic stimulation for refractory partial epilepsy. Seizure 2017;45:133–41; https://doi.org/10.1016/j.seizure.2016.12.014.

[58] Yan H, Toyota E, Anderson M, et al. A systematic review of deep brain stimulation for the treatment of drug-resistant epilepsy in childhood. J Neurosurg Pediatr 2018;23(3):274–84.
[59] Jain P, Arya R. Vagus nerve stimulation and seizure outcomes in pediatric refractory epilepsy: systematic review and meta-analysis. Neurology 2021; https://doi.org/10.1212/WNL.0000000000012030.
[60] Nagahama Y, Zervos TM, Murata KK, et al. Real-world preliminary experience with responsive neurostimulation in pediatric epilepsy: a multicenter retrospective observational study. Neurosurgery 2021; https://doi.org/10.1093/neuros/nyab343.

Advances in Pediatrics 69 (2022) 75–93

ADVANCES IN PEDIATRICS

Chronic and Recurrent Sinusitis in Children, as Manifestation of Immune Dysfunction and Atopic Background

Farn-Hsuan Tseng, MD[a], Marissa Newman[b], Charles H. Song, MD[a,*]

[a]Harbor-University of California, Los Angeles, Torrance, CA 90509, USA; [b]University of California, Los Angeles, Los Angeles, CA 90095, USA

Keywords

• Acute rhinosinusitis • Chronic rhinosinusitis • Immune deficiency • Allergy

Key points

- Acute rhinosinusitis (ARS) is defined as upper respiratory infection symptoms increasing after 5 days or persisting after 10 days.
- Among patients with ARS, signs of potential acute bacterial rhinosinusitis include at least 3 of the 5 criteria: fever, discolored mucus, worsening symptoms, Table 1 severe pain, and raised ESR/CRP.
- Chronic rhinosinusitis (CRS) in children is defined as presence of 2 or more symptoms, one of which should be either nasal obstruction or nasal discharge), plus facial pressure or cough, for more than or equal to 12 weeks.
- Pathology of CRS is not completely understood, and treatment includes nasal irrigation, nasal and oral steroid, and remedial approaches for allergy and immune defect.
- The most common immune deficiency in CRS is the low levels of pneumococcal antibodies, which must be corrected by vaccination.

INTRODUCTION

Rhinosinusitis is a common problem in the general population, both adults and children, involving infectious and inflammatory pathology. In children,

*Corresponding author. *E-mail address:* Chucksong209@gmail.com

https://doi.org/10.1016/j.yapd.2022.03.012

Abbreviations

ARS	acute rhinosinusitis
CRS	chronic rhinosinusitis
ABRS	acute bacterial rhinosinusitis
CRSwNP	chronic rhinosinusitis with nasal polyposis
CF	cystic fibrosis
IEI	inborne errors of immunity

distinction between allergic rhinitis, acute viral and bacterial rhinosinusitis (ARS), chronic rhinosinusitis (CRS), and adenoid hypertrophy/adenoiditis can be difficult. When rhinosinusitis recurs or becomes chronic, it poses a significant challenge to patients and providers, prompting them to investigate the predisposing factors, including allergy and immune or anatomic defects. The authors discuss some new approaches for diagnosis besides traditional imaging studies and for the detection of causative pathogens. The most important aspect of management is the implementation of disease-modifying approaches in consideration of cause and pathogenesis that go beyond the pharmacologic treatment. This should include the correction of defects in immune function, microbiome, and anatomy, using biologics, probiotics, and surgical approach. Once these defects are rectified, as demonstrated in the following case history, the patients' conditions may be completely resolved.

A CASE HISTORY

A 5-year-old toddler was seen for persistent wet cough in the last 4 months. The patient has a persistent stuffy nose and occasional colored nasal discharge. The patient was treated with nebulized albuterol and budesonide (0.5 mg q 12 hours) for 2 weeks without symptom relief. Chest radiographs a week before the visit were normal. Allergy skin testing showed moderate sensitivity to dust mite. Pertinent physical findings include bilateral edematous nasal turbinates and normal ear and chest findings. Laboratory findings showed elevated eosinophils (10%, 610/uL), normal levels of immunoglobulins, decreased levels of pneumococcal antibodies (2 out of 23 serotypes in protective range), nasal dipstick score of 6 [1], and predominance of *Streptococcus pneumoniae* by nasal DNA-polymerase chain reaction (PCR). Nasal endoscopy showed thick purulent drainage in the bilateral middle meatus and in the choana. The patient was treated with amoxicillin-clavulanate for 14 days and vaccinated with Pneumovax 23. On his return visit a month later, the repeat nasal endoscopy showed total clearance of the drainage in the nasal cavity. The nasal dipstick score decreased to 2. Post-vaccination pneumococcal serotypes were protective in 19 out of 23. The patient has remained asymptomatic since then.

CLINICAL MANIFESTATION AND DIAGNOSIS

The common clinical symptoms of sinusitis include nasal obstruction, cough, facial pain/pressure, purulent rhinorrhea, and hyposmia. Some of these symptoms may become dominant as the disease progresses. In young children, who may not be able to verbalize their complaints, coughing may become the major and only symptom. The signs and symptoms may occur alone or in the context of other diseases, as these symptoms in some combinations may also be present in common upper airway infections without sinus involvement. If a child has existing respiratory conditions including asthma and rhinitis, or chronic disease such as cystic fibrosis or primary immune deficiency, it may not be easy to isolate the symptoms of sinusitis unless one maintains a high index of suspicion.

To aid providers in sorting out the complexity of the clinical presentation and arriving at the diagnosis, the diagnostic guidelines of sinusitis for children and adults were published in the United States and Europe based on these clinical manifestations (Table 1) [2,3]. These guidelines offer the clinical criteria for primary care providers and additional procedure-based criteria for specialists. It should be noted that in contrast to adult criteria, pediatric guidelines do not

Table 1
Diagnostic guidelines of acute rhinosinusitis

	Adult	Children
EPOS 2020	2 or more symptoms: • One of which must be nasal obstruction or discharge (anterior or posterior) ± facial pressure ± hyposmia <12 wk AND (for specialists) • endoscopic signs of nasal polyps, and/or purulent discharge from middle meatus, and/or edema/mucosal obstruction in middle meatus and/or • CT changes: mucosal changes within the osteomeatal complex and/or sinuses	2 or more symptoms: • One of which must be nasal obstruction or discharge (anterior or posterior) ± facial pressure ± cough <12 wk Same as adults
Practice Parameter 2014	• URI lasting longer than 10 d • Symptoms including congestion, purulent rhinorrhea, facial-dental pain, postnasal drainage, headache, and cough • Signs including sinus tenderness, mucosal erythema, and discolored nasal and oropharyngeal secretions • Imaging studies not essential except in complicated cases	Same as adults

include imaging studies unless surgery is scheduled due to the high chance of false-positive findings and radiation risks for the vulnerable age group.

Nasal endoscopy is considered a very useful tool that can be used even for young children. The presence of purulent drainage from the osteomeatal complex or in the choana strongly suggests sinusitis. Identification of responsible pathogens may not be easy or accurate unless one resorts to a sinus aspiration, which cannot be obtained in the office setting. Nasal cultures are not recommended due to its unreliability resulting from the contamination by nasal flora [4]. There are reports that the dipstick analyses of the nasal secretion from the osteomeatal complex correlate very closely with imaging studies of sinusitis and DNA-PCR analysis of the secretion [1,5]. Although this approach has not been adopted widely, this simple method is very practical and deserves further consideration for the diagnosis of bacterial sinusitis in the primary care setting.

EPIDEMIOLOGY

In the general population, CRS is potentially the most prevalent chronic disease in the United States, with an estimated prevalence of 13% by National Health Interview Surveys [6]. In children it may not be as common, with 2 estimates placing the prevalence between 2.1% and 4% [7,8]. Although it can occur during infancy, pediatric CRS most commonly occurs between 4 to 7 years of age, usually following viral upper respiratory infections (URIs). Children are reported to have 6 to 8 URIs per year, about 8% of which are complicated by bacterial sinusitis [9]. The breakdown between pediatric chronic versus acute sinusitis is reported to favor chronic sinusitis (2.1% vs 0.6%) in patients up to 20 years of age in outpatient clinic settings [7].

CLASSIFICATION

Sinusitis is classified by phenotypes defined by duration, anatomical location, and infectious etiology, and endotypes, which entail the different pathological mechanisms and management approaches.

A. PHENOTYPES

- **Duration:** Sinusitis is classified based on the symptom duration which varies slightly by different guidelines.
  - European Position Paper on Rhinosinusitis and Nasal Polyps 2020 (EPOS) [3]: acute- $\leq$ 12 weeks, chronic- >12 weeks, recurrent$\geq$4/year.
  - Practice Parameters by American College of Allergy, Asthma, and Immunology [2]: acute and chronic – same as EPOS, recurrent- acute episodes $\geq$3 times/year.
  - Clinical Practice Guidelines [10]: acute - <30 days, subacute - $\geq$30 days and <90 days, and recurrent – 3 acute episodes $\geq$3/6 months or $\geq$4/year.
- **Anatomical location:** frontal, ethmoid, sphenoid, maxillary; unilateral vs. bilateral.

  It is important to consider the timeline of sinus development when interpreting the location of sinus pain/pressure; maxillary and ethmoid sinuses are radiologically visible before 1 year, sphenoid by 5 years, and frontal sinus by age 6-8 [2,11].

- **Infectious etiology:** virus vs. bacteria vs. fungal vs. mixed

  Due to the unreliability of nasal cultures, direct aspirations from sinus cavities or middle ear have been used for analysis in experimental settings. As a practical approach, DNA-PCR sampling of the secretion from the osteomeatal complex has yielded reliable results and will be more commonly available to the generalists in the future [5]. Viruses, bacteria, and fungi very often coexist as part of commensal microbiomes, but one of them may become dominant as the cavities get infected [12]. Fungi become pathogenic generally in patients with immune deficiency or deviation [13].

ACUTE RHINOSINUSITIS (ARS): POST-VIRAL & BACTERIAL

ARS is defined as symptoms increasing after 5 days or persisting after 10 days with less than 12 weeks duration, and includes post-viral and bacterial subtypes [3]. In most instances, acute post-viral or bacterial sinusitis follows viral URI. The duration of symptoms serves as a practical and useful diagnostic aid in which viral URI is expected to resolve in 7-10 days. Signs of potential acute bacterial rhinosinusitis (ABRS) include at least 3 of the 5 criteria: fever >38°C, persistent and worsening symptoms, unilateral disease, severe pain, and raised ESR/CRP [3].

CHRONIC RHINOSINUSITIS (CRS)

Chronic rhinosinusitis (with or without nasal polyps) in children is defined as the presence of two or more symptoms: one of which should be either nasal blockage/obstruction/congestion or nasal discharge (anterior/posterior nasal drip), plus facial pain/pressure or cough, for ≥12 weeks[3]. When referred, specialists can employ CT/MRI scan or endoscopy for confirmation of the diagnosis and an exact anatomical location of abnormalities, especially before the procedures. These symptoms may overlap and present concomitantly with persistent allergic rhinitis and non-allergic rhinitis although itching and sneezing may be more prevalent in the latter two conditions (Table 2).

B. ENDOTYPES

With the advance in research for pathophysiology, sinusitis can be divided by its endotypes as in asthma and other inflammatory diseases (Table 3, Fig. 1). More detailed discussion will follow in the pathophysiology section.

PATHOPHYSIOLOGY

Microbiome of the sinus cavities

The evolutionary history of sinuses points to their emerging role as that of a respiratory organ rather than olfactory. One of their main functions is to produce mucus that moisturizes the inside of the nose and to protect it from pollutants and microorganisms. Normal sinus and nasal cavities are populated by diverse commensal organisms [14]. Commensal bacteria are considered

Table 2
Differential diagnosis of chronic rhinosinusitis

	Chronic rhinosinusitis	Allergic rhinitis	Nonallergic rhinitis
Symptoms	Nasal obstruction Purulent rhinorrhea Cough Facial pain (hyposmia)	Nasal itching Sneezing Nasal obstruction Rhinorrhea Seasonal variation	Nasal itching Sneezing Nasal obstruction Rhinorrhea Specific triggers (smoke, mist, and so on)
Nasal endoscopy	Purulent drainage	Clear mucus	Clear mucus
Nasal dipstick score [1]	>3, very often	≤3	≤3
PCR finding	+/− Dominance of *Staphylococcus aureus*, Pseudomonas, or other bacteria or fungi	Mixed	Mixed
CT scan	Opacification	+/− opacification	+/− opacification
Presence of atopy (by skin test or sIgE)	+/−	+	−

Abbreviations: sIgE:serum IgE.

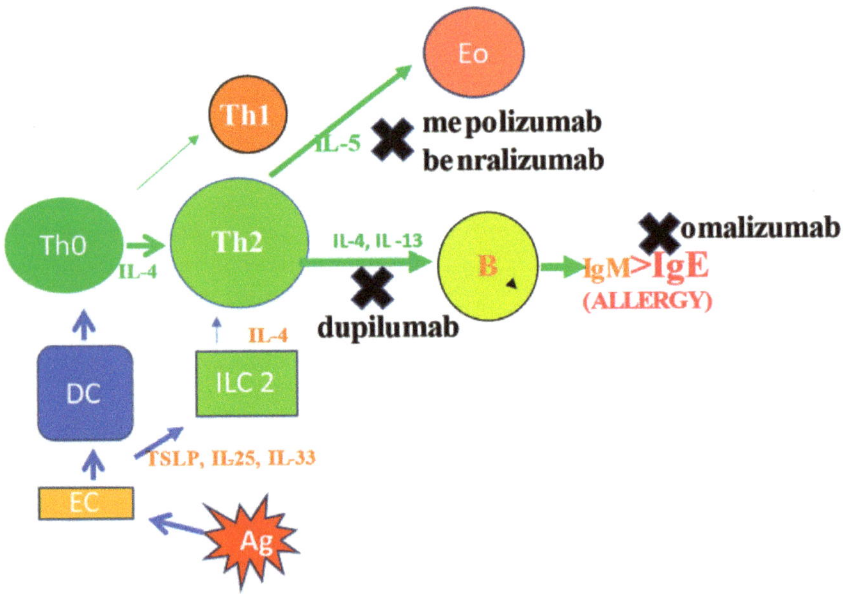

Fig. 1. Type 2 (Th2 and ILC2) endotype and biologics. Epithelial cells (EC), on interaction with antigens (bacteria, virus, allergens), produce alarmins (TSLP [thymic stromal lymphopoetin], IL-25, IL-33), which induce type 2 cells (Th2 and ILC2 [type2 innate lymphocytes]). The type 2 cells secrete IL-4 and IL-13, which act on B cells to produce IgE molecules. Type 2 cells also secrete IL-5, which attracts and activates eosinophils. Mepolizumab and benralizumab block IL-5 activities. Dupilumab blocks IL-4 and IL-13 together, resulting in inhibition of IgE production from B cells. Omalizumab interacts with Fc region of circulating IgE molecules, blocking their adherence to IgE receptors on the mast cells and other immune cells.

Table 3
Classification of endotypes in chronic rhinosinusitis

Endotype	Pathology	Phenotypes	Laterality
Type 2[a]	IgE and eosinophil associated	Allergic sinusitis AFRS (allergic fungal rhinosinusitis) CRSwNP (CRS with nasal polyps) EGPA (eosinophilic granulomatosis with polyangiitis, Churg-Strauss syndrome)	Unilateral or bilateral
Type 1[a]	Interferon-γ associated	Nonallergic sinusitis	Often bilateral
Type 3[a]	IL-17A associated	Nonallergic sinusitis	Often bilateral
Mixed (type 2 + 3, type 1 + 2)	—	Nonallergic sinusitis	Often bilateral

[a]Type 2: Th2 and ILC-2 (type 2 innate lymphoid cells) induced; type 1: Th1 and ILC-1 (type 1 innate lymphoid cells) induced; type 3: Th17 and ILC-3 (type 3 innate lymphoid cells) induced.

nonpathogenic or even protective and include Propionibacterium acnes, Streptococcus viridans, and coagulase-negative staphylococcus and sometimes potentially pathogenic bacteria associated with ABRS[15,16]. Corynebacterium has been reported in both pathogenic and nonpathogenic roles [17–19]. Sinus infection may ensue if this microbial balance is disturbed in favor of dominance of a single (or few) bacteria, often in the presence of immunologic dysfunction including allergic conditions [20].

ARS: In most cases, viral respiratory disease precedes sinusitis. Viral infection increases the adherence of bacteria to the epithelial tissues in the nasal and sinus cavity [21]. Occasionally, viruses may propagate in the sinus cavities for a prolonged time, leading to increased bacterial adhesion to the epithelial layer. An acute infection ensues with dominance of a potentially pathogenic bacterium including *Streptococcus pneumoniae*, *Haemophilus influenzae*, and *Moraxella catarrhalis* [22,23].

CRS: It is considered a chronic inflammatory process, probably originating from ABRS, that is associated with persistent opacification of the cavities and thickening of membranes in imaging studies. The role of bacteria is less clearly understood in CRS. Biofilm has been detected in most of the patients with CRS and may play a significant role in the persistence of bacteria in the mucous layer [24]. This viscous biofilm is shared by different parts of the respiratory tract and blocks the diffusion of antibiotics to the deeper layer of the matrix [25].

Commonly detected bacteria include aerobes–*Staphylococcus aureus, Streptococcus species, Haemophilus influenzae, Pseudomonas aeruginosa*, and *Moraxella catarrhalis*–and anaerobes–*Prevotella species, anaerobic streptococci*, and *Fusobacterium species* [20,26].

Table 4
Complication of chronic rhinosinusitis

	AFRS (allergic fungal rhinosinusitis)	CRSwNP (CRS with nasal polyposis)
Demographics	Younger, female	Adults, children with cystic fibrosis
Comorbidity	AR, asthma	AR, asthma
Fungal colonization	Aspergillus	Alternaria and Cladosporium
Secretion	"Peanut butter"	Thick mucous
Bacterial colonization	*Staphylococcus aureus* common	Pseudomonas, *S aureus*
CT scan	Bony erosion	Bony erosion, less likely
Serum IgE	High	Variable
Immune response	Endotype type 2 (Th2 and ILC2)	Endotype type 2 and CD8 (cytotoxic cells)

There are 3 subtypes: CRS without nasal polyps, CRS with nasal polyps, and allergic fungal sinusitis. In children, the latter 2 subtypes are rare and will be described as complications (Table 4).

ASSOCIATED CONDITIONS

Allergy (immunoglobulin E–mediated)

Allergic disorders affect 30% to 35% of children and affect the sinus cavities in various ways [27]. Children with allergic rhinitis produce increased amounts of mucus with biofilm formation in most instances in the nasal and sinus cavities, where pathogenic microbes may become dominant and infectious [2]. The major underlying mechanism for this mucous overproduction is stimulation of the mucous glands by mediators from activated mast cells resulting from the interaction between allergens and immunoglobulin E (IgE) molecules occupying IgE receptors on the mast cell surface. IgE receptors are also present on macrophages/dendritic cells. When these IgE receptors are occupied, macrophages fail to produce sufficient amounts of type 1 interferons to eradicate viruses on the sinus biofilm [28]. This defective mechanism contributes to the persistence of viruses, which enhances bacterial adherence to the biofilm. However, the pathology of CRS is more complicated and not completely understood, as it is a chronic inflammatory process that affects nonallergic subjects as well.

Immune deficiencies

Recurrent sinusitis or CRS may be an early manifestation of immune deficiencies, both primary and secondary. For primary immune deficiencies, more than 400 monogenic mutations are listed in the table of inborne errors of immunity (IEI) published in 2020 and interested readers are referred to the table for further detail [29]. Among these, antibody deficiencies (common variable immune disease [CVID], X-linked agammaglobulinemia, etc.) are more likely to lead to bacterial rhinosinusitis. Other entities involving T-cell and innate immune deficiencies may lead to fungal rhinosinusitis. Human immunodeficiency virus infection and protein losing gastroenteritis are examples of secondary immune deficiency.

But the most common defect is low levels of pneumococcal antibodies not associated with known genetic defects. When the levels of pneumococcal antibodies are normalized in these patients by vaccinations, sinus infections stop recurring in most instances. If pneumococcal antibody levels do not respond to vaccinations, the condition is defined as specific antibody deficiency. It is noteworthy that specific antibody deficiency is also part of many IEI. In a study of patients aged 6 to 70 years with recurrent respiratory symptoms and without other health issues, 81% had low baseline pneumococcal antibodies [30]. Of these patients, 76% responded to the vaccination (Pneumovax23 and/or Prevnar13). The recurrence rate of sinusitis within the next year among the vaccine responders was significantly lower compared with nonresponders (40% vs 76%), demonstrating the impact the normalization of pneumococcal antibodies by vaccination has on the recurrence of sinusitis. Overall, the rate of specific antibody deficiency among patients with CRS was 26%. It was reported that patients with allergic rhinitis/asthma have a lower prevalence of adequate baseline pneumococcal antibody compared with nonallergic patients (6–70 years 15% vs 24%, $P<.05$; 2–5 years 20% vs 36%, $P = .29$) [30]. This association between allergy and low pneumococcal antibody level presents a double jeopardy for sinusitis.

Cystic fibrosis

Up to 50% of cystic fibrosis (CF) patients have CRS and/or nasal polyps and greater than 90% show CT evidence of upper airway abnormalities [31]. CF is typically diagnosed within the first 2 years of life by pulmonary and gastrointestinal symptoms, although sinusitis may rarely be the initial presentation [32]. Onset of nasal polyposis usually occurs between ages 5 and 14 years, with the prevalence seemingly increasing with age through adolescence [33]. Therefore, CF should be considered in any children presenting with nasal polyposis or nasal/sinus culture growing *Pseudomonas aeruginosa* [2]. It is important to note that carriers of the cystic fibrosis mutation have higher prevalence of CRS [34].

Gastroesophageal/oropharyngeal reflux

Symptoms of GERD including heartburn, throat clearing, hoarseness, and cough mimic CRS and may masquerade, as 1 or the 2 conditions may coexist. Although the overall link between CRS and GERD is not strong, one study involving 30 children showed the incidence of pH probe–proven GERD was higher in children with CRS compared with healthy controls (63% vs 5%), and that CRS symptoms improved with antiacid treatment [35,36].

Primary ciliary dyskinesia (Kartagener syndrome)

Kartagener syndrome is associated with the triad of CRS, bronchiectasis, and situs inversus. Primary ciliary dyskinesia may occur with nasal discharge in the absence of situs inversus starting at birth or during early infancy [37].

LAB STUDIES

The following laboratory studies are recommended: CBC, IgG, IgA, IgM, IgE, specific IgE for environmental allergens, allergen skin test, pneumococcal antibody levels, tetanus antibody levels, and CRP/procalcitonin.

COMPLICATIONS

Warning signs in rhinosinusitis that require immediate attention are vomiting and headache persisting longer than 24 hours, reduced consciousness, periorbital edema, double vision, ophthalmoplegia, reduced visual acuity, severe headache, signs of meningitis, and neurologic signs. These signs indicate that the infection may be spreading to adjacent tissues or is a manifestation of some systemic disease.

Preseptal/periorbital cellulitis

Preseptal/periseptal cellulitis is an infection of the anterior portion of the eyelid not involving the orbit or other ocular structures. Preseptal cellulitis is generally a milder condition than orbital cellulitis and is characterized by edema and erythema of the lids and periorbital area that rarely leads to serious complications.

Orbital cellulitis

Although an uncommon complication of ABRS, orbital cellulitis occurs more commonly in young children and is a danger sign that will require immediate referral to an ophthalmologist to rule out entrapment of the ocular muscles. Characterized by periorbital edema, eyelid erythema, proptosis, and eye movement impairment, it may cause loss of vision and even loss of life, unless treated aggressively [38,39].

Intracranial complications

Intracranial complications may result from frontal or sphenoidal sinusitis and may even be the initial presentation in 5% of patients hospitalized for rhinosinusitis [40]. Subdural empyema is the most common intracranial complication. Extradural empyema, brain abscess, meningitis, cavernous sinus thrombophlebitis, and sphenoid osteomyelitis are other less frequent complications that can be diagnosed by imaging studies [41,42].

Fungal involvement

Although not common in children, fungi may play a role in CRS. There are different manifestations of fungal involvement in the sinus cavity, detailed discussion of which is beyond the scope of this article. Patients with unusual presentations including an intractable course, green/brown nasal discharge, persistent imaging abnormalities (thickened membrane, opacified cavities), and increased allergic laboratory markers (high IgE, eosinophilia) must be referred to specialists for further workup. Allergic fungal sinusitis is considered a distinct subtype of CRS resulting from a strong chronic allergic reaction to colonizing fungi (mostly Aspergillus species) in the sinus cavities of immunocompetent adolescents and young adults in the southern United States (see

Table 4). Invasive fungal rhinosinusitis is a more serious disease with fungi invading the mucosal tissue and often spreading to the adjacent tissue and is very often associated immunocompromised status [13].

Nasal polyps

CRS with nasal polyps (CRSwNP) is common in among adults (20%) and is associated with the type 2 pathway (see Table 4). In children younger than 12 years, the incidence rate is low and if present, CF should be ruled out (10%–32% prevalence) [43].

DIFFERENTIAL DIAGNOSIS

Allergic rhinitis

It may be hard to distinguish sinus infection from allergic rhinitis especially when a patient has a strong allergic background (atopic dermatitis and asthma). Eliminating other diagnostic entities including sinusitis can be accomplished by following the diagnostic guidelines (see Table 1).

Protracted bacterial bronchitis

One of the most common causes of persistent cough in children younger than 5 years is protracted bacterial bronchitis, which is associated with the presence of bacterial pathogens in the biofilm of the lower airway [44]. Although not reported in the literature, it is conceivable that CRS is a precursor of protracted bacterial bronchitis or both conditions coexist, as the biofilm in the airway may extend from the upper airway to the lower airway.

Nasal foreign body

Radiographic imaging is recommended for unilateral CRS to exclude anatomic defect, foreign body, or tumor. Unilateral nasal drainage in young children especially suggests nasal foreign body or unilateral choanal atresia [2].

Pertussis

Nasal symptoms (catarrhal stage) usually improve by 10 days after which the severity of cough increases with whoop (paroxysmal stage), which distinguishes it from sinusitis.

Migraine/facial pain syndrome

Chronic facial pain may be incorrectly attributed to "sinus headache" by patients and generalists but may reflect migraine [45,46]. Migraine symptoms include unilateral headache, sinus pressure, nasal congestion, rhinorrhea, and ophthalmic findings due to the involvement of 3 different branches of trigeminal nerves and so may resemble acute sinusitis.

MANAGEMENT

Management approach includes symptomatic and etiologic treatments for both acute and CRS. The efficacy of various treatment modalities for sinusitis is summarized in Table 5.

Table 5
Management of rhinosinusitis

	ARS		
	Postviral	ABRS	CRS
Nasal irrigation	–	–	+
Nasal steroid	+	+	+
Nasal steroid rinse	...	...	+
Oral steroid	+/–	+/–	+/–
Oral antihistamines	–	–	–
Oral antibiotics	–	+	+/–
Antibiotic rinse	–	–	+
Biologics	–	–	+
Surgery	–	–	+/-
Allergen immunotherapy (allergy shots)	–	+/–	+/–

Nasal irrigation

Irrigation of the nasal and sinus cavity with normal clean saline solution (using boiled or distilled water) has been used for adults and children with CRS and allergic rhinitis, and most studies indicate its efficacy. [47–49]. Studies of baby shampoo rinses report improvement in symptoms and olfaction; however, uncomfortable side effects, primarily nasal burning and headache, are noted and biofilm growth is only inhibited, not eradicated [50,51]. Clinical benefits of mupirocin (and other antiotics) rinses including eradication of Stapylococcus aureus and improvement in nasal endoscopy findings, are generally short-lived [52], [53].

Nasal steroids (inhaler and steroid solution rinse)

A Cochrane review found that inhaled nasal steroids are beneficial as a monotherapy or an adjunctive therapy for ABRS. Although there are no randomized controlled trials to support the efficacy of nasal steroids for CRS in children, its current recommendation is based on the safety study for children and their efficacy in adults [54,55]. There are studies indicating that a dilute steroid sinus rinse is safe and more effective than nasal spray and saline irrigation in postsurgical patients, although not approved by Food and Drug Administration (FDA) [56]. An exhalation-driven delivery system for fluticasone (Xhance) may be beneficial for older children [50,57,58].

Systemic corticosteroid

ARS: one study shows the efficacy of oral steroid (15-day taper) as an adjunct to oral antibiotics in reducing the symptoms and CT scan score. Cochrane analysis showed a short-term benefit of symptom relief but no long-term benefit [59].

CRS: it is common practice to use a "burst" of steroid (eg, Prednisone, 0.5 mg/kg qd x 5), intramuscular solumedrol, or prolonged oral steroid for CRS, and its efficacy and tolerability in children has been reported [60–62].

But one should weigh the potential benefits against the risks associated with accumulative side effects such as weight gain, Cushingoid features, and growth retardation associated with long-term or recurrent systemic steroid use [63].

Antibiotics

ARS: antibiotics are not indicated for viral or postviral ARS. In ABRS, antibiotics have demonstrated efficacy in the treatment of ABRS. The most common bacterial pathogens causing acute sinusitis in children are *Streptococcus pneumonia, H influenzae,* and *M catarrhalis* [64]. Initial empirical treatment with antibiotics covering all these bacteria is recommended for 10 to 14 days in children: Amoxicillin-clavulanate is preferred, but cephalosporins (cefpodoxime, ceftriaxone, cefdinir), azithromycin, trimethoprim-sulfamethoxazole, and clindamycin are alternate drugs for penicillin-sensitive or -resistant patients [10,65,66]. One may also attempt to find a causative pathogen by obtaining a DNA-PCR of nasal secretions from the opening of the osteomeatal complex, especially, in recurrent ABRS.

CRS: although children with CRS are commonly treated with antibiotics of various duration, there is currently no strong evidence to support its use, including prolonged use of macrolide antibiotics [3]. However, there is an earlier study showing that a combination of amoxicillin/clavulanic acid and methylprednisolone taper for 30 days was efficacious [60].

Oral and nasal antihistamines, decongestants, and oral antileukotrienes

These agents are for temporary allergy symptom relief but not useful for the treatment of sinusitis. It may be used as an adjunctive therapy once sinusitis is successfully treated. Use of nasal decongestant should be restricted to less than 3 days per week to prevent rebound nasal congestion.

Allergen and irritant control measures as an adjunctive therapy

Avoidance of exposures to allergens and irritants including smoke and allergen immunotherapy can reduce rhinitis symptoms, which may indirectly decrease the incidence of sinusitis.

Biologics

CRS: biologics are increasingly being used for treatment of type 2 immune(allergic) disorders, including severe persistent asthma and CRSwNP. Although no biologics are approved by the FDA for use in sinusitis, anecdotal reports show the improvement of CRS when type 2 immune antagonists were used for concomitant severe asthma or atopic dermatitis (see Fig. 1) [67–69]. These biologics are now approved for patients with CRSwNP with strong type 2 immune background who did not respond to surgical interventions and repeated systemic steroid courses (see Fig. 1) [70,71]. Commonly used biologics for type 2 immune diseases include the following:

- Omalizumab: monoclonal antibody (mAb) against the Fc portion of IgE, thus blocking its interaction with FcER. Has been approved for treatment of moderate and severe asthma and CRSwNP.

- Dupilumab: mAb against the common γ chain of interleukin-13 (IL-13) and IL-4. Has been approved for treatment of severe atopic dermatitis, asthma, and CRSwNP [67].
- Mepolizumab: mAb against IL-5 molecules from Th2 cells. Has been approved for eosinophil-dominant asthma and CRSwNP.

Vaccination with pneumococcal vaccines

Responders

Most of these patients with low pneumococcal antibody levels respond to polysaccharide or conjugated pneumococcal vaccination. Among responders, the rate of recurrent sinusitis is significantly reduced [30]. Many of these nonresponders (specific antibody deficiency) continue to have recurrent or persistent sinusitis.

Nonresponders (specific antibody deficiency)

Children with specific antibody deficiency and recurrent sinusitis need to be treated with continuous prophylactic antibiotics for a year or immunoglobulin replacement [72]. Commonly used antibiotics are amoxicillin daily or azithromycin twice a week [73]. After a year, antibiotic prophylaxis is stopped, and unconjugated pneumococcal vaccine is given again. Some patients do show protective responses, presumably because their B-cell immunity has finally matured. Immunoglobulin replacement therapy may be initiated first or after prophylactic antibiotics failed. After a year, immune status can be tested similarly as in patients with prophylactic antibiotic therapy. Specific antibody deficiency may be an early manifestation of more serious primary immunodeficiency including CVID; these patients must be observed closely [74].

Probiotics

Studies show that most subjects with CRS have an abnormal array of microbiota in the nasal cavity [75]. Research is ongoing to find out if "normalizing" the nasal microbiome with protective microbiota would be therapeutic for CRS. Some probiotic nasal applications were reported to play a protective role, but currently such products are not available in the United States [76,77].

SURGERY

Surgery is less frequently used in pediatrics compared with adults. Adenoidectomy is considered the first-line approach.

Adenoidectomy

Adenoid hypertrophy is a common finding associated with CRS or recurrent sinusitis. Adenoid tissue may become enlarged as the result of recurrent URI, and in turn a large adenoid may obstruct the drainage of nasal mucus, further increasing the mucous pool, which may serve as a medium where pathogenic bacteria may persist. In addition, adenoid tissue, through its crevices, may become a reservoir for the pathogens [78]. For this reason, adenoidectomy may benefit, especially, younger children with CRS, noisy breathing, and sleep apnea [79,80]. Additional maxillary antral irrigation at the time of surgery may yield additional benefit [81].

Sinus surgery: balloon sinuplasty (balloon ostial dilation) versus functional endoscopic sinus surgery

Patients who do not respond to medical therapy and adenoidectomy must be evaluated for sinus surgery, the goal of which is to clean the sinus cavities and create a larger opening. Balloon sinuplasty is the simpler of 2 outpatient procedures. Although it is approved by FDA for use in children in the United States, its efficacy and cost-effectiveness has no supporting evidence, and it is not endorsed by the American Academy of Otolaryngologist [55]. Functional endoscopic sinus surgery (FESS) is a minimally invasive endoscopic procedure in which nasal and sinus cavities are viewed and obstructing tissue can be removed with minimal damage to the surrounding tissue. Studies have demonstrated a positive outcome in 71% to 100% of operated children after FESS and parental satisfaction with symptom improvement on 10-year follow-up [82,83].

SUMMARY

Sinusitis may result from various common and uncommon causes, but most often it is a complication of persistent rhinitis due to URI and/or allergic sensitization. Once the diagnosis is made based on the clinical criteria and laboratory studies including the dipstick method, patients need to be managed with medical therapies and, if all fails, with surgical interventions. When the sinusitis persists or recurs, one must consider immune defects. The most common immune defects are the presence of persistent allergic rhinitis and low levels of pneumococcal antibodies. Allergic conditions need to be treated vigorously, including allergen immunotherapy and biologics. Allergic conditions may suppress the baseline pneumococcal antibody levels, which can be corrected by immunization with the polysaccharide and conjugate vaccines. Patients who do not respond to the vaccines may continue to have chronic and recurrent sinusitis. These nonresponders may be treated with prophylactic antibiotics or immunoglobulin replacement.

Disclosure

The authors have nothing to disclose.

Reference

[1] Huang S-W, Small PA. Rapid diagnosis of bacterial sinusitis in patients using a simple test of nasal secretions. Allergy Asthma Proc 2008;29(6):640–3.
[2] Peters AT, Spector S, Hsu J, et al. Diagnosis and management of rhinosinusitis: a practice parameter update. Ann Allergy Asthma Immunol 2014;113(4); https://doi.org/10.1016/j.anai.2014.07.025.
[3] Fokkens WJ, Lund VJ, Hopkins C, et al. European Position Paper on Rhinosinusitis and Nasal Polyps 2020. Rhinology 2020;58:1–464.
[4] Gordts F, Abu Nasser I, Clement PAR, et al. Bacteriology of the middle meatus in children. Int J Pediatr Otorhinolaryngol 1999;48(2):163–7.
[5] Song C, Chorath J, Pak Y, et al. Use of Dipstick Assay and Rapid PCR-DNA Analysis of Nasal Secretions for Diagnosis of Bacterial Sinusitis in Children With Chronic Cough. Allergy Rhinol 2019;10:215265671882128.

[6] Blackwell DL, Lucas JW, Clarke TC. Summary health statistics for U.S. adults: national health interview survey, 2012. Vital Health Stat 10 2021;260:1–161.
[7] Gilani S, Shin JJ. The Burden and Visit Prevalence of Pediatric Chronic Rhinosinusitis. Otolaryngol Neck Surg 2017;157(6); https://doi.org/10.1177/0194599817721177.
[8] Sidell D, Shapiro NL, Bhattacharyya N. Obesity and the risk of chronic rhinosinusitis, allergic rhinitis, and acute otitis media in school-age children. Laryngoscope 2013; https://doi.org/10.1002/lary.24038.
[9] Marom T, Alvarez-Fernandez PE, Jennings K, et al. Acute Bacterial Sinusitis Complicating Viral Upper Respiratory Tract Infection in Young Children. Pediatr Infect Dis J 2014;33(8); https://doi.org/10.1097/INF.0000000000000278.
[10] Wald ER, Applegate KE, Bordley C, et al. Clinical Practice Guideline for the Diagnosis and Management of Acute Bacterial Sinusitis in Children Aged 1 to 18 Years. Pediatrics 2013;132(1):e262–80.
[11] Wolf G, Anderhuber W, Kuhn F. Development of the Paranasal Sinuses in Children: Implications for Paranasal Sinus Surgery. Ann Otol Rhinol Laryngol 1993;102(9):705–11.
[12] Kumpitsch C, Koskinen K, Schöpf V, et al. The microbiome of the upper respiratory tract in health and disease. BMC Biol 2019;17(1); https://doi.org/10.1186/s12915-019-0703-z.
[13] Chakrabarti A, Denning DW, Ferguson BJ, et al. Fungal rhinosinusitis. Laryngoscope 2009;119(9); https://doi.org/10.1002/lary.20520.
[14] Meltzer EO, Hamilos DL, Hadley JA, et al. Rhinosinusitis: Establishing definitions for clinical research and patient care. J Allergy Clin Immunol 2004;114(6):155–212.
[15] Brugger SD, Bomar L, Lemon KP. Commensal–Pathogen Interactions along the Human Nasal Passages. PLoS Pathog 2016;12(7); https://doi.org/10.1371/journal.ppat.1005633.
[16] Boase S, Foreman A, Cleland E, et al. The microbiome of chronic rhinosinusitis: culture, molecular diagnostics and biofilm detection. BMC Infect Dis 2013;13(1):210.
[17] Abreu NA, Nagalingam NA, Song Y, et al. Sinus Microbiome Diversity Depletion and Corynebacterium tuberculostearicum Enrichment Mediates Rhinosinusitis. Sci Transl Med 2012;4(151); https://doi.org/10.1126/scitranslmed.3003783.
[18] Kanmani P, Clua P, Vizoso-Pinto MG, et al. Respiratory Commensal Bacteria Corynebacterium pseudodiphtheriticum Improves Resistance of Infant Mice to Respiratory Syncytial Virus and Streptococcus pneumoniae Superinfection. Front Microbiol 2017;8; https://doi.org/10.3389/fmicb.2017.01613.
[19] Funke G, von Graevenitz A, Clarridge JE, et al. Clinical microbiology of coryneform bacteria. Clin Microbiol Rev 1997;10(1):125–59.
[20] Feazel LM, Robertson CE, Ramakrishnan VR, et al. Microbiome complexity and Staphylococcus aureus in chronic rhinosinusitis. Laryngoscope 2012;122(2):467–72.
[21] Heath J, Hartzell L, Putt C, et al. Chronic Rhinosinusitis in Children: Pathophysiology, Evaluation, and Medical Management. Curr Allergy Asthma Rep 2018;18(7); https://doi.org/10.1007/s11882-018-0792-8.
[22] Wald ER. Microbiology of Acute and Chronic Sinusitis in Children and Adults. Am J Med Sci 1998;316(1):13–20.
[23] Gwaltneyjr J, Scheld W, Sande M, et al. The microbial etiology and antimicrobial therapy of adults with acute community-acquired sinusitis: A fifteen-year experience at the University of Virginia and review of other selected studies. J Allergy Clin Immunol 1992;90(3):457–62.
[24] Cryer J, Schipor I, Perloff JR, et al. Evidence of Bacterial Biofilms in Human Chronic Sinusitis. ORL 2004;66(3):155–8.
[25] Fastenberg JH, Hsueh WD, Mustafa A, et al. Biofilms in chronic rhinosinusitis: Pathophysiology and therapeutic strategies. World J Otorhinolaryngol Head Neck Surg 2016;2(4):219–29.
[26] Finegold SM, Flynn MJ, Rose FV, et al. Bacteriologic Findings Associated with Chronic Bacterial Maxillary Sinusitis in Adults. Clin Infect Dis 2002;35(4):428–33.

[27] Chad Z. Allergies in children. Paediatr Child Health 2001;6(8); https://doi.org/10.1093/pch/6.8.555.
[28] Gonzales-van Horn SR, Farrar JD. Interferon at the crossroads of allergy and viral infections. J Leukoc Biol 2015;98(2); https://doi.org/10.1189/jlb.3RU0315-099R.
[29] Bousfiha A, Jeddane L, Picard C, et al. Human Inborn Errors of Immunity: 2019 Update of the IUIS Phenotypical Classification. J Clin Immunol 2020;40(1):66–81.
[30] Song CH, Estevez D, Chernikova D, et al. Low Baseline Pneumococcal Antibody Titers Predict Specific Antibody Deficiency, Increased Upper Respiratory Infections, and Allergy Sensitization. Allergy Rhinol 2020;11:215265671990033.
[31] Mainz JG, Koitschev A. Management of chronic rhinosinusitis in CF. J Cyst Fibros 2009;8:S10–4.
[32] Wiatrak BJ. Cystic Fibrosis Presenting With Sinus Disease in Children. Arch Pediatr Adolesc Med 1993;147(3); https://doi.org/10.1001/archpedi.1993.02160270020006.
[33] Schraven SP, Wehrmann M, Wagner W, et al. Prevalence and histopathology of chronic polypoid sinusitis in pediatric patients with cystic fibrosis. J Cyst Fibros 2011;10(3); https://doi.org/10.1016/j.jcf.2011.01.003.
[34] Wang X, Kim J, McWilliams R, et al. Increased Prevalence of Chronic Rhinosinusitis in Carriers of a Cystic Fibrosis Mutation. Arch Otolaryngol Neck Surg 2005;131(3):237.
[35] Barbero GJ. Gastroesophageal reflux and upper airway disease. Otolaryngol Clin North Am 1996;29(1):27–38.
[36] Flook EP, Kumar BN. Is there evidence to link acid reflux with chronic sinusitis or any nasal symptoms? A review of the evidence. Rhinol J 2011;49(1):11–6.
[37] PEDERSEN M, MYGIND N. Rhinitis, sinusitis and otitis media in Kartagener's syndrome (primary ciliary dyskinesia). Clin Otolaryngol 1982;7(6); https://doi.org/10.1111/j.1365-2273.1982.tb01400.x.
[38] Jackson K, Baker SR. Periorbital cellulitis. Head Neck Surg 1987;9(4); https://doi.org/10.1002/hed.2890090406.
[39] MILLS RP, KARTUSH JM. Orbital wall thickness and the spread of infection from the paranasal sinuses. Clin Otolaryngol 1985;10(4); https://doi.org/10.1111/j.1365-2273.1985.tb00243.x.
[40] Brook I. Microbiology and antimicrobial treatment of orbital and intracranial complications of sinusitis in children and their management. Int J Pediatr Otorhinolaryngol 2009;73(9); https://doi.org/10.1016/j.ijporl.2009.01.020.
[41] Bayonne E, Romain K, Patrice T, et al. Intracranial complications of rhinosinusitis. A review, typical imaging data and algorithm of management. Rhinology 2009;47(1):59–65.
[42] Chaiyasate S, Fooanant S, Navacharoen N, et al. The Complications of Sinusitis in a Tertiary Care Hospital: Types, Patient Characteristics, and Outcomes. Int J Otolaryngol 2015;2015; https://doi.org/10.1155/2015/709302.
[43] Ramsey B, Richardson M. Impact of sinusitis in cystic fibrosis. J Allergy Clin Immunol 1992;90(3):547–52.
[44] Chang AB, Upham JW, Masters IB, et al. Protracted bacterial bronchitis: The last decade and the road ahead. Pediatr Pulmonol 2016;51(3):225–42.
[45] Eross E, Dodick D, Eross M. The Sinus, Allergy and Migraine Study (SAMS). Headache J Head Face Pain 2007;47(2); https://doi.org/10.1111/j.1526-4610.2006.00688.x.
[46] Schreiber CP, Hutchinson S, Webster CJ, et al. Prevalence of Migraine in Patients With a History of Self-reported or Physician-Diagnosed "Sinus" Headache. Arch Intern Med 2004;164(16); https://doi.org/10.1001/archinte.164.16.1769.
[47] Brown CL, Graham SM. Nasal irrigations: good or bad? Curr Opin Otolaryngol Head Neck Surg 2004;12(1); https://doi.org/10.1097/00020840-200402000-00004.
[48] Pham V, Sykes K, Wei J. Long-term outcome of once daily nasal irrigation for the treatment of pediatric chronic rhinosinusitis. Laryngoscope 2014;124(4); https://doi.org/10.1002/lary.24224.

[49] Wei JL, Sykes KJ, Johnson P, et al. Safety and efficacy of once-daily nasal irrigation for the treatment of pediatric chronic rhinosinusitis. Laryngoscope 2011;121(9); https://doi.org/10.1002/lary.21923.
[50] Chiu AG, Palmer JN, Woodworth BA, et al. Baby Shampoo Nasal Irrigations for the Symptomatic Post-functional Endoscopic Sinus Surgery Patient. Am J Rhinol 2008;22(1); https://doi.org/10.2500/ajr.2008.22.3122.
[51] Farag AA, Deal AM, McKinney KA, et al. Single-blind randomized controlled trial of surfactant vs hypertonic saline irrigation following endoscopic endonasal surgery. Int Forum Allergy Rhinol 2013;3(4); https://doi.org/10.1002/alr.21116.
[52] Jervis-Bardy J, Wormald P-J. Microbiological outcomes following mupirocin nasal washes for symptomatic, Staphylococcus aureus-positive chronic rhinosinusitis following endoscopic sinus surgery. Int Forum Allergy Rhinol 2012;2(2); https://doi.org/10.1002/alr.20106.
[53] Jervis-Bardy J, Boase S, Psaltis A, et al. A randomized trial of mupirocin sinonasal rinses versus saline in surgically recalcitrant staphylococcal chronic rhinosinusitis. Laryngoscope 2012;122(10); https://doi.org/10.1002/lary.23486.
[54] Allen DB, Meltzer EO, Lemanske RF Jr, et al. No Growth Suppression in Children Treated with the Maximum Recommended Dose of Fluticasone Propionate Aqueous Nasal Spray for One Year. Allergy Asthma Proc 2002;23(6):407–13.
[55] Brietzke SE, Shin JJ, Choi S, et al. Clinical Consensus Statement. Otolaryngol Neck Surg 2014;151(4); https://doi.org/10.1177/0194599814549302.
[56] Aukema A, Mulder P, Fokkens W. Treatment of nasal polyposis and chronic rhinosinusitis with fluticasone propionate nasal drops reduces need for sinus surgery. J Allergy Clin Immunol 2005;115(5):1017–23.
[57] Sachanandani NS, Piccirillo JF, Kramper MA, et al. The Effect of Nasally Administered Budesonide Respules on Adrenal Cortex Function in Patients With Chronic Rhinosinusitis. Arch Otolaryngol Neck Surg 2009;135(3):303.
[58] Palmer JN, Messina JC, Biletch R, et al. A cross-sectional, population-based survey of U.S. adults with symptoms of chronic rhinosinusitis. Allergy Asthma Proc 2019;40(1):48–56.
[59] Venekamp RP, Thompson MJ, Hayward G, et al. Systemic corticosteroids for acute sinusitis. Cochrane Database Syst Rev 2014; https://doi.org/10.1002/14651858.CD008115.pub3.
[60] Ozturk F, Bakirtas A, Ileri F, et al. Efficacy and tolerability of systemic methylprednisolone in children and adolescents with chronic rhinosinusitis: A double-blind, placebo-controlled randomized trial. J Allergy Clin Immunol 2011;128(2); https://doi.org/10.1016/j.jaci.2011.04.045.
[61] Lal D, Scianna JM, Stankiewicz JA. Efficacy of Targeted Medical Therapy in Chronic Rhinosinusitis, and Predictors of Failure. Am J Rhinol Allergy 2009;23(4):396–400.
[62] Skorpinski EW, Vannelli PM, Yousef E, et al. Radiologic outcomes in children with chronic rhinosinusitis and ostiomeatal complex obstruction after medical management. Ann Allergy Asthma Immunol 2008;100(6):529–32.
[63] Hox V, Lourijsen E, Jordens A, et al. Benefits and harm of systemic steroids for short- and long-term use in rhinitis and rhinosinusitis: an EAACI position paper. Clin Transl Allergy 2020;10(1); https://doi.org/10.1186/s13601-019-0303-6.
[64] Brook I. Bacteriology of Acute and Chronic Frontal Sinusitis. Arch Otolaryngol Neck Surg 2002;128(5); https://doi.org/10.1001/archotol.128.5.583.
[65] Chow AW, Benninger MS, Brook I, et al. Executive Summary: IDSA Clinical Practice Guideline for Acute Bacterial Rhinosinusitis in Children and Adults. Clin Infect Dis 2012;54(8); https://doi.org/10.1093/cid/cir1043.
[66] Ikeda K, Tamura G, Shimomura A, et al. Endoscopic Sinus Surgery Improves Pulmonary Function in Patients with Asthma Associated with Chronic Sinusitis. Ann Otol Rhinol Laryngol 1999;108(4):355–9.

[67] Bachert C, Han JK, Desrosiers M, et al. Efficacy and safety of dupilumab in patients with severe chronic rhinosinusitis with nasal polyps (LIBERTY NP SINUS-24 and LIBERTY NP SINUS-52): results from two multicentre, randomised, double-blind, placebo-controlled, parallel-group phase 3 trials. Lancet 2019;394(10209); https://doi.org/10.1016/S0140-6736(19)31881-1.
[68] Tiotiu A, Oster J, Roux P, et al. Effectiveness of Omalizumab in Severe Allergic Asthma and Nasal Polyposis: A Real-Life Study. J Investig Allergol Clin Immunol 2020;30(1); https://doi.org/10.18176/jiaci.0391.
[69] Weinstein SF, Katial RK, Bardin P, et al. Effects of Reslizumab on Asthma Outcomes in a Subgroup of Eosinophilic Asthma Patients with Self-Reported Chronic Rhinosinusitis with Nasal Polyps. J Allergy Clin Immunol Pract 2019;7(2); https://doi.org/10.1016/j.jaip.2018.08.021.
[70] Fokkens WJ, Lund V, Bachert C, et al. EUFOREA consensus on biologics for CRSwNP with or without asthma. Allergy 2019;74(12); https://doi.org/10.1111/all.13875.
[71] Gevaert P, Nouri-Aria KT, Wu H, et al. Local receptor revision and class switching to IgE in chronic rhinosinusitis with nasal polyps. Allergy 2013;68(1):55–63.
[72] Paris K, Sorensen RU. Assessment and clinical interpretation of polysaccharide antibody responses. Ann Allergy Asthma Immunol 2007;99(5); https://doi.org/10.1016/S1081-1206(10)60572-8.
[73] Wolpert J, Knutsen AP. Natural History of Selective Antibody Deficiency to Bacterial Polysaccharide Antigens in Children. Pediatr Asthma Allergy Immunol 1998;12(3):183–91.
[74] Wilson SP, Ballas ZK. Progression of Specific Antibody Deficiency (SAD) to Common Variable Immunodeficiency (CVID). J Allergy Clin Immunol 2010;125(2); https://doi.org/10.1016/j.jaci.2009.12.287.
[75] Dimitri-Pinheiro S, Soares R, Barata P. The Microbiome of the Nose—Friend or Foe? Allergy Rhinol 2020;11; https://doi.org/10.1177/2152656720911605.
[76] Cervin AU. The Potential for Topical Probiotic Treatment of Chronic Rhinosinusitis, a Personal Perspective. Front Cell Infect Microbiol 2018;7; https://doi.org/10.3389/fcimb.2017.00530.
[77] Kramer MF, Heath MD. Probiotics in the Treatment of Chronic Rhinoconjunctivitis and Chronic Rhinosinusitis. J Allergy 2014;2014:1–7.
[78] Coticchia J, Zuliani G, Coleman C, et al. Biofilm Surface Area in the Pediatric Nasopharynx. Arch Otolaryngol Neck Surg 2007;133(2); https://doi.org/10.1001/archotol.133.2.110.
[79] Brietzke SE, Brigger MT. Adenoidectomy outcomes in pediatric rhinosinusitis: A meta-analysis. Int J Pediatr Otorhinolaryngol 2008;72(10); https://doi.org/10.1016/j.ijporl.2008.07.008.
[80] Shin KS, Cho SH, Kim KR, et al. The role of adenoids in pediatric rhinosinusitis. Int J Pediatr Otorhinolaryngol 2008;72(11); https://doi.org/10.1016/j.ijporl.2008.07.016.
[81] Ramadan HH, Cost JL. Outcome of Adenoidectomy Versus Adenoidectomy With Maxillary Sinus Wash for Chronic Rhinosinusitis in Children. Laryngoscope 2008;118(5); https://doi.org/10.1097/MLG.0b013e3181653422.
[82] Lusk RP, Bothwell MR, Piccirillo J. Long-Term Follow-Up for Children Treated With Surgical Intervention for Chronic Rhinosinusitis. Laryngoscope 2006;116(12); https://doi.org/10.1097/01.mlg.0000244387.11129.a0.
[83] Vlastarakos PV, Fetta M, Segas JV, et al. Functional Endoscopic Sinus Surgery Improves Sinus-Related Symptoms and Quality of Life in Children With Chronic Rhinosinusitis. Clin Pediatr (Phila) 2013;52(12); https://doi.org/10.1177/0009922813506489.

Advances in Pediatrics 69 (2022) 95–105

ADVANCES IN PEDIATRICS

Management of Pediatric Obstructive Sleep Apnea After Failed Tonsillectomy and Adenoidectomy

Abhay Varun Sharma, MD[a,*], Tapan Padhya, MD[a], Sagarika Nallu, MD[b]

[a]Department of Otolaryngology Head and Neck Surgery, University of South Florida Morsani College of Medicine, 12901 Bruce B Downs Boulevard, MDC 73 Tampa, FL 33612, USA; [b]USF Health Department of Pediatrics, Division of Neurology, 13101 Bruce B Downs Boulevard, Tampa, FL 33612, USA

Keywords

• Adenotonsillectomy • Obstructive sleep apnea • Drug-induced sleep endoscopy • Cine MRI • Pharyngoplasty • Lingual tonsillectomy • Tongue base

Key points

- The reasons adenotonsillectomy (AT) fails to improve obstructive sleep apnea (OSA) are diverse and include increased severity of OSA, obesity, craniofacial syndromes, and neuromuscular syndromes.
- Evaluation of patients after failed AT includes repeat polysomnography (PSG), physical examination, drug-induced sleep endoscopy (DISE), and cine magnetic resonance imaging (MRI).
- Surgical therapy should be directed at specific sites of obstruction, including the nose, palate, tongue base, and supraglottis.
- Close follow-up and repeat PSG are important after salvage treatment.

INTRODUCTION

The field of pediatric sleep has been growing over the last 2 decades. Obstructive sleep apnea (OSA) has a high prevalence in the pediatric population, ranging from 2% to 4% of American children. The severe metabolic, neurocognitive, and cardiovascular consequences make it important to effectively treat OSA [1,2].

*Corresponding author. *E-mail address:* asharma1521@gmail.com

https://doi.org/10.1016/j.yapd.2022.03.006
0065-3101/22/Published by Elsevier Inc.

Children with OSA present differently than adults. The typical syndrome of daytime sleepiness is absent and replaced by hyperactivity, restlessness, and learning difficulties [3]. Polysomnography (PSG) typically shows continuous snoring with hypopneas rather than alternating snoring seen in adults with obstructive apneas [3]. The definition of pediatric OSA, as outlined by the International Classification of Sleep Disorders 3rd Edition, (ICSD-3) is: (1) clinical criteria with observed obstruction during sleep or daytime consequences such as hyperactivity and learning difficulties, and (2) PSG criteria defined as apnea-hypopnea index (AHI) > 1. An AHI of 1 to 5 events/h is considered mild, 5 to 10 events/h is moderate, and > 10 events/hr is severe [4].

The Childhood Adenotonsillectomy Trial (CHAT) results published in 2013 showed that adenotonsillectomy (AT) had a definitive benefit for children with OSA, with multiple objective and subjective parameters significantly improving after surgery compared with watchful waiting [5]. However, 20% of patients after AT had persistent OSA on PSG. While an AHI > 1 implies there is at least mild OSA, the definition of residual OSA varies. In the context of performing repeat interventions, some define residual OSA as persistent severe disease (AHI > 10 events/h) or an AHI between 2 and 10 events/h with continuing daytime or nighttime symptoms [6]. More complex pediatric patients (morbid obesity, craniofacial syndromes, Down syndrome, neuromuscular disorders) have a much lower success rate than healthy patients with enlarged tonsils and adenoids [7]. The subset of the pediatric population whose OSA is not cured after AT can be particularly difficult to evaluate and treat. OSA treatments, once confined to AT, have now expanded to include a wide variety of new pathways for evaluation and treatment. We review treatment options for pediatric patients who have persistent OSA after AT.

Reasons for the failure of adenotonsillectomy

Predictors for the failure of AT include severe OSA, craniofacial anomalies, age > 7, black race, and obesity [5,8]. Studies of follow-up PSGs have demonstrated that residual disease is more common than previously recognized. A systematic review of cure rates after AT in children showed 34% had respiratory disturbance index (RDI) > 5, with nonresolution in 61% of patients with comorbidities (morbid obesity, severe OSA, younger than 3 years of age) [7]. Studies have shown that 27% of obese children with no sleep symptoms have OSA, and 25% to 40% of obese children with sleep symptoms will be found to have OSA [9,10]. In a 2009 meta-analysis by Costa and colleagues of AT for obese children, AHI decreased by 18.3 events/h, but only 49% of children achieved an AHI < 5. Using an AHI < 1 as the success criteria, up to 88% of obese children will have residual OSA [9]. Given the risk of residual disease, follow-up and repeat PSG are necessary to ensure improvement after surgery.

Evaluation

History and physical examination

Although history and physical can provide strong evidence that a child has OSA, its ability to accurately predict the presence of OSA is not strong. A systematic review by Brietzke and colleagues in 2004 showed that the clinical examination alone is not sufficient to diagnose OSA based on a gold standard evaluation of PSG [11]. In patients who have failed AT, clinical evaluation alone is not sufficient. Awake flexible endoscopy examination findings do not correlate with those found during sleep [12,13].

Drug-induced sleep endoscopy

Drug-induced sleep endoscopy (DISE) is an effective method for evaluating pediatric patients with OSA. However, one of the main issues with the evaluation is the variety of scoring methods. A recent study by Lam and colleagues describes one of the many effective methods to score DISE, termed the sleep endoscopy rating scale (SERS). This 12-point scale scoring system using 6 anatomic levels (nose, nasopharynx, velum, oropharynx, hypopharynx, arytenoids) correlated well with OSA severity. A score > 6 had a sensitivity and specificity of 81.8% and 87.5%, respectively, for severe OSA.

A systematic review of children with persistent OSA after AT by Manickam and colleagues showed the most common site of obstruction on DISE to be the tongue base, adenoids, inferior turbinates, velum, and lateral oropharyngeal walls [12,14]. In addition, children with severe OSA were more likely to have multi-level obstruction. There is evidence that DISE-directed surgery may be effective, though studies are limited [15,16]. For example, DISE can impact the surgical approach in 35% to 61% of cases, but whether it improves outcomes is still debated. Wooten and colleagues studied 34 consecutive children with residual OSA after AT and found that DISE improved outcomes, with mean AHI falling from 7 to 3 [17].

A recent clinical consensus statement on DISE provides some clarification for pressing questions. Specifically, there was agreement that DISE is indicated for patients with residual OSA and for children at risk for residual disease. In addition, they determined that DISE-directed surgery does improve outcomes in children with residual OSA after AT [6,16]. Whether DISE should be performed in surgically naïve patients is also controversial, but it can be helpful in patients with small tonsils or those at risk for residual OSA [6]. However, the fact that DISE-directed surgery does not always lead to complete resolution of apnea shows that it may not reveal every site of obstruction [17].

Cine magnetic resonance imaging

Cine magnetic resonance imaging (MRI), though less commonly used, is a useful adjunct for the evaluation of pediatric patients with OSA. It is used less than DISE due to the need to sedate children with severe OSA, who may not have a secure airway, while in the MRI scanner. In the meta-analysis noted earlier, 3 of the 14 studies used cine MRI to evaluate upper airway collapse in pediatric patients with OSA, and the site of obstruction could be identified in 93% of patients [12]. A retrospective study by Clark and colleagues showed similar efficacy of cine MRI and DISE in determining the site of obstruction in pediatric patients who had failed AT [18]. Most of the cases show similar areas of obstruction during both evaluations, though a few cases showed differences between evaluation methods. The advantages of using cine MRI are the ability to concurrently assess multiple sites of obstruction and to quantify lingual tonsillar hypertrophy volumetrically, neither of which is possible with DISE. These advantages are especially helpful in patients with Down syndrome, as they generally have more complex OSA [1,19].

Medical treatment

Continuous positive airway pressure (CPAP) is second-line therapy for children with OSA due to low tolerance in the pediatric population and the risk that chronic pressure from mask use can affect the facial structure. However, there is clear evidence of its effectiveness [20,21]. Tolerance for CPAP in one systematic review by Watach and colleagues showed an adherence rate of only 56.9%. Female sex, younger age, and developmental delays were predictors of higher adherence rates [22]. Some studies have also shown maternal education and family history of CPAP used to be predictors of success [23].

Anti-inflammatory drugs have shown mixed effectiveness for pediatric OSA. An updated Cochrane review by Kuhle and colleagues in 2020 showed uncertain efficacy of intranasal steroids. There seemed to be an improvement in oxygen desaturation index and oxygen saturation, but uncertainty regarding the effect on AHI. Montelukast improved the AHI for healthy, nonobese, surgically naive patients [24]. A study by Wang and colleagues demonstrated montelukast significantly improved AHI in pediatric patients with mild residual OSA after AT, but cure (AHI < 1) was only obtained in 5 of the 58 patients [25].

Conservative dental treatments include mandibular advancement devices (MAD) and myofunctional therapy. Though a few prospective trials have shown improvement in respiratory parameters with MADs, currently there is limited evidence to support long-term use in pediatric OSA [26]. Myofunctional therapy has shown some effectiveness in a limited number of studies. These techniques are meant to strengthen the Oral (eg, tongue) and oropharyngeal structures (eg, soft palate, lateral pharyngeal wall).A prospective case-control study by Villa and colleagues showed improvement in residual OSA after AT in the myofunctional therapy group (mean AHI of 4.8–1.8) compared with control (mean AHI of 4.5–4.1). However, the small size of this cohort and inability to analyze long-term effects make it difficult to draw significant conclusions about this therapy for residual OSA.

Surgical treatment

There are a variety of surgical treatments available after a failed primary AT. This section describes these techniques based on anatomic abnormalities. Fig. 1 summarizes this information.

Nose

Though nasal surgery is not used to treat OSA, there is evidence that it improves AHI and quality of life outcomes in children. Cheng and colleagues compared combined inferior turbinate reduction with AT to AT alone. The combined procedure resulted in lower mean postoperative AHI (0.8 vs 3.5) and greater reduction in OSA-18 scores, a quality-of-life questionnaire [27]. Septoplasty can be considered in older children as there is a risk of affecting nasal structure with the developing septal cartilage [1]. No studies have analyzed nasal surgery on its own as a treatment of pediatric OSA, though it can be a useful adjunctive technique.

Palate

Palate surgeries for residual OSA after AT have shown success. Modified uvulopalatopharyngoplasty (UPPP) techniques, such as the expansion palatopharyngoplasty (ESP), have improved AHI in patients after AT. Ulualp retrospectively compared his modified ESP technique to AT in surgically naïve patients with severe OSA. He showed greater improvement in the ESP group–despite children in the ESP group having higher BMI and smaller tonsils [28]. More extensive pharyngoplasty techniques should be used with caution in patients prone to hypernasality (Down syndrome, submucous clefts) as these conditions can cause significant velopharyngeal insufficiency [13]. Though definitive conclusions on the efficacy of palate surgery are not possible due to the paucity of data, it provides a good option for patients who have lateral pharyngeal wall collapse on DISE.

Tongue

Phenotypic abnormalities of the tongue are one of the most common causes of residual obstruction in this patient population, occurring in 35% to 85% of these patients [12]. Three phenotypes seen in tongue base obstruction are glossoptosis, lingual tonsillar hypertrophy, and macroglossia [1]. Lingual tonsillectomy currently has the most evidence of success and is the most commonly performed. Techniques include sharp dissection, microdebrider, laser, and coblation-assisted methods [8]. A meta-analysis by Kang and colleagues showed an overall decrease in AHI by 8.9, which corresponded to complete resolution ($AHI < 1$) in 17% and improvement to mild OSA ($AHI < 5$) in 51% [28–31]. Postoperative bleeding rates are slightly higher than with AT. If performed as part of a multi-level surgery, care should be taken to avoid connecting the incisions with the palate, as oropharyngeal stenosis can be a devastating complication [1,12,32].

Posterior midline glossectomy is used to treat glossoptosis and macroglossia. Coblation is a commonly used technique, though transoral robotic surgery (TORS) is also an option. In these cases, ultrasound can be used to map out the lingual arteries. If the ultrasound is not conducted, care must be taken to remain 1.5 cm from the midline posterior to the foramen cecum and within 1 cm of the midline anterior to this point [17,19]. Other techniques include tongue base suspension and hyoid suspension. Evidence of success for these surgeries are limited to small case series [12,17].

There has been a large increase In frenuloplasty for ankyloglossia in the last decade, and its role as a treatment of OSA is controversial. The mechanism of treatment stems from the idea that a tethered tongue leads to a narrow palatal

Site of Obstruction	Intervention
Nasal cavity	
Septum	Septoplasty
Inferior turbinates	SMR, coblation
Hard palate	RME, DOG of maxilla
Nasopharynx	
Adenoids	Adenoidectomy
Oropharynx	
Tonsillar hypertrophy	Revision tonsillectomy Partial tonsillectomy
Lateral wall collapse	ESP, UPPP
Tongue	
Lingual tonsillar hypertrophy	Lingual tonsillectomy
Glossoptosis	Tongue base suspension Hyoid myotomy and suspension Posterior midline glossectomy
Micrognathia	MAD, DOG of mandible
Larynx	
Laryngomalacia	Supraglottoplasty
Epiglottis	Epiglottopexy

Fig. 1. Sites of obstruction and their respective surgical treatments. DOG, distraction osteogenesis; ESP, expansion sphincter pharyngoplasty; MAD, mandibular advancement device; RME, rapid maxillary expansion; SMR, submucous resection; UPPP, uvulopalatopharyngoplasty.

arch and abnormal maxillary growth. Only one retrospective analysis of 150 patients by Guilleminault and colleagues noted an association between pediatric patients with sleep-disordered breathing and short lingual frenulum [33]. High-level evidence for this is lacking, and a recent consensus statement in 2020 determined ankyloglossia does not cause OSA [34].

Hypoglossal nerve stimulation has shown encouraging results in pediatric patients with Down syndrome, 80% of whom have OSA. AT remains first-line treatment of children with Down syndrome, but OSA only resolves in 16% to 33% of these patients. Though currently hypoglossal nerve stimulator surgery is only approved for adults, there is an ongoing trial assessing its effectiveness in the pediatric Down syndrome population. A recent update on the first 20 patients in this trial revealed that in 45% of patients, AHI was reduced to <5; this reduction was defined as therapy response as these patients would not have to continue CPAP use. The mean age of the population was 15.5 years, with a baseline AHI of 24.2. Though it seems difficult to achieve complete resolution of OSA for pediatric Down syndrome patients, the reduction in apneas and significant subjective improvements suggest a role for hypoglossal nerve stimulation for this population in the future [35,36].

Supraglottis

Supraglottoplasty is another common procedure performed for residual OSA in children. Awake laryngomalacia and sleep-state-dependent laryngomalacia are both indications to perform supraglottoplasty. The increasing frequency of DISE in children has led to increased diagnosis of sleep-state dependent laryngomalacia, also known as occult laryngomalacia [37]. The estimated prevalence of occult laryngomalacia in children with sleep-disordered breathing is 3.9%, and a recent meta-analysis showed significant improvement in AHI as well as lowest oxygen saturation for patients undergoing isolated supraglottoplasty without prior AT [37,38]. Epiglottopexy can also be helpful in children with an independently collapsing epiglottis noted on DISE. This procedure entails demucosalizing the epiglottis, vallecula, and adjacent base of tongue, followed by anchoring the epiglottis to the tongue base [1]. Given the nature of this type of surgery, there can be a concern for dysphagia in children postoperatively. Kanotra and colleagues retrospectively evaluated 5 children who had undergone epiglottopexy and found no significant dysphagia based on functional endoscopic evaluation of swallow (FEES) [39].

Craniofacial abnormalities

Craniofacial surgery has been shown to be effective in treating resistant OSA [40,41]. For patients with craniofacial abnormalities, mandibular or maxillary distraction osteogenesis can be successful. For patients with Pierre Robin sequence, this can avert the need for tracheostomy. Rapid maxillary expansion (RME) is performed with an oral appliance and can be performed into the teenage years as the full fusion of the midpalatal suture line does not occur until this age. RME for children with high arched palates or narrow hard palates significantly improves AHI. A meta-analysis of RME showed an improvement in AHI from a mean of 4.9 to 0.9 in children who had residual OSA after AT (46 patients). However, cure rates (AHI < 1) were low, at 25.6% for the population studied ($n = 90$) [40]. Older children with skeletal deficiencies can be considered for maxillomandibular advancement (MMA).

Obesity

In morbidly obese children, residual OSA after AT is common, as described earlier [42,43]. This population is becoming increasingly important as the prevalence of obesity in children increases. A meta-analysis by Scheffler and colleagues described the outcomes of different surgeries on this population. In addition to a 51% to 66% success rate of AT in obese children, they also reviewed the limited data on other surgeries. UPPP alone had a success rate, defined as an AHI < 1.5, of 13%. Obese patients undergoing lingual tonsillectomy had higher preoperative (15 vs 10 events/h) and postoperative (9 vs 4 events/h) AHI. Given the high rates of failure despite more extensive and multilevel surgeries, maintaining close follow-up is important as further interventions may be necessary.

For adolescents who have failed nonsurgical weight loss and who have developed significant comorbidities, bariatric surgery is now a consideration. The techniques used in the pediatric population include gastric bypass surgery, gastric banding, and sleeve gastrectomy. A retrospective review of 38 patients, 89% of whom had OSA and 47% of whom were on CPAP, revealed significant

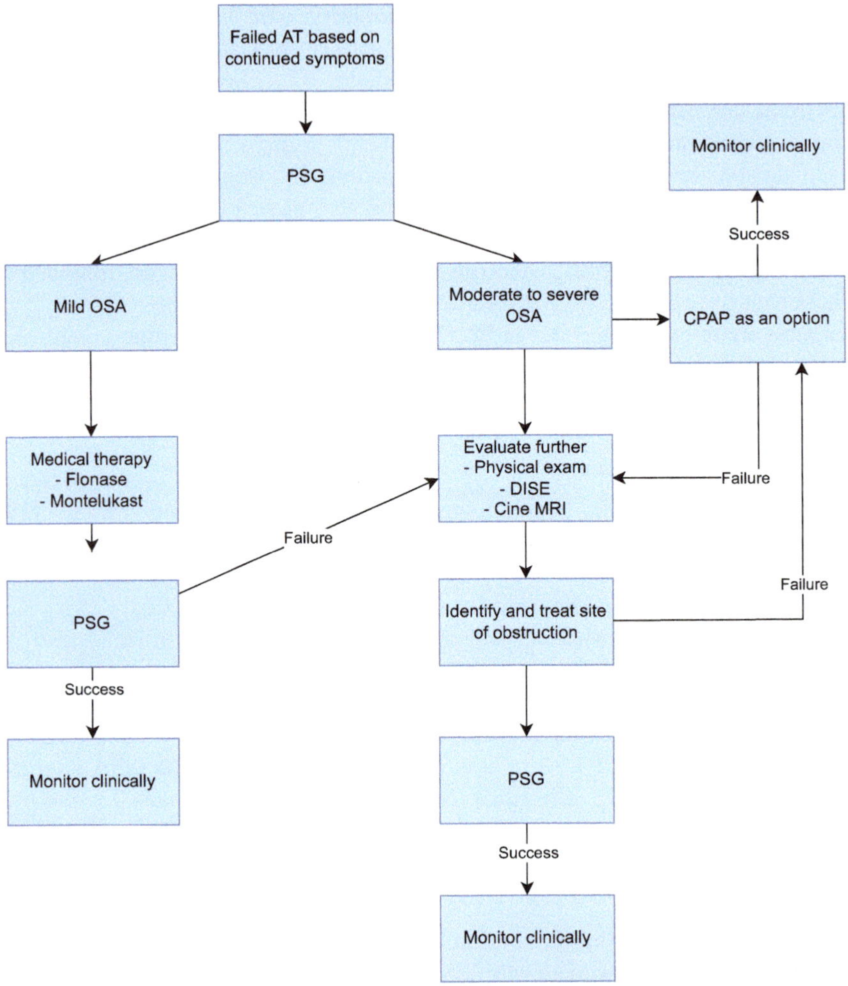

Fig. 2. Algorithm for evaluation and treatment after failed adenotonsillectomy. CPAP, continuous positive airway pressure; OSA, obstructive sleep apnea; PSGY, polysomnogram.

improvement in symptoms. Though postoperative PSG was not performed, at 1 year there was complete resolution of symptoms in those that did not require CPAP. In addition, 16 of 18 patients who previously required CPAP were able to discontinue it [44,45]. Overall, interventions other than AT for OSA in the obese pediatric patient result in some improvement, but residual disease is still exceedingly common even after multiple procedures [43].

SUMMARY

Pediatric OSA is a complex disorder. Patients who have failed the primary treatment of AT can be difficult to manage. This is especially true in patients with comorbidities such as Down syndrome, obesity, neuromuscular disorders, and craniofacial deformities. Evaluation requires multiple repeat polysomnograms as well as labor and time-intensive drug-induced sleep endoscopies or cine MRIs. Even when these methods elucidate clear sites of obstruction, residual OSA can still occur. Fig. 2 demonstrates an approach for these types of patients. Further studies are needed to determine the effectiveness of different upper airway surgeries, both acutely and long term. However, our knowledge of OSA in the last decade has progressed significantly. These improvements will continue as we advance our understanding of the pathophysiology of pediatric OSA and develop new techniques for treatment.

CLINICS CARE POINTS

- Polysomnography is an essential part of the initial work up for patients with residual symptoms after adenotonsillectomy.
- For those patients with moderate to severe OSA, drug induced sleep endoscopy or CINE MRI can be helpful to determine the next step in treatment.
- CPAP should be a consideration for patients with persistent OSA despite its low adherence in children.
- Higher level studies are needed to evaluate the effectiveness of surgical approaches in children after failed adenotonsillectomy.

Disclosure

The authors have no financial or commercial conflicts of interest to disclose.

References

[1] Bluher AE, Ishman SL, Baldassari CM. Managing the child with persistent sleep apnea. Otolaryngol Clin North Am 2019;52(5):891–901.
[2] Tan HL, Gozal D, Kheirandish-Gozal L. Obstructive sleep apnea in children: a critical update. Nat Sci Sleep 2013;5:109–23.
[3] Leung TN, Cheng JW, Chan AK. Paediatrics: how to manage obstructive sleep apnoea syndrome. Drugs Context 2021;10:2020-12-5.
[4] Benedek P, Balakrishnan Karthik, Cunningham Michael, et al. International Pediatric Otolaryngology group (IPOG) consensus on the diagnosis and management of pediatric obstructive sleep apnea (OSA). Int J Pediatr Otorhinolaryngol 2020;138:110276.
[5] Marcus CL, Moore Reneé, Rosen Carol, et al. A randomized trial of adenotonsillectomy for childhood sleep apnea. N Engl J Med 2013;368(25):2366–76.
[6] Baldassari CM, Lam Derek, Ishman Stacey, et al. Expert consensus statement: pediatric drug-induced sleep endoscopy. Otolaryngol Head Neck Surg 2021;165(4):578–91.
[7] Friedman M, Wilson Meghan, Lin Hsin-Ching, et al. Updated systematic review of tonsillectomy and adenoidectomy for treatment of pediatric obstructive sleep apnea/hypopnea syndrome. Otolaryngol Head Neck Surg 2009;140(6):800–8.
[8] Sulman CG. Pediatric sleep surgery. Front Pediatr 2014;2:51.
[9] Costa DJ, Mitchell R. Adenotonsillectomy for obstructive sleep apnea in obese children: a meta-analysis. Otolaryngol Head Neck Surg 2009;140(4):455–60.

[10] Xu Z, Jiaqing An, Yuchuan Li, et al. A case-control study of obstructive sleep apnea-hypopnea syndrome in obese and nonobese chinese children. Chest 2008;133(3):684–9.
[11] Brietzke SE, Katz ES, Roberson DW. Can history and physical examination reliably diagnose pediatric obstructive sleep apnea/hypopnea syndrome? a systematic review of the literature. Otolaryngol Head Neck Surg 2004;131(6):827–32.
[12] Manickam PV, Shott Sally, Boss Emily, et al. Systematic review of site of obstruction identification and non-CPAP treatment options for children with persistent pediatric obstructive sleep apnea. Laryngoscope 2016;126(2):491–500.
[13] Ehsan Z, Ishman SL. Pediatric obstructive sleep apnea. Otolaryngol Clin North Am 2016;49(6):1449–64.
[14] Wilcox LJ, Bergeron Mathieu, Reghunathan Saranya, et al. An updated review of pediatric drug-induced sleep endoscopy. Laryngoscope Investig Otolaryngol 2017;2(6):423–31.
[15] He S, Peddireddy Nithin, Smith David, et al. Outcomes of drug-induced sleep endoscopy-directed surgery for pediatric obstructive sleep apnea. Otolaryngol Head Neck Surg 2018;158(3):559–65.
[16] Socarras MA, Landau BP, Durr ML. Diagnostic techniques and surgical outcomes for persistent pediatric obstructive sleep apnea after adenotonsillectomy: a systematic review and meta-analysis. Int J Pediatr Otorhinolaryngol 2019;121:179–87.
[17] Wootten CT, Chinnadurai S, Goudy SL. Beyond adenotonsillectomy: outcomes of sleep endoscopy-directed treatments in pediatric obstructive sleep apnea. Int J Pediatr Otorhinolaryngol 2014;78(7):1158–62.
[18] Clark C, Ulualp SO. Multimodality assessment of upper airway obstruction in children with persistent obstructive sleep apnea after adenotonsillectomy. Laryngoscope 2017;127(5):1224–30.
[19] Ishman SL, Chang KW, Kennedy AA. Techniques for evaluation and management of tongue-base obstruction in pediatric obstructive sleep apnea. Curr Opin Otolaryngol Head Neck Surg 2018;26(6):409–16.
[20] Marcus CL, Radcliffe Jerilynn, Konstantinopoulou Sofia, et al. Effects of positive airway pressure therapy on neurobehavioral outcomes in children with obstructive sleep apnea. Am J Respir Crit Care Med 2012;185(9):998–1003.
[21] Beebe DW, Byars KC. Adolescents with obstructive sleep apnea adhere poorly to positive airway pressure (PAP), but PAP users show improved attention and school performance. PLoS One 2011;6(3):e16924.
[22] Watach AJ, Xanthopoulos Melissa, Afolabi-Brown Olufunke, et al. Positive airway pressure adherence in pediatric obstructive sleep apnea: a systematic scoping review. Sleep Med Rev 2020;51:101273.
[23] DiFeo N, Meltzer Lisa, Beck Suzanne, et al. Predictors of positive airway pressure therapy adherence in children: a prospective study. J Clin Sleep Med 2012;8(3):279–86.
[24] Kuhle S, Hoffmann Dorle, Mitra Souvik, et al. Anti-inflammatory medications for obstructive sleep apnoea in children. Cochrane Database Syst Rev 2020;1(1):Cd007074.
[25] Wang B, Liang J. The effect of montelukast on mild persistent OSA after adenotonsillectomy in children: a preliminary study. Otolaryngol Head Neck Surg 2017;156(5):952–4.
[26] Nazarali N, Altalibi Mostafa, Nazarali Samir, et al. Mandibular advancement appliances for the treatment of paediatric obstructive sleep apnea: a systematic review. Eur J Orthod 2015;37(6):618–26.
[27] Cheng PW, Fang Kai-Min, Su Huang-Wei, et al. Improved objective outcomes and quality of life after adenotonsillectomy with inferior turbinate reduction in pediatric obstructive sleep apnea with inferior turbinate hypertrophy. Laryngoscope 2012;122(12):2850–4.
[28] Ulualp S. Outcomes of tongue base reduction and lingual tonsillectomy for residual pediatric obstructive sleep apnea after adenotonsillectomy. Int Arch Otorhinolaryngol 2019;23(4):e415–21.

[29] Kang KT, Koltai Peter, Lee Chia-Hsuan, et al. Lingual tonsillectomy for treatment of pediatric obstructive sleep apnea: a meta-analysis. JAMA Otolaryngol Head Neck Surg 2017;143(6):561–8.
[30] Rivero A, Durr M. Lingual tonsillectomy for pediatric persistent obstructive sleep apnea: a systematic review and meta-analysis. Otolaryngol Head Neck Surg 2017;157(6):940–7.
[31] DeMarcantonio MA, Senser E, Meinzen-Derr J, et al. The safety and efficacy of pediatric lingual tonsillectomy. Int J Pediatr Otorhinolaryngol 2016;91:6–10.
[32] Prager JD, Hopkins Brandon, Propst Evan, et al. Oropharyngeal stenosis: a complication of multilevel, single-stage upper airway surgery in children. Arch Otolaryngol Head Neck Surg 2010;136(11):1111–5.
[33] Guilleminault C, Huseni S, Lo L. A frequent phenotype for paediatric sleep apnoea: short lingual frenulum. ERJ Open Res 2016;2(3):00043–2016.
[34] Messner AH, Walsh Jonathan, Rosenfeld Richard, et al. Clinical Consensus Statement: Ankyloglossia in Children. Otolaryngol Head Neck Surg 2020;162(5):597–611.
[35] Yu PK, Jayawardena Asitha, Stenerson Matthew, et al. Redefining success by focusing on failures after pediatric hypoglossal stimulation in down syndrome. Laryngoscope 2020;131(7):1663–9.
[36] Caloway CL, Diercks Gillian, Keamy Donald, et al. Update on hypoglossal nerve stimulation in children with down syndrome and obstructive sleep apnea. Laryngoscope 2020;130(4):e263–7.
[37] Camacho M, Dunn Brandyn, Torre Carlos, et al. Supraglottoplasty for laryngomalacia with obstructive sleep apnea: a systematic review and meta-analysis. Laryngoscope 2016;126(5):1246–55.
[38] Thevasagayam M, Rodger Kirsty, Cave Dominic, et al. Prevalence of laryngomalacia in children presenting with sleep-disordered breathing. Laryngoscope 2010;120(8):1662–6.
[39] Kanotra SP, Givens VB, Keith B. Swallowing outcomes after pediatric epiglottopexy. Eur Arch Otorhinolaryngol 2020;277(1):285–91.
[40] Camacho M, Chang Edward, Song Sungjin, et al. Rapid maxillary expansion for pediatric obstructive sleep apnea: a systematic review and meta-analysis. Laryngoscope 2017;127(7):1712–9.
[41] Templier L, Rossi Cecilia, Miguez Manuel, et al. Combined surgical and orthodontic treatments in children with OSA: a systematic review. J Clin Med 2020;9(8):2387.
[42] Andersen IG, Holm JC, Homøe P. Obstructive sleep apnea in obese children and adolescents, treatment methods and outcome of treatment - A systematic review. Int J Pediatr Otorhinolaryngol 2016;87:190–7.
[43] Scheffler P, Wolter Nikolaus, Narang Indra, et al. Surgery for obstructive sleep apnea in obese children: literature review and meta-analysis. Otolaryngol Head Neck Surg 2019;160(6):985–92.
[44] Jaramillo JD, Snyder Elizabeth, Farrales Susan, et al. A multidisciplinary approach to laparoscopic sleeve gastrectomy among multiethnic adolescents in the United States. J Pediatr Surg 2017;52(10):1606–9.
[45] Kanney ML, Harford Kelli-Lee, Raol Nikhila, et al. Obstructive sleep apnea in pediatric obesity and the effects of sleeve gastrectomy. Semin Pediatr Surg 2020;29(1):150887.

Advances in Pediatrics 69 (2022) 107–121

ADVANCES IN PEDIATRICS

The Antiphospholipid Syndrome in the Pediatric Population

Elizabeth E. Sloan, MD[a,*], Deborah McCurdy, MD[b]

[a]Department of Pediatrics, Division of Rheumatology, University of Texas Southwestern Medical Center, Scottish Rite for Children and Children's Medical Center Dallas, 2222 Welborn Street, Dallas, TX 75219, USA; [b]Department of Pediatrics, Division of Allergy/Immunology/Rheumatology, David Geffen School of Medicine, UCLA, Mattel Children's Hospital, 10833 Le Conte Avenue, Los Angeles, CA 90095, USA

Keywords

• Antiphospholipid antibodies (aPL) • Antiphospholipid syndrome (APS) • Procoagulant state • Hypercoagulability • Thromboembolism • Thrombosis • Bleeding diathesis • Chronic/recurrent

Key points

- Antiphospholipid syndrome is rare in childhood but can be life threatening and needs to be identified quickly.
- Children with thrombosis should be screened for antiphospholipid antibodies. If positive, persistence should be confirmed.
- Treatment of children with antiphospholipid syndrome is complex and often requires the use of anticoagulants and immunosuppression.
- The use of estrogen contraceptives is contraindicated in the antiphospholipid syndrome and can lead to increased risk of thrombosis, limiting the choices for contraceptive use.

INTRODUCTION

The antiphospholipid syndrome (APS) is a systemic immune-mediated disease process characterized by thrombotic or obstetric complications in the presence of pathogenic antiphospholipid antibodies (aPL) [1,2]. These autoantibodies target anionic phospholipids and protein-phospholipid complexes and result in a proinflammatory and prothrombotic state [3]. Pediatric APS is defined as APS that occurs in someone less than 18 years of age.

*Corresponding author. *E-mail address:* elizabeth.sloan@utsouthwestern.edu

https://doi.org/10.1016/j.yapd.2022.03.013

APS is the most common cause of acquired thrombophilia [4]. Unfortunately, it can often lead to significant morbidity and mortality depending on the type and extent of thrombotic event. In addition, patients with APS often require long-term anticoagulation, which can be challenging to manage in an active child.

Definitions and classification criteria

The current classification criteria for APS were developed in 2006 to standardize the identification of APS in adult patients for clinical trials [1]. At least one clinical criterion and one laboratory criterion are required to meet classification of APS. Clinical criteria require a confirmed vascular thrombotic event and/or pregnancy morbidity. To meet laboratory criteria, at least one persistently positive aPL must be present in moderate to high titers. Criteria aPL include lupus anticoagulant (LA), anticardiolipin (aCL) immunoglobulin G (IgG) or IgM, and anti-beta 2 glycoprotein I (aβ2GPI) IgG or IgM. To demonstrate persistence, a positive finding should be present at least twice and at least 12 weeks apart (Box 1).

These criteria are used to identify children with APS even though they were not developed for pediatric APS and have not been validated in the pediatric population. It should also be noted that these are classification criteria, not diagnostic criteria. There are currently no pediatric-specific diagnostic or classification criteria, which poses several challenges. For one, children are less likely to meet the obstetric clinical criteria. In addition, nonthrombotic manifestations of APS are not considered in the criteria, yet they are commonly seen in pediatric APS. In children, APS most often presents with thrombosis, but it may present with other manifestations, such as hematologic or neurologic manifestations.

APS can be either primary, in which it is independent of other autoimmune disease, or secondary, in which it occurs in the presence of other autoimmunity. The most common cause of secondary APS is systemic lupus

Box 1: Revised Sapporo criteria used for diagnosis of the antiphospholipid syndrome [1]

Clinical criteria

- Vascular thrombosis: Venous, arterial, or small vessel
- Pregnancy morbidity: Unexplained fetal death after 10 weeks' gestation, premature birth owing to eclampsia or placental insufficiency, or at least 3 consecutive spontaneous abortions before 10 weeks' gestation without other explanation

Laboratory criteria: The laboratory tests must be positive on 2 occasions, 12 weeks apart

- Lupus anticoagulant
- Anticardiolipin IgG or IgM in moderate to high titer; >40 GPL or MPL
- Anti-β2-glycoprotein 1 IgG or IgM antibody in high titer, >99th percentile

erythematosus (SLE), but secondary APS may also occur in the presence of other autoimmune conditions. APS can sometimes be a child's initial presentation of an autoimmune disease, and it is important to screen for additional evidence of autoimmunity to make the diagnosis as accurate as possible.

Epidemiology

Fortunately, APS is rare in children, but it is important to recognize because it is associated with a hypercoagulable state that can be life threatening. In adults, the estimated incidence of APS is 2 to 5 cases per 100,000 per year with a prevalence of 40 to 50 cases per 100,000 [48]. Although the incidence and prevalence are not established in children, in a study of 1000 patients with APS, it was estimated that only 2.8% presented at 15 years old or younger [5]. In part, this reflects the fact that children have fewer risk factors contributing to thrombosis, such as atherosclerosis, smoking, hypertension, and medications. Conversely, this may also suggest the children who experience thrombotic events could have a higher genetic risk or other molecular drivers contributing to their hypercoagulable state.

To date, the largest published study of children with APS is the international Ped-APS Registry, which described 121 patients. In this cohort, APS onset occurred at a mean age of 10.7 years, and about half of the patients had an additional autoimmune disease. Girls and boys were affected almost equally. Most patients experienced venous thrombosis, although arterial events were not uncommon. Rarely, some patients had both arterial and venous thrombosis. Unfortunately, many cases were also complicated by recurrent thromboses and/or nonthrombotic manifestations. Interestingly, in this cohort, primary APS progressed to secondary APS associated with SLE at 4 times the rate observed in adult populations [6,7].

Pathogenesis

Cell membranes are composed of a bilayer of phospholipids in which the negatively charged hydrophilic phosphate group faces outward to the extracellular and intracellular aqueous interface, while the hydrophobic fatty acid tail faces inward (Fig. 1). Different cell types may have different phospholipids in their membranes; thus, there is not just one antiphospholipid antibody but many. The antibodies may be directed against phospholipid complexes on the endothelial cells of blood vessels, platelets, red blood cells, and others. Multiple tests are required to adequately evaluate for the different types of antibodies.

Although the cause is multifactorial and not yet completely understood, as with most autoimmune diseases, there are genetic and environmental components. There are rare reports of familial APS, but aPL can be found in first-degree relatives of patients with SLE or APS. The HLA are most strongly associated, and HLA-DR and HLA-DQ alleles have been associated with both primary and secondary APS. There are at least 22 other genes that have been associated with primary APS, but none as strongly as the HLA locus [8].

Environmental factors are also implicated. In the APS literature, the "two-hit" hypothesis is widely accepted as a mechanism for the development of

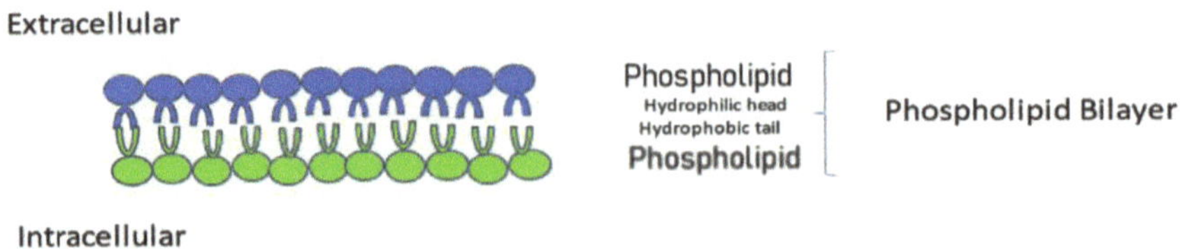

Fig. 1. Cell membrane.

thrombosis [9]. This theory suggests that a person with APS has pathogenic aPL persistently circulating in their blood vessels. The presence of these antibodies tips the scale toward hypercoagulability and lowers the threshold for a thrombotic event. A "second-hit" then causes a disruption of the cellular membrane that allows the circulating aPL to bind and subsequently inhibit membrane repair and promote thrombosis. The cellular membrane may be disrupted by many factors, such as atherosclerosis in adults, vasculitis in those with autoimmune disease, or perhaps a viral infection. Once the membrane is activated, more negatively charged phosphate groups become exposed. β2GPI, also known as apolipoprotein H, is a phospholipid binding protein that is a member of the complement control protein family and usually has a natural anticoagulant property. However, it has affinity for negatively charged phospholipids. Antibodies to the phospholipid alone may bind but may not be pathologic. When the β2GPI binds to the phospholipid, there is a new epitope created that is associated with pathologic changes leading to thrombosis.

A myriad of effects downstream of aPL-epitope binding have been identified in animal and human models [8,10,11]. Several mechanisms that lead to the disease pathogenesis include complement activation; inhibition of physiologic anticoagulants, such as protein C, antithrombin III, and the annexin A5 anticoagulant shield; and impaired fibrinolysis. Neutrophils have also been implicated, and there is growing evidence for the role of neutrophil extracellular trap (NET) formation (NETosis) [12]. Platelets primed by lipopolysaccharides or cytokines have increased expression of apolipoprotein ER2 receptor and bind aPL and β2GPI, which leads to platelet activation and thromboxane release. Once the aPL bind to the phospholipid/β2GPI epitope, there is impaired synthesis of the vasodilator nitric oxide, increased expression of intracellular adhesion molecule, ICAM-1, and vascular adhesion molecules, VCAM-1 and E-selectin, thus increasing adhesiveness of leukocytes and platelets. Pathogenic aPL also increase cytokine expression by endothelial cells and leukocytes, leading to ongoing inflammation and coagulation [2,11].

Spectrum of disease

aPL are associated with a wide spectrum of clinical presentations. In some children, aPL may be present but remain nonpathologic or asymptomatic [13]. B cells can produce antibodies to phospholipids that bind with a low affinity or are transient and do not result in ongoing activation of the immune system.

Following infections, aPL antibodies may be noted without a clinical correlation. Certainly, there are many reports of aPL following COVID-19 infections, some of which have been implicated in COVID-related thrombosis, but in many patients, these antibodies may be short-lived and inconsequential [14,15]. For reasons such as this, aPL must persist over a 12-week period to make a diagnosis of APS.

Conversely, children with aPL may develop a full APS picture with thromboses in the venous and/or arterial systems [16,17]. This distinguishes APS from other procoagulant states whereby only the venous system is involved. Different aPL profiles also vary in risk. Triple positivity, or having positive LA, aCL, and aβ2GPI, confers the greatest thrombotic risk [18]. In patients with SLE, there may be other signs of immune activation, but in primary APS the patient may not have any other clinical signs or risk factors of an autoimmune disease.

In rare cases, there are patients who clearly appear to have APS clinically, but they have consistently negative results for the common aPL assays. These patients are termed "seronegative," and additional studies may demonstrate antibodies to specific phospholipids or phospholipid binding proteins, which are known as "extra-criteria aPL."

More frequently than adults, children with aPL may experience nonthrombotic clinical manifestations, including cytopenias, skin involvement with livedo reticularis and/or cutaneous necrosis, and neurologic manifestations, including movement disorders, epilepsy, and migraine headaches [7,19].

The most severe and life-threatening presentation is catastrophic antiphospholipid syndrome (CAPS). This is associated with widespread thrombotic disease with rapid development of multiorgan failure characterized by small vessel occlusions in the presence of aPL. Despite improvements in recognition and therapy, the mortality is still high [20,21].

MANIFESTATIONS

Thrombosis

aPL may be present and persist for years without a clinical event. In the children who do have thrombotic events, the most common initial event is deep vein thrombosis, and about half of these patients are at risk for a pulmonary embolism. Other venous sites include cerebral sinus veins, the portal vein, deep veins of the upper extremities, and superficial veins of the skin. Arterial thrombosis occurs in about 30% of patients with APS, with ischemic stroke being the most common followed by peripheral arterial thrombosis [7]. Arterial thromboses are more common in those with primary APS than those with secondary APS [10,18]. Sneddon syndrome, which is characterized by stroke or other neurologic features and livedo reticularis, is associated with aPL in about 50% of patients [22] (Figs. 2 and 3). Small vessel thromboses occur in the skin or kidneys and can present with digital ischemia or thrombotic microangiopathy noted on renal biopsy, respectively.

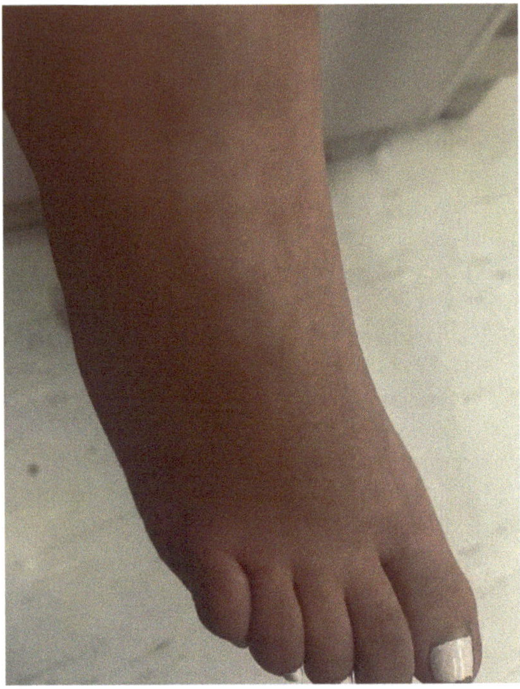

Fig. 2. Livedo reticularis with net-like, lacy reticular pattern.

Obstetric antiphospholipid syndrome

Complications in adolescent pregnancies are not uncommon, and these complications may be further exacerbated if pathogenic aPL are present [23,24]. During pregnancy, there are changes in the hemostatic system that result in increased risk of thrombosis. With APS, risks during pregnancy are heightened with increased rates of venous or arterial thrombotic events, preeclampsia/eclampsia, and HELLP syndrome (hemolysis, elevated liver enzymes, and low platelets). Each of these is potentially life threatening to the mother and the fetus. There are increased rates of fetal loss after the 10th week of gestation. This is secondary to inflammation, complement activation, and clots in the placental decidual arteries that lead to placental failure and miscarriage or preterm birth [2,25]. Obstetric care is based on combined medical-obstetric high-risk management, and patients are often managed with aspirin and heparin.

Catastrophic antiphospholipid syndrome

CAPS is characterized by rapid progression of multiple small vessel occlusions resulting in multiorgan failure over the course of a week [20,26,27] (Box 2). Not infrequently, it is the first presentation in children with primary APS and can be the first presentation of autoimmune disease. Most often the inciting factor is sepsis, but surgery, disseminated intervascular coagulation, underlying

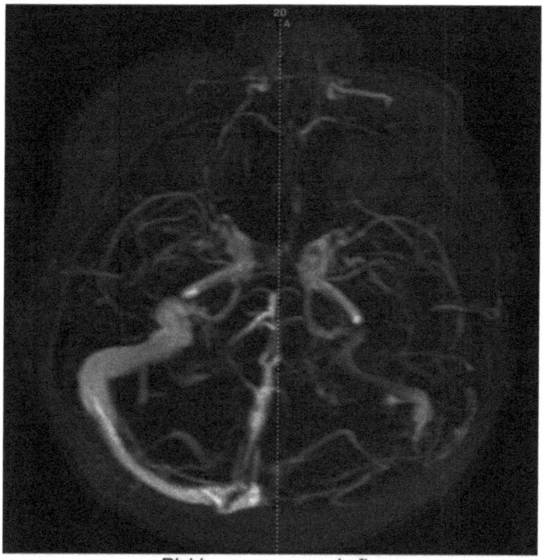

Fig. 3. Left-sided dural venous sinus thrombosis on magnetic resonance venography (MRV).

autoimmune disease, or malignancy may be implicated. In these cases, children may present with neurologic symptoms, including somnolence, confusion, and irritability, and may be combative. If they have pulmonary involvement, they may present with acute respiratory failure or pulmonary hemorrhage. Renal involvement is common and can manifest as severe hypertension, proteinuria, acute renal failure, and possibly a need for continuous renal replacement therapy. Cardiac involvement may cause heart failure or myocardial infarction. All other organs may be involved, and there may be thromboses in the peripheral extremities. The mortality remains high, between 24% and 33%.

Microangiopathic disease

Microangiopathic antiphospholipid-associated syndrome refers to children with thrombotic microangiopathy, such as hemolytic uremic syndrome and thrombotic thrombocytopenic purpura, who also have aPL. Because aPL are thought to be an immune response to exposure of phospholipids after injury, the aPL may not be the cause or contribute to the disease pathogenesis.

Hematologic

aPL may bind to platelets, red blood cells, and white blood cells, leading to autoimmune thrombocytopenia (ITP), hemolytic anemia that may be Coomb positive, and autoimmune neutropenia. In the setting of SLE, lymphopenia may also be present. It is important to recognize that isolated onset of ITP in teenagers can be the initial presentation of APS and/or SLE.

Box 2: Criteria used for diagnosis of the catastrophic antiphospholipid syndrome [27]

- Clinical evidence of vessel occlusions affecting three or more organ systems
- Rapid onset of manifestations concurrently or within one week
- Confirmed small vessel occlusion in at least one organ on histopathology
- Serologic confirmation of presence of aPL positivity (LA and/or moderate to high titers of other criteria aPL); persistence should be demonstrated

Definite CAPS: All 4 criteria

Probable CAPS: 1, 2, 4

Other diagnoses should be excluded

Acquired lupus anticoagulant-hypoprothrombinemia syndrome

Rarely, in the presence of the LA, patients may present with a bleeding diathesis. This is more common in children than in adults and is associated with antibodies to antiprothrombin with decreased plasma prothrombin and consequent bleeding. This may be mild with bruising and gingival bleeding, but female patients often have prolonged menstrual periods. Of note, the prothrombin time, in addition to the partial thromboplastin time (PTT), is usually prolonged in these patients [28].

Skin manifestations

Livedo reticularis and livedo racemosa may be associated with aPL, and patients with significant Raynaud's phenomenon or livedoid rashes should be tested for aPL. These are the most common skin manifestations, but other manifestations may include small vessel thromboses and cutaneous necrosis.

Neurologic

Many neurologic presentations may be associated with aPL from movement disorders, epilepsy, migraines, to many other manifestations. Other neurologic findings associated with APS may include multiple sclerosis–like lesions, transverse myelitis, and cognitive dysfunction. The association of aPL with these nonthrombotic presentations is now clearer, but the exact pathophysiology may be more related to immune dysregulation, antibody binding to neurons and glial cells, and/or breakdown of the blood-brain barrier [29].

Other manifestations

APS in children may also affect other organ systems and cause end-organ damage, although this occurs less commonly than hematologic, dermatologic, and neurologic manifestations. Cardiac involvement may contribute to cardiac valve abnormalities or cardiomyopathy. Renal involvement may manifest as thrombotic microangiopathy or glomerulonephritis. Obstetric complications can include late preeclampsia, late preterm birth, and unexplained miscarriages. aPL have also been implicated in musculoskeletal complications, such as avascular necrosis.

Table 1
Laboratory tests to confirm the diagnosis of antiphospholipid syndrome

Antibodies to phospholipids	Detection method
Lupus anticoagulant (LA)	Combination of screening tests, mixing test, and a confirmatory test, measured by PTT-LA, dilute Russell viper venom time (dRVVT), or other recommended assays [32]
Anticardiolipin (aCL) IgG and/or IgM in moderate to high titer >40 GPL or MPL	ELISA
Anti-β2-glycoprotein 1 (aβ2GPI) IgG and/or IgM in high titer, >99%	ELISA

Other noncriteria aPL, including IgA isotypes of aCL and aβ2GPI, antiphosphatidylserine/prothrombin IgG/IgM, anti-domain I of β2-glycoprotein, and others may provide supporting evidence or assist with risk-stratification in APS [31].

LABORATORY INVESTIGATIONS

In the 1940s, it was noted that patients with SLE with thrombotic events frequently had a false positive test for syphilis. This test, known as the Wassermann test, relies on antibodies known as reagin to bind a substance. Graham Hughes [30] noted the substance bound was cardiolipin and first described the association with thrombosis. The aCL test is done by an enzyme-linked immunosorbent assay (ELISA) (Table 1). The higher the titer on ELISA, the more specific the test. Antibodies to β2GPI are tested in the same way. IgG, IgM, and IgA antibodies are tested and read out in IgG phospholipid units (GPL), IgM phospholipid units (MPL), or IgA phospholipid units (APL). A titer of greater than 20 is considered positive. Low titers may be nonspecific, but titers more than 40 units, especially if they are of the IgG or IgM isotype, are more likely related to thrombosis. Thus, many APS experts use a cutoff value of 40 units to define aPL positivity. In addition, antibodies to β2GPI, especially of the IgG isotype, at moderate to high titers are associated with increased pathogenicity.

There are a number of tests for the LA, which is a functional assay that can indicate the presence of aPL (see Table 1). To correctly determine LA positivity, the laboratory must first run a screening test to determine if there is prolongation of a phospholipid-dependent clotting assay. This can be ascertained with screening tools such as a prolonged PTT. The second step is a mixing study. This can be done by activating the PTT and adding back serum, which will replace the missing clotting factors. If the PTT does not return to normal when mixed with healthy serum, this suggests the presence of an inhibitor rather than other causes of PTT prolongation, such as a clotting factor deficiency. A confirmatory test is then performed where excess phospholipids are added to overcome inhibition from aPL, thus correcting the PTT. LA may also be measured by similar studies using the dilute Russell viper venom, the Kaolin clotting time, and others. It may be necessary to do several of these tests to determine the presence of aPL antibodies. This correlates more strongly with thrombosis risk than a single positive test for aCL and/or β2GPI [31,32].

Other tests may support another autoimmune disease, and most patients with primary antiphospholipid antibody syndrome should be evaluated for additional autoimmune phenomena at initial diagnosis and in the presence of new clinical manifestations. Over half of children with SLE may have aPL positivity [17,33]. The presence of aPL in children with SLE is associated with increased odds of thrombosis as well as a higher risk of organ damage, suggesting that aPL positivity may portend a poor prognosis or be associated with more severe forms of SLE [16,17].

IMAGING AND BIOPSY

To make a diagnosis of thrombotic APS, it is important to document a thrombotic event by imaging or biopsy. Depending on the site, ultrasound or Doppler studies may be helpful, especially for peripheral sites in the upper or lower extremities. Magnetic resonance imaging with angiography and/or venography or computed tomography angiography are helpful in evaluating deeper thromboses, such as pulmonary emboli, cerebral sinus venous thrombosis, or arterial stroke. For microvascular thromboses, including cutaneous involvement or renal thrombotic microangiopathy, biopsy may be necessary for definitive diagnosis.

MANAGEMENT

Goals of management

The management of children with aPL and those with full criteria for APS is complex and challenging [2,34–36]. Patients require a full evaluation with laboratory tests and imaging to confirm the presence of thrombosis and adequate anticoagulation to treat the acute thrombosis. Often, pediatric subspecialists, including rheumatologists, hematologists, nephrologists, and neurologists, help direct the evaluation, especially if there are other clinical manifestations related to their expertise. Once the diagnosis of APS is established, the goal is to prevent future thrombotic events. If there is an underlying autoimmune disease, treatment goals also include adequate control of that disease.

Anticoagulation and antiplatelet therapy

In children with aPL and an acute thrombotic event, heparin is started and gradually transitioned to warfarin in most cases, although some patients may opt for low-molecular-weight heparin for long-term therapy. If the thrombotic event was a single event in a peripheral site, the warfarin is adjusted to target an international normalized ratio (INR) of 2 to 3. In more severe cases, such as with an arterial thrombotic event, a pulmonary embolism, in cases with triple-positive aPL, and recurrent thrombotic events despite anticoagulation, some physicians may target a higher INR, although practices vary. In cases of recurrent thrombosis or an arterial event, aspirin or other antiplatelet therapy is often added.

Direct oral anticoagulants (DOACs), such as rivaroxaban, directly inhibit specific proteins in the coagulation cascade. For many, they are more desirable than traditional anticoagulation given the oral administration and reduced need for laboratory monitoring. However, in adult patients with APS, some studies have shown concern for increased risk of recurrent thrombosis when compared with standard-of-care therapy with warfarin [37–40]. Thus, DOACs should be used with caution in patients with APS, especially those with triple aPL positivity or refractory disease.

In 2017, European evidence-based recommendations for diagnosis and treatment of pediatric APS were published, and these may provide further guidance for clinicians caring for a child with APS [35].

Adjunctive therapies

Apart from anticoagulation, evidence to guide additional management in pediatric APS is mostly based on adult experience, limited cohort studies, preclinical mechanistic data, and case reports. When the aPL antibodies remain high, rituximab or other immunomodulatory therapy may be considered to decrease the aPL titers, although data are limited to guide these treatments. Other adjunctive therapies for refractory disease may include hydroxychloroquine (especially in the presence of concurrent SLE), statins, other B-cell targeting therapies like belimumab, and other immunomodulatory medications [36].

Primary prophylaxis

aPL may also be present in the absence of a thrombotic event. This most often occurs in children with SLE. Although these patients are concerning in regard to potential thrombotic risk, long-term prophylaxis with anticoagulation is also not without risk. In cases with persistent but asymptomatic aPL, it can be challenging to know what, if any, treatment may be necessary. Clinicians can evaluate the child and family for thrombotic risk factors and nonthrombotic APS manifestations. In the absence of other concerns, there may be no specific therapy started, but the child and family should be counseled appropriately. In a high-risk situation, such as decreased mobility after surgery or during a severe illness, some clinicians may consider transient anticoagulation if there is concern for aPL-induced hypercoagulability.

In patients with autoimmune disease, such as SLE, patients are often prescribed hydroxychloroquine. Many rheumatologists will additionally recommend low-dose aspirin for primary prophylaxis of thrombosis in an aPL-positive patient, although data are limited [41–44]. In one small retrospective cohort of children with lupus and persistently positive aPL, hypertension and Raynaud phenomena were associated with increased odds of thrombotic events [45]. More studies are needed to further delineate thrombotic risk factors associated with aPL positivity and how best to prevent thrombosis.

Birth control and pregnancy considerations

Estrogen-containing contraceptives carry an increased risk for thrombosis and are not recommended in patients with APS or high-titer aPL [46]. Often, progestin-only contraceptives have been used and, in general, are not associated with a significant increase in blood clots. Concern was raised however when a meta-analysis indicated that there was an increased risk of deep vein thrombosis and pulmonary embolism in women using progesterone injections [47]. Those taking progesterone-only pills and use of the progesterone intrauterine device (IUD) did not significantly increase the risk of clots. The increased risk of clotting in those using progesterone-only injections may be due to other factors, however, such as obesity and smoking. Long-acting forms of contraception, such as the progesterone IUD or subdermal implant, are used for patients with APS. The levonorgestrel IUD is a good alternative for many patients with APS and often decreases menstrual blood loss.

In patients with SLE complicated by APS, safe contraceptive methods will allow planning for pregnancy during a period when the disease is not active. During pregnancy, patients with APS are treated with prophylactic-dose heparin and low-dose aspirin. In those with the concern for thrombosis, additional therapies are considered, including hydroxychloroquine, steroids, intravenous immunoglobulin, and plasma exchange.

SUMMARY

Pediatric APS is a challenging and complex disease that requires a high index of suspicion to diagnose. Screening for aPL positivity in a child with thrombosis is imperative to reach the diagnosis, and aPL positivity should be confirmed 12 weeks later. Furthermore, thrombosis in a pediatric patient can lead to significant long-term sequelae, including complications such as postthrombotic syndrome and stroke-related deficits. Thus, prevention of future thromboses is of utmost importance in managing these patients, and long-term anticoagulation is often necessary. For refractory disease or disease complicated by other autoimmunity, immunosuppression and/or adjunctive therapies may be necessary as well. A multidisciplinary approach is key to optimizing the recognition, treatment, and outcomes of children with APS.

CLINICS CARE POINTS

- A thrombotic event is an unusual occurrence in children, and antiphospholipid syndrome should be considered in a child with a thrombotic event.
- Multidisciplinary care and a comprehensive approach are essential when diagnosing and managing a child with antiphospholipid syndrome.
- Anticoagulation is the primary treatment approach for acute thrombosis, and most patients with antiphospholipid syndrome require continuation of long-term therapeutic anticoagulation to prevent further thrombotic events.

- Immunosuppressive therapy and adjunctive agents may be necessary to treat antiphospholipid syndrome, especially in the presence of an underlying autoimmune disease.
- Adolescents with autoimmune diseases, such as lupus or immune-mediated cytopenias, should be screened for antiphospholipid antibodies.
- Estrogen-containing contraceptives should be avoided in those with persistently positive antiphospholipid antibodies.

Disclosure

The authors have nothing to disclose.

References

[1] Miyakis S, Lockshin MD, Atsumi T, et al. International consensus statement on an update of the classification criteria for definite antiphospholipid syndrome (APS). J Thromb Haemost 2006;4(2):295–306.
[2] Garcia D, Erkan D. Diagnosis and Management of the Antiphospholipid Syndrome. N Engl J Med 2018;378(21):2010–21.
[3] McIntyre JA, Wagenknecht DR, Faulk WP. Antiphospholipid antibodies: discovery, definitions, detection and disease. Prog Lipid Res 2003;42(3):176–237.
[4] Pierangeli SS, Chen PP, Raschi E, et al. Antiphospholipid antibodies and the antiphospholipid syndrome: pathogenic mechanisms. Semin Thromb Hemost 2008;34(3):236–50.
[5] Cervera R, Piette JC, Font J, et al. Antiphospholipid syndrome: clinical and immunologic manifestations and patterns of disease expression in a cohort of 1,000 patients. Arthritis Rheum 2002;46(4):1019–27.
[6] Avcin T, Cimaz R, Rozman B. The Ped-APS registry: the antiphospholipid syndrome in childhood. Lupus 2009;18(10):894–9.
[7] Avcin T, Cimaz R, Silverman ED, et al. Pediatric antiphospholipid syndrome: clinical and immunologic features of 121 patients in an international registry. Pediatrics 2008;122(5):e1100–7.
[8] Moulton VR, Suarez-Fueyo A, Meidan E, et al. Pathogenesis of human systemic lupus erythematosus: a cellular perspective. Trends Mol Med 2017;23(7):615–35.
[9] Chaturvedi S, McCrae KR. Diagnosis and management of the antiphospholipid syndrome. Blood Rev 2017;31(6):406–17.
[10] Arachchillage DRJ, Laffan M. Pathogenesis and management of antiphospholipid syndrome. Br J Haematol 2017;178(2):181–95.
[11] Giannakopoulos B, Krilis SA. The pathogenesis of the antiphospholipid syndrome. N Engl J Med 2013;368(11):1033–44.
[12] Meng H, Yalavarthi S, Kanthi Y, et al. *In Vivo* role of neutrophil extracellular traps in antiphospholipid antibody-mediated venous thrombosis. Arthritis Rheumatol 2017;69(3):655–67.
[13] Favaloro EJ, Henry BM, Lippi G. COVID-19 and antiphospholipid antibodies: time for a reality check? Semin Thromb Hemost 2021;48(1):72–92.
[14] Zuo Y, Estes SK, Ali RA, et al. Prothrombotic autoantibodies in serum from patients hospitalized with COVID-19. Sci Transl Med 2020;12(570):eabd3876.
[15] Borghi MO, Beltagy A, Garrafa E, et al. Anti-phospholipid antibodies in COVID-19 are different from those detectable in the anti-phospholipid syndrome. Front Immunol 2020;11:584241.
[16] Driest KD, Sturm MS, O'Brien SH, et al. Factors associated with thrombosis in pediatric patients with systemic lupus erythematosus. Lupus 2016;25(7):749–53.

[17] Descloux E, Durieu I, Cochat P, et al. Paediatric systemic lupus erythematosus: prognostic impact of antiphospholipid antibodies. Rheumatology (Oxford) 2008;47(2):183–7.

[18] Sciascia S, Amigo MC, Roccatello D, et al. Diagnosing antiphospholipid syndrome: 'extra-criteria' manifestations and technical advances. Nat Rev Rheumatol 2017;13(9):548–60.

[19] Wincup C, Ioannou Y. The differences between childhood and adult onset antiphospholipid syndrome. Front Pediatr 2018;6:362.

[20] Berman H, Rodríguez-Pintó I, Cervera R, et al. Pediatric catastrophic antiphospholipid syndrome: descriptive analysis of 45 patients from the "CAPS Registry". Autoimmun Rev 2014;13(2):157–62.

[21] Meroni PL, Argolini LM, Pontikaki I. What is known about pediatric antiphospholipid syndrome? Expert Rev Hematol 2016;9(10):977–85.

[22] Francès C, Papo T, Wechsler B, et al. Sneddon syndrome with or without antiphospholipid antibodies. a comparative study in 46 patients. Medicine (Baltimore) 1999;78(4):209–19.

[23] Di Prima FA, Valenti O, Hyseni E, et al. Antiphospholipid syndrome during pregnancy: the state of the art. J Prenat Med 2011;5(2):41–53.

[24] De Carolis S, Tabacco S, Rizzo F, et al. Antiphospholipid syndrome: An update on risk factors for pregnancy outcome. Autoimmun Rev 2018;17(10):956–66.

[25] de Jesus GR, Agmon-Levin N, Andrade CA, et al. 14th international congress on antiphospholipid antibodies task force report on obstetric antiphospholipid syndrome. Autoimmun Rev 2014;13(8):795–813.

[26] Rosina S, Chighizola CB, Ravelli A, et al. Pediatric antiphospholipid syndrome: from pathogenesis to clinical management. Curr Rheumatol Rep 2021;23(2):10.

[27] Go EJL, O'Neil KM. The catastrophic antiphospholipid syndrome in children. Curr Opin Rheumatol 2017;29(5):516–22.

[28] Pilania RK, Suri D, Jindal AK, et al. Lupus anticoagulant hypoprothrombinemia syndrome associated with systemic lupus erythematosus in children: report of two cases and systematic review of the literature. Rheumatol Int 2018;38(10):1933–40.

[29] Ricarte IF, Dutra LA, Abrantes FF, et al. Neurologic manifestations of antiphospholipid syndrome. Lupus 2018;27(9):1404–14.

[30] Hughes GR. Hughes' syndrome: the antiphospholipid syndrome. a historical view. Lupus 1998;7(Suppl 2):S1–4.

[31] Devreese KMJ, Zuily S, Meroni PL. Role of antiphospholipid antibodies in the diagnosis of antiphospholipid syndrome. J Transl Autoimmun 2021;4:100134.

[32] Devreese KMJ, de Groot PG, de Laat B, et al. Guidance from the scientific and standardization committee for lupus anticoagulant/antiphospholipid antibodies of the international society on thrombosis and haemostasis: update of the guidelines for lupus anticoagulant detection and interpretation. J Thromb Haemost 2020;18(11):2828–39.

[33] Madison JA, Zuo Y, Knight JS. Pediatric antiphospholipid syndrome. Eur J Rheumatol 2019;7(Suppl 1):1–10.

[34] Tektonidou MG, Andreoli L, Limper M, et al. EULAR recommendations for the management of antiphospholipid syndrome in adults. Ann Rheum Dis 2019;78(10):1296–304.

[35] Groot N, de Graeff N, Avcin T, et al. European evidence-based recommendations for diagnosis and treatment of paediatric antiphospholipid syndrome: the SHARE initiative. Ann Rheum Dis 2017;76(10):1637–41.

[36] Madison JA, Duarte-García A, Zuo Y, et al. Treatment of thrombotic antiphospholipid syndrome in adults and children. Curr Opin Rheumatol 2020;32(3):215–27.

[37] Pengo V, Denas G, Zoppellaro G, et al. Rivaroxaban vs warfarin in high-risk patients with antiphospholipid syndrome. Blood 2018;132(13):1365–71.

[38] Ordi-Ros J, Sáez-Comet L, Pérez-Conesa M, et al. Rivaroxaban versus vitamin K antagonist in antiphospholipid syndrome: a randomized noninferiority trial. Ann Intern Med 2019;171(10):685–94.

[39] Malec K, Góralczyk T, Undas A. The use of direct oral anticoagulants in 56 patients with antiphospholipid syndrome. Thromb Res 2017;152:93–7.

[40] Dufrost V, Risse J, Zuily S, et al. Direct oral anticoagulants use in antiphospholipid syndrome: are these drugs an effective and safe alternative to warfarin? a systematic review of the literature. Curr Rheumatol Rep 2016;18(12):74.
[41] Bala MM, Paszek E, Lesniak W, et al. Antiplatelet and anticoagulant agents for primary prevention of thrombosis in individuals with antiphospholipid antibodies. Cochrane Database Syst Rev 2018;7:Cd012534.
[42] Erkan D, Harrison MJ, Levy R, et al. Aspirin for primary thrombosis prevention in the antiphospholipid syndrome: a randomized, double-blind, placebo-controlled trial in asymptomatic antiphospholipid antibody-positive individuals. Arthritis Rheum 2007;56(7):2382–91.
[43] Zuo Y, Barbhaiya M, Erkan D. Primary Thrombosis Prophylaxis in Persistently Antiphospholipid Antibody-Positive Individuals: Where Do We Stand in 2018? Curr Rheumatol Rep 2018;20(11):66.
[44] Arnaud L, Mathian A, Devilliers H, et al. Patient-level analysis of five international cohorts further confirms the efficacy of aspirin for the primary prevention of thrombosis in patients with antiphospholipid antibodies. Autoimmun Rev 2015;14(3):192–200.
[45] Sloan E, Wright T, Zuo Y. Identifying additional risk factors for arterial and venous thrombosis among pediatric antiphospholipid antibodies carriers. Lupus 2021;30(5):828–32.
[46] Sammaritano LR. Which hormones and contraception for women with APS? exogenous hormone use in women with APS. Curr Rheumatol Rep 2021;23(6):44.
[47] Mantha S, Karp R, Raghavan V, et al. Assessing the risk of venous thromboembolic events in women taking progestin-only contraception: a meta-analysis. BMJ 2012;345:e4944.
[48] Duarte-García A, Pham MM, Crowson CS, et al. The Epidemiology of Antiphospholipid Syndrome: A Population-Based Study. Arthritis Rheumatol 2019;71(9):1545–52.

Advances in Pediatrics 69 (2022) 123–132

ADVANCES IN PEDIATRICS

Pediatric Chronic Kidney Disease

Valerie Panzarino, MD[a,*], Jake Lesser, MD[b], Frank Ayestaran Cassani, MD[c]

[a]Department of Pediatrics, Division of Pediatric Nephrology, University of South Florida Health, 2 Tampa General Circle, Fifth Floor, Tampa, FL 33606, USA; [b]University of South Florida Health, 2 Tampa General Circle, Fifth Floor, Tampa, FL 33606, USA; [c]Department of Pediatrics, Division of Pediatric Nephrology, University of South Florida Health, 2 Tampa General Circle, Fifth Floor, Tampa, FL 33606, USA

Keywords

• Chronic kidney disease • End-stage renal disease • Pediatrics

Key points

- General renal protective measures, such as avoiding potential nephrotoxic agents, effectively treating high blood pressure, and avoiding excessive protein supplementation, should be used in all children with chronic kidney disease.
- Central lines and peripherally inserted central lines should be avoided in children with advanced stage chronic kidney disease.
- Based on the stage of chronic kidney disease, comorbid conditions should be anticipated and appropriately treated, including metabolic acidosis, bone disease, anemia, cardiovascular complications, malnutrition and electrolyte abnormalities, growth failure, and psychosocial issues.
- Effective management of children with chronic kidney disease requires a specialized multidisciplinary team approach.

Pediatric chronic kidney disease (CKD) is a complex disorder that has a lifelong impact and is associated with a decreased quality of life [1–3]. Potential adverse outcomes of CKD can be delayed or prevented by early identification and treatment. Common causes of CKD in childhood (Table 1) vary by age, race, and geography. Congenital abnormalities of the kidneys and urinary tract are the most common cause of CKD in younger children. The incidence of glomerulonephritis increases with age [4–7]. Identifying and appropriately treating the underlying cause is essential to preventing or delaying the progression of the CKD.

*Corresponding author. *E-mail address:* vpanzari@usf.edu

https://doi.org/10.1016/j.yapd.2022.03.008
0065-3101/22/

Table 1
Chronic kidney disease in children

• Congenital Anomalies of the Kidneys and Urinary Tract (CAKUT) o Aplasia, hypoplasia, dysplasia o Obstructive uropathy o Reflux nephropathy o Prune belly syndrome • Focal segmental glomerulosclerosis • Polycystic kidney disease	• Chronic glomerulonephritis • Medullary cystic renal disease • Hemolytic uremic syndrome • Congenital nephrotic syndrome • Familial nephritis/Alport syndrome Cystinosis • Chronic interstitial nephritis

Progression of CKD, regardless of the underlying cause, is also affected by comorbidities, such as hypertension, obesity, prematurity, and persistent microalbuminuria or proteinuria [8–11]. Low-birth-weight and small for gestational age infants have an increased risk of developing end-stage renal disease in adolescence [12,13]. General renal protective measures (Box 1) should be implemented in all children with CKD [14,15]. Angiotensin-converting enzyme inhibitors and angiotensin receptor blockers may be preferentially prescribed in patients with CKD for their antihypertensive and renal protective properties, especially in proteinuric renal diseases. However, these agents may increase serum creatinine levels and may cause hyperkalemia, necessitating judicious use and careful monitoring of serum electrolytes and renal function in children with CKD [16,17].

Determining the degree of renal dysfunction in CKD can be complex. One widely accepted method of estimating renal function is to calculate the glomerular filtration rate (GFR). In pediatric patients, GFR can be calculated using the serum creatinine or serum cystatin C, or a combination of both [18,19]. Cystatin C is a protein that is fully catabolized in the proximal renal tubule after glomerular filtration and is not reabsorbed to the blood. Unlike serum creatinine, cystatin C it is not affected by gender, age, race, protein intake, and muscle mass [20]. In most clinical settings, however, obtaining results for serum cystatin C versus serum creatinine takes longer, costs more, and may not be reimbursed by all insurance companies. In children, the Bedside Schwartz formula (Box 2) has been a widely accepted, simple method of estimating GFR that requires the patient's serum creatinine and height in centimeters for the calculation [21,22]. It is important to recognize that small changes in GFR, especially when calculated using serum creatinine alone, are expected and that they may not always indicate true progression of CKD.

Estimated GFR is used to stage and track progression of CKD, as well as to adjust dosing of renally excreted medications [23]. The Kidney Disease Outcomes and Quality Initiative (NKF-KDOQI) Clinical Practical Guidelines for Chronic

Box 1: General renal protective measures

- General renal protective measures that should be used in all children with CKD include avoiding potential nephrotoxic agents, treating high blood pressure, and avoiding excessive protein supplementation.

Box 2: Bedside Schwartz formula

- To estimate GFR in children using the bedside Schwartz formula: multiply the height (in centimeters) by 0.413 and divide by the serum creatinine (in mg/dL).

Data from [Schwartz GJ and Work DF. Measurement and estimation of GFR in children and adolescents. J Am Soc Nephrol. 2009; Nov; 4(11): 1832-643].

Kidney Disease: Evaluation, Classification, and Stratification includes pediatric considerations. CKD is defined as the presence of kidney damage with either a normal or increased GFR greater than 90 mL/min/1.73 m^2 or decreased GFR less than 90 mL/min/1.73 m^2 for greater than 3 months. Kidney damage is defined as pathologic abnormalities or markers of damage, including abnormalities in blood or urine tests or imaging studies [24]. The KDOQI guidelines include a classification or staging system (Box 3). This staging system allows for a more complete picture of each patient's condition, directs testing and treatment decisions, and identifies the patient's risks for progression and complications [25,26]. Progression of CKD and prognosis depend on many factors that include the cause of the CKD, GFR, degree of albuminuria, and other comorbid conditions. Pediatric nephrologists can use these factors to estimate a patient's time to requiring renal replacement therapy [27]. The stages of the CKD can be used to guide the care of children with CKD including the timing of referral for preemptive renal transplantation and anticipation of the development of certain comorbidities, such as metabolic acidosis, secondary hyperparathyroidism and renal mineral-bone disease, anemia of CKD, and electrolyte abnormalities [26]. In addition, central lines or peripherally inserted central lines should not be placed in children with advanced CKD (stages 3–5) without consultation with pediatric nephrology in an effort to preserve long-term vascular access.

Metabolic acidosis usually occurs later in the course of the CKD [28] and is known to contribute to growth failure, weakness and fatigue, electrolyte disturbance, and bone disease [29]. Metabolic acidosis is treated with alkali supplementation. There are numerous commercially available forms of alkali supplements that are typically either bicarbonate or citrate based and contain

Box 3: Stages of chronic kidney disease in mL/min/1.73

- Stage 1: kidney damage with GFR $\geq$ 90
- Stage 2: kidney damage with GFR 60–89
- Stage 3a: GFR 45–59
- Stage 3b: GFR 30–44
- Stage 4: GFR 15–29
- Stage 5: GFR < 15

Data from [Hogg, Ronald J., et al. "National Kidney Foundation's Kidney Disease Outcomes Quality Initiative clinical practice guidelines for chronic kidney disease in children and adolescents: evaluation, classification, and stratification." *Pediatrics* 111.6 (2003): 1416-1421].

varying degrees of sodium or potassium [30]. These are available in solution or tablet and may be associated with gastrointestinal intolerance and lack of palatability. A long-acting microgranular formulation of alkali containing K + -citrate and K + -bicarbonate was introduced in Europe in 2017 and has the potential advantages of reduced frequency of intake and better tolerability [31]; it is currently under investigation in the United States.

Bone disease in children with CKD is multifactorial and complex with positive and negative feedback loops. In CKD, phosphorous levels increase secondary to decreased renal excretion. There is also dysfunctional hydroxylation of 25 hydroxy vitamin D to 1,25 hydroxy vitamin D, which leads to decreased overall vitamin D activity; this leads to decreased calcium absorption from the gut and contributes to hypocalcemia [32–35]. Elevated phosphorous levels and elevated parathyroid hormone levels typically occur early in the CKD course [36]. 1,25 hydroxy vitamin D inhibits parathyroid hormone synthesis. Hypocalcemia and hyperphosphatemia are triggers that lead to increased parathyroid hormone levels. Increased parathyroid hormone results in increased bone resorption and an overall decrease in bone deposition [33–35]. Patients with CKD may also have concomitant 25 hydroxy vitamin D deficiency that contributes to worsening bone disease. Ensuring bone health in children with CKD requires close monitoring of serum calcium, serum phosphorous, 25 hydroxy vitamin D, and parathyroid hormone levels [36]. Treatment of bone disease in CKD requires a multifaceted approach (Box 4) [32–40]. Serum phosphorous levels should be maintained in the normal range for age by avoiding foods containing high amounts of phosphorous (Box 5) [35,37] and with dietary phosphorous binders, if needed. Adherence to the phosphorous binder regimen is a challenge, as it requires medication administration 3 to 4 times a day. If hypocalcemia is present, calcium supplementation can be used alone or in combination with vitamin D supplementation. Elevated parathyroid levels are maintained in the target range using vitamin D analogues or calcimimetics and by maintaining normal phosphorous and calcium levels [38–40].

Box 4: Prevention of renal bone disease

- Maintain phosphorous in normal range
  - Dietary phosphorous restriction
  - Utilization of phosphorous binders
- Maintain calcium levels in normal range
  - Calcium supplementation
  - Vitamin D analogues

Supplement vitamin D if 25 OH vitamin D deficiency is present

- Maintain parathyroid hormone levels in the target range
  - Maintain normal calcium and phosphorous levels
  - Vitamin D analogues
  - Calcimimetic agents

Box 5: Foods with high phosphorous content

- Dairy products
- Beans
- Lentils
- Nuts
- Bran cereals
- Oatmeal
- Dark sodas

Anemia is another frequent comorbidity in children with CKD. Erythropoietin production in the kidney is decreased, which leads to decreased red blood cell production. In addition, the intestinal absorption of iron and the release of iron stores for erythropoiesis are downregulated [41,42]. Treatment of anemia in CKD uses both erythropoiesis-stimulating agents and routine iron supplementation. Erythropoiesis-stimulating agents can be administered by intravenous or subcutaneous routes with typical dosing windows ranging from twice monthly to 3 times a week. The optimal target hemoglobin level for children with CKD is debated, but a widely accepted range is 10 to 12 g/dL [43,44]. Lower levels of hemoglobin in children with CKD can be associated with progression of disease, increased cardiovascular disease risk, increased hospitalization and mortality, and a decreased quality of life [45].

Cardiovascular disease is the leading cause of death in children with CKD [46,47]. Current strategies for reducing cardiovascular risk in children with CKD include close monitoring of blood pressure with most recommendations for target blood pressures at or less than the 90%ile; the utilization of ambulatory blood pressure monitors with 24-hour mean arterial pressure target at or less than the 50%ile; identifying and treating dyslipidemia; promoting a healthy weight and diet; and increased physical activity [48–50].

Children with CKD are at risk for malnutrition as well as electrolyte abnormalities. Caloric requirements, protein intake targets, and specific electrolyte needs vary with age, underlying condition, and severity of CKD. Children with hypertension or edema may require sodium restriction, whereas children with renal dysplasia may waste sodium and require sodium supplementation. Potassium restriction may be required especially in those with lower GFRs, but potassium supplementation may be required in children with tubulopathies who have potassium wasting, such as Bartter syndrome. Hyperkalemia can be exacerbated by the use of angiotensin-converting enzyme inhibitors or angiotensin receptor blockers, whereas hypokalemia and hyponatremia can be exacerbated by diuretic use. If potassium restriction alone does not control the hyperkalemia, pretreatment of formula with sodium polystyrene sulfate to reduce the potassium content [51,52] or intermittent dosing with sodium polystyrene sulfate may be needed. Children with CKD are often at risk for fluid retention and typically require fluid restriction, especially as their CKD progresses. However, some

Box 6: Poor growth in chronic kidney disease

- Causes of poor growth in CKD include inadequate nutritional intake, metabolic acidosis, renal bone disease, persistent anemia, and a relative resistance to growth hormone.

children with CKD are unable to concentrate their urine and have polyuria, and this may be seen in tubulopathies and those with renal dysplasia [53]. This polyuria and its associated increased thirst results in children drinking water or other fluids in lieu of calorie dense foods, thus contributing to malnutrition. Infants with CKD are at particular risk for malnutrition and growth failure and may require specific formulas and nasogastric or gastrostomy tube feeds [53]. The care team for children with CKD should include a registered dietician with specific knowledge of the complex dietary issues faced by these children.

Poor growth in CKD is often multifactorial (Box 6) and is associated with decreased quality of life [54–57]. The relative resistance to growth hormone (GH) in children with CKD is related to multiple factors involving the GH and insulinlike growth factor (IGF) pathway. One factor involves a relative increase in the circulating IGF-binding protein 3 (IGF BP3), which results in more IGF being bound to the IGF 3 and less IGF being unbound or free in its active form. This relative resistance can be overcome by supplementing with exogenous GH, resulting in increased circulating IGF to overcome the increase in IGF BP3 [58,59]. Exogenous GH therapy is a safe and effective treatment of children with growth deficiency due to CKD with or without renal transplantation [59] One accepted guideline is to first optimize other risk factors for growth failure and then to start GH therapy if their height is less than the third percentile and height velocity is less than the 25th percentile for more than 3 months in infants and for more than 6 months in children and adolescents [59,60]. However, GH treatments are expensive and may have insurance restrictions; treatment involves repeated subcutaneous injections, which some children and families cannot tolerate; concomitant steroid therapy may decrease its effectiveness; and growth velocity may slow after discontinuation of GH therapy.

In addition to supportive care and treating the underlying cause of the CKD, chronic renal replacement therapy may be needed. Clinically available renal replacement therapies are peritoneal dialysis, hemodialysis, and renal transplantation. The timing of chronic renal replacement therapy and the preferred modality should be anticipated by the pediatric nephrologist with choices made in

Box 7: Infections secondary to an impaired immune response and have specific vaccine requirements

- Children with CKD should receive the influenza vaccine yearly and may have additional specific pneumococcal, meningococcal, hepatitis B, and COVID-19 vaccine requirements based on the underlying cause and stage of their chronic kidney disease.

Box 8: Primary care pearls

- Implement renal protective measures, including avoiding nephrotoxic medications
- Dose medications based on renal function
- Check blood pressures at all visits with target range based on sex, age, and height with lower blood pressure goals for children with CKD
- Provide 23 valent pneumococcal vaccine, meningococcal vaccine, higher dose hepatitis B vaccine, and influenza and COVID 19 vaccines as indicated based on the specific renal disease and stage of CKD
- Close monitoring of growth and attention to specific nutritional needs
- Close monitoring of psychosocial well-being and attention to specific educational needs
- Avoid placement of central lines and peripherally inserted central catheters in children with advanced CKD

conjunction with the patient and family with consideration to medical and social issues [61,62]. In addition, children with CKD are at increased risk for infections secondary to an impaired immune response and have specific vaccine requirements (Box 7) based on the severity of the CKD and underlying cause [63,64].

Children with CKD are at risk for developmental delay, learning and behavioral issues, sleep disturbance, adjustment disorder, and depression. Their care should involve screening for these issues with appropriate resources provided to their families and prompt referral for specific therapies and psychosocial services as needed. Treatment of children with CKD requires close monitoring not only of their medical issues but also of their psychosocial needs [65,66].

CKD in children is a complex disorder optimally managed through a patient-centered and family centered approach by a specialized multidisciplinary team. As key members of the multidisciplinary team, primary care providers should be knowledgeable of specific issues pertinent to the care of children with CKD and the integral role they play in the care of children with CKD (Box 8).

CLINICS CARE POINTS

- Bedside Schwartz formula is used in children to estimate GFR and requires the patient's serum creatinine and height in centimeters.
- Metabolic acidosis contributes to growth failure and bone disease.
- Hypocalcemia and hyperphosphatemia are triggers that lead to increased parathyroid hormone levels.
- Erythropoietin production may decrease in CKD.
- Cardiovascular disease is the deading cause of death in children with CKD.
- The care team for children with CKD should include a registered dietician.
- The timing of chronic renal replacement therapy and the preferred modality should be anticipated.

Disclosure

V. Panzarino, J. Lesser, and F.A. Cassini do not have any commercial or financial conflicts of interest or related funding sources relevant to the authorship of this article.

References

[1] Goldstein S, Gerson A, Goldman C, et al. Quality of life for children with chronic kidney disease. Semin Nephrol 2006;18(2):114–7.
[2] Gerson A, Wentz A, Abraham A, et al. Health-related quality of life of children with mild to moderate chronic kidney disease. Pediatrics 2010;125:e349–57.
[3] Tjaden L, Tong A, Henning P, et al. Children's experiences of dialysis: a systematic review of qualitative studies. Arch Dis Child 2012;97:395.
[4] Baum M. Overview of chronic kidney disease in children. Curr Opin Pediatr 2010;22: 158–60.
[5] Wong C, Moxey-Mims M, Jerry-Fluker J, et al. CKiD (CKD in children) prospective cohort study: a review of current findings. Am J Kidney Dis 2012;60(6):1002–11.
[6] Harambat J, et al. Epidemiology of chronic kidney disease in children. Pediatr Nephrol 2012;27:363–73.
[7] Warady BA, Chadha V. Chronic kidney disease in children: the global perspective. Pediatr Nephrol 2007;22(12):1999–2009.
[8] Ding W, Cheung W, Mak R. Impact of obesity on kidney function and blood pressure in children. World J Nephrol 2015;4:223–9.
[9] Staples A, Wong C. Risk factors for progression of chronic kidney disease. Curr Opin Pediatr 2010;22(2):161–9.
[10] Fuhrman D, Schneider M, Dell K, et al. Albuminuria, Proteinuria, and renal disease progression in children with CKD. Clin J Am Soc Nephrol 2017;12(6):912–20.
[11] Wühl E, Schaefer F. Therapeutic strategies to slow chronic kidney disease progression. Pediatr Nephrol 2008;23:705.
[12] Vikse B, Irgens L, Leivestad T, et al. Low birth weight increases risk for end-stage renal disease. J Am Soc Nephrol 2008;19(1):151–7.
[13] Carmody J, Charlton J. Short-term gestation, long-term risk: prematurity and chronic kidney disease. Pediatrics 2013;131:1168–79.
[14] Moffett B, Goldstein S. Acute kidney injury and increasing nephrotoxic-medication exposure in noncritically-ill children. Clin J Am Soc Nephrol 2011;6(4):856–63.
[15] Dionne J. Evidence-based guidelines for the management of hypertension in children with chronic kidney disease. Pediatr Nephrol 2015;30:1919–27.
[16] Webb N, Shahinfar S, Wells T, et al. Losartan and enalapril are comparable in reducing proteinuria in children. Kidney Int 2012;82(7):819–26.
[17] Abraham A, Betoko A, Fadrowski J, et al. Renin-angiotensin II-aldosterone system blockers and time to renal replacement therapy in children with CKD. Pediatr Nephrol 2017;32(4): 643–9.
[18] Ng D, Levey A, Shlipak M, et al. Validation of a simple equation for glomerular filtration rate measurement based on plasma iohexol disappearance. Clin Kidney J 2019;13(3): 397–401.
[19] Schwartz G, Schneider M, Maier P, et al. Improved equations estimating GFR in children with chronic kidney disease using an immunonephelometric determination of cystatin C. Kidney Int 2012;82(4):445–53.
[20] Ferguson T, Komenda P, Tangri N. Cystatin C as a biomarker for estimating glomerular filtration rate. Curr Opin Nephrol Hypertens 2015;24(3):295–300.
[21] Schwartz G, Munoz A, Schneider M, et al. New equations to estimate GFR in children with CKD. J Am Soc Nephrol 2009;20:629–37.
[22] Schwartz G, Work D. Measurement and estimation of GFR in children and adolescents. J Am Soc Nephrol 2009;4(11):643–1832.

[23] Wong H, Mylrea K, Feber J, et al. Prevalence of complications in children with chronic kidney disease according to KDOQI. Kidney Int 2006;70(3):585–90.
[24] Levin A, Stevens P, Bilous R, et al. Kidney disease: improving global outcomes (KDIGO) CKD work group. KDIGO 2012 clinical practice guideline for the evaluation and management of chronic kidney disease. Kidney Int S 2013;3(1):1–150.
[25] Hogg R, Furth S, Lemley K, et al. National Kidney Foundation's Kidney Disease Outcomes Quality Initiative clinical practice guidelines for chronic kidney disease in children and adolescents: evaluation, classification, and stratification. Pediatrics 2003;111(6):1416–21.
[26] Becherucci F, Roperto R, Materassi M, et al. Chronic kidney disease in children. Clin Kidney J 2016;9(4):583–91.
[27] Furth SL, Pierce C, Wui W, et al. Estimating time to ESRD in children with CKD. Am J Kidney Dis 2018;71(6):783–92.
[28] Michal L, Melamed K, Raphael L. Metabolic acidosis in CKD: A review of recent findings. Kidney Med 2021;3(2):267–77.
[29] Chen W, Abramowitz M. Metabolic acidosis and the progression of chronic kidney disease. BMC Nephrol 2014;15(55).
[30] Harambat J, Kunzmann K, Azukaitis K, et al. Metabolic acidosis is common and associates with disease progression in children with chronic kidney disease. Kidney Int 2017;92(6): 1507–14.
[31] Bertholet-Thomas A, Guittet C, Manso-Silvan M, et al. Efficacy and safety of an innovative prolonged-release combination drug in patients with distal renal tubular acidosis: an open-label comparative trial versus standard of care treatments. Pediatr Nephrol 2021;36(1): 83–91.
[32] Wesseling-Perry K. Bone disease in pediatric chronic kidney disease. Pediatr Nephrol 2013;28(4):569–76.
[33] National Kidney Foundation. K/DOQI. Clinical practice guidelines for bone metabolism and disease in children with chronic kidney disease. Am J Kidney Dis 2005;46:S12.
[34] Martin K, González E. Metabolic bone disease in chronic kidney disease. J Am Soc Nephrol 2007;18(3):875–85.
[35] D'Alessandro C, Piccoli G, Cupisti A. The "phosphorus pyramid": a visual tool for dietary phosphate management in dialysis and CKD patients. BMC Nephrol 2015;16(9).
[36] McAlister L, Pugh P, Greenbaum L, et al. The dietary management of calcium and phosphate in children with CKD stages 2-5 and on dialysis-clinical practice recommendation from the pediatric renal nutrition taskforce. Pediatr Nephrol 2020;35:501–18.
[37] Hahn D, Hodson E, Craig J. Interventions for metabolic bone disease in children with chronic kidney disease. Cochrane Database Syst Rev 2015;11.
[38] Klaus G, Watson A, Edefonti A, et al. Prevention and treatment of renal osteodystrophy in children on chronic renal failure: European guidelines. Pediatr Nephrol 2006;21(2): 151–9.
[39] Moe S, Drüeke T. Management of secondary hyperparathyroidism: the importance and the challenge of controlling parathyroid hormone levels without elevating calcium, phosphorus, and calcium-phosphorus product. Am J Nephrol 2003;23:369–79.
[40] Warady B, Ng E, Bloss L, et al. Cinacalcet studies in pediatric subjects with secondary hyperparathyroidism receiving dialysis. Pediatr Nephrol 2020;35:1679–97.
[41] Greenbaum LA. Anemia in children with chronic kidney disease. Adv Chronic Kidney Dis 2005;12(4):385–96.
[42] Atkinson MA, White CT. Hepcidin in anemia of chronic kidney disease: review for the pediatric nephrologist. Pediatr Nephrol 2012;27(1):33–40.
[43] Schaefer F, Hoppe B, Jungraithmayr T, et al. Safety and usage of darbepoetin alfa in children with chronic kidney disease: prospective registry study. Pediatr Nephrol 2016;31: 443–53.
[44] K/DOQI; National Kidney Foundation. Clinical practice recommendations for anemia in chronic kidney disease in children. Am J Kidney Dis 2006;47(Suppl 3):S86–108.

[45] Gerson A, Hwang W, Fiorenza J, et al. Anemia and health-related quality of life in adolescents with chronic kidney disease. Am J Kidney Dis 2004;44(6):1017–23.
[46] Mitsnefes M. Cardiovascular complications of pediatric chronic kidney disease. Pediatr Nephrol 2008;23(1):27–39.
[47] Rinat C, Becker-Cohen R, Nir A, et al. A comprehensive study of cardiovascular risk factors, cardiac function and vascular disease in children with chronic renal failure. Nephrol Dial Transpl 2010;25(3):785–93.
[48] Sethna C, Merchant K, Reyes A. Cardiovascular disease risk in children with kidney disease. Semin Nephrol 2018;38(3):298–313.
[49] Brady T, Schnieder M, Flynn J, et al. Carotid intima-media thickness in children with CKD: results from the CKiD study. Clin J Am Soc Nephrol 2012;7(12):1930–7.
[50] Brady T, Roem J, Cox C, et al. Adiposity, sex, and cardiovascular disease risk in children with CKD: a longitudinal study of youth enrolled in the Chronic Kidney Disease in Children (CKiD) study. Am J Kidney Dis 2020;76(2):166–73.
[51] Le Palma K, Rampolla Pavlick E, Copelovitch L. Pretreatment of enteral nutrition with sodium polystyrene sulfonate: effective, but beware the high prevalence of electrolyte derangements in clinical practice. Clin Kidney J 2018;11(2):166–71.
[52] Sgambat K, Amatya K, Moudgil A. Nutritional challenges across the spectrum of chronic kidney disease. Asian J Pediatr Nephrol 2019;2:2–15.
[53] Ledermann S, Spitz L, Moloney J, et al. Gastrostomy feeding in infants and children on peritoneal dialysis. Pediatr Nephrol 2002;17(4):246–50.
[54] Al-Uzri A, Matheson M, Gipson D, et al. The impact of short stature on health-related quality of life in children with chronic kidney disease. J Pediatr 2013;163(3):736–41.
[55] Brown D, Dauber A. Growth hormone and insulin-like growth factor dysregulation in pediatric chronic kidney disease. Horm Res Paediatr 2021;94:105–14.
[56] Stonebrook E, Mahan J. Treatment of growth retardation in a child with CKD. Clin J Am Soc Nephrol 2019;14(11):1658–60.
[57] Mahan J, Warady B, et al. Assessment and treatment of short stature in pediatric patients with chronic kidney disease: a consensus statement. Pediatr Nephrol 2006;21:917–30.
[58] Mahesh S, Kaskel F. Growth hormone axis in chronic kidney disease. Pediatr Nephrol 2008;23(1):41–8.
[59] K/DOQI, National Kidney Foundation. Clinical practice guidelines for nutrition in chronic renal failure. Am J Kidney Dis 2000;35:S1.
[60] Drube J, Wan M, Bonthuis M, et al. Clinical practice recommendations for growth hormone treatment in children with chronic kidney disease. Nat Rev Nephrol 2019;15(9):577–89.
[61] Van der Heijden B, Van Dijk P, Verrier-Jones K, et al. Renal replacement therapy in children: data from 12 registries in Europe. Pediatr Nephrol 2004;19:213–21.
[62] Chesnaye NC, Schaefer F, Bonthuis M, et al. Mortality risk disparities in children receiving chronic renal replacement therapy for the treatment of end-stage renal disease across Europe: an ESPN-ERA/EDTA registry analysis. Lancet 2017;389:2128.
[63] Esposito S, Mastrolia M, Prada E, et al. Vaccine administration in children with chronic kidney disease. Vaccine 2014;32(49):6601–6.
[64] Neu A. Immunizations in children with chronic kidney disease. Pediatr Nephrol 2012;27(8):1257–63.
[65] Groothoff J, Grootenhuis M, Offringa M, et al. Social consequences in adult life of end-stage renal disease in childhood. J Pediatr 2005;146:512.
[66] Tjaden L, Maurice-Stam H, Grootenhuis M, et al. Impact of renal replacement therapy in childhood on long-term socioprofessional outcomes: a 30-year follow-up study. J Pediatr 2016;171:189.

Advances in Pediatrics 69 (2022) 133–147

ADVANCES IN PEDIATRICS

Advances in Hemophilia A Management

Sukjoo Cho, MD[a], Ashley M. Perry, MD[a], Anna M. Cheng, MD[b], Carrie Wang, BA[c], Juan Felipe Rico, MD[d,*]

[a]Division of Hematology/Oncology, Department of Pediatrics, University of South Florida Morsani College of Medicine, 2 Tampa General Circle, 5th Floor, Tampa, FL 33606, USA; [b]Department of Pediatrics, University of Texas Southwestern Medical Center, 5323 Harry Hines Boulevard, Dallas, TX 75390, USA; [c]University of South Florida Morsani College of Medicine, 560 Channelside Drive, Tampa, FL 33602, USA; [d]Division of Hematology/Oncology, Department of Pediatrics, University of South Florida Morsani College of Medicine, 2 Tampa General Circle, 5th Floor, Tampa, FL 33606, USA

Keywords

• Hemophilia A • Management • Prophylaxis • Clotting factor concentrates • Extended half-life • Inhibitor • Emicizumab • Gene therapy

Key points

- Prophylaxis using regular replacement therapy with clotting factor concentrates is the gold standard for the management of moderate to severe hemophilia A.
- Extended half-life products can reduce the burden of frequent factor replacement injections.
- Up to 30% of patients with hemophilia A on prophylaxis therapy develop "inhibitors," neutralizing anti-Factor VIII (FVIII) autoantibodies.
- Therapeutic options for hemophilia A with inhibitors include the immune tolerance induction (ie, inhibitor eradication) and the management of acute bleeds with bypassing agents and/or emicizumab.
- Emicizumab is a biphasic monoclonal antibody mimicking activated FVIII, approved for patients with hemophilia A with/without inhibitors.

*Corresponding author. Division of Hematology/Oncology, Department of Pediatrics, University of South Florida Morsani College of Medicine, 2 Tampa General Cir, 5th Floor, Tampa, FL 33606. *E-mail address:* jrico@usf.edu

https://doi.org/10.1016/j.yapd.2022.03.009

INTRODUCTION

Hemophilia A is a clotting disorder characterized by an inherited insufficiency of Factor VIII (FVIII), one of the critical clotting factors of the coagulation cascade [1]. As a cofactor of Factor IX (FIX), FVIII plays an indispensable role in increasing the optimal activation of Factor X (FX), required for both the intrinsic and extrinsic coagulation cascades [2]. The lack of FVIII therefore prevents FX from adequately mediating the transformation of prothrombin to thrombin. Thrombin subsequently mediates the transformation of fibrinogen to fibrin, an insoluble protein, which in combination with platelets forms the clot itself. Therefore, the interruption of the clotting cascade at the level of FVIII can lead to serious hemorrhage.

The Centers for Disease Control and Prevention asserts that the prevalence of hemophilia A, although considered rare, has been grossly underestimated [3], with a report finding the prevalence may be as high as 1 in 5000 male births [4]. Because of its X-linked recessive inheritance pattern, the misconception that women cannot present with hemophilia A persists; this has been disproven, as up to 50% of female carriers of the gene may present with FVIII levels low enough to qualify for mild hemophilia [5–7].

Hemophilia A can be further classified into mild, moderate, and severe subtypes, depending on the concentration of functional FVIII in the patient's plasma: mild if 5% to 40%, moderate if 1% to 5%, and severe if less than 1% of normal [8]. Individuals with mild hemophilia generally do not experience spontaneous bleeding and can even tolerate invasive medical procedures with delayed bleeding; those with severe hemophilia, however, not only experience profuse bleeding with trauma but may also suffer from spontaneous joint and muscle bleeds [9].

To prevent bleeding, particularly hemarthrosis that would lead to arthropathy and disability, prophylaxis with regular administration of therapeutic products is strongly recommended [10,11]. Fortunately, during the past few years, there has been unprecedented progress in the development of novel therapeutics as well as acknowledged paradigm shifts in the principles of hemophilia care [10]. Herein, we review recent advances in the management of hemophilia A including newer clotting factor concentrates (CFCs) with extended half-life and emicizumab, an innovative nonfactor replacement therapy.

Comprehensive care

Management of hemophilia A is best provided by comprehensive care consisting of multidisciplinary medical services, typically offered by hemophilia treatment centers [12]. Such integrated care promotes physical fitness and psychosocial wellness and reduces morbidity, mortality, and hospitalization [13–15]. Therefore, comprehensive care should be initiated shortly after the diagnosis of hemophilia is made [12].

Newborn care

Newborns with hemophilia A may present with persistent bleeding after circumcision, routine heel pokes, or intracranial hemorrhage as a direct result of labor and delivery [16]. Providers should therefore counsel pregnant women who are carriers to opt for unassisted vaginal deliveries if possible, avoiding the use of vacuum or forceps.

Immunization

Children and adults with hemophilia A should receive the same standard immunizations as the general population [10,17]. The finest needle available (ie, 23 gauge or smaller) should be used and the application of firm pressure on the injection site for at least 2 minutes after administration is recommended. Some experts prefer subcutaneous administration to reduce the risk of intramuscular hematoma [10], although evidence of equal efficacy is only available for a few vaccines such as pneumococcal polysaccharide, inactivated polio, and hepatitis A and B vaccines [17].

Physical activity

Although regular physical activity for fitness is encouraged for people with hemophilia A, sports with high risk of frequent collisions (eg, soccer) or high velocity (eg, skiing) are not advised given the risk for life-threatening injuries, unless the individual is on a proper prophylactic regimen to cover such activities [10]. Therefore, noncontact sports such as swimming [18,19] are encouraged.

Oral and dental care

Optimal oral hygiene is important in people with hemophilia A, not only to prevent gum and tooth disease that may cause serious gum bleeding but also to avoid any needs for major dental surgery [20–22]. Thus, access to regular dental care is critical as a part of comprehensive hemophilia care [10]. To ensure plaque removal, it is recommended that patients brush teeth twice daily with a soft-to-medium textured toothbrush and fluoridated toothpaste and use dental floss or interdental brushes [10].

Pain management

For individuals with hemophilia A who have acute or chronic pain, NSAIDs should be avoided given the potential risk of bleeding [17,23]. Acetaminophen can be a safe first choice. If it is not effective, cyclooxygenase-2 (COX-2) inhibitors (eg, celecoxib [24], etoricoxib [25]) or acetaminophen plus codeine or acetaminophen plus tramadol should be considered as a next step, although codeine should be avoided in children aged younger than 12 years. If the pain persists, morphine would be a next option.

Planning for elective surgery

Elective surgery for people with hemophilia A is most effectively undertaken by a multidisciplinary team that includes a hematologist [26]. For people with mild hemophilia A undergoing surgery, desmopressin, a synthetic analog of vasopressin that increases FVIII and von Willebrand Factor (vWF) levels, can be used once the response is confirmed in the preoperative testing [27,28]. FVIII should be used for people with moderate-to-severe hemophilia A who need surgery.

Preventive care

Prophylaxis

Prophylaxis is regarded as the gold standard for the management of moderate-to-severe hemophilia A because it prevents bleeding and delays joint damage development in pediatric and adult populations. Prophylaxis reduces bleeding and long-term complications of bleeding such as chronic arthropathy in patients with severe hemophilia [29]. There are 3 main types of prophylaxis, defined by the International Society on Thrombosis and Hemostasis [8]. Primary prophylaxis is a continuous therapy that starts in early childhood before the age of 3 years and after the first evident joint bleed. Secondary prophylaxis begins either after the age of 3 years or after 2 or more joint bleeds but before evidence of joint disease appears; it can be continuous or intermittent therapy. Tertiary prophylaxis is therapy that starts after the onset of joint disease with the goal of slowing the progression of joint disease; it is mainly used in adults with hemophilia.

Primary prophylaxis is most efficient when initiated before the age of 2 years because it reduces long-term joint damage compared with the initiation of primary prophylaxis after 6 years of age [11,30,31]. It has also been suggested by multiple studies that early prophylaxis treatment may reduce FVIII inhibitor development [32–34]. Ultimately, the current practice of prophylaxis in hemophilia is based on clinical presentation and severity, risks, and personal factors such as cost, time, patient values, and preferences [29].

Extended half-life products: factor VIII and factor IX

In 2014, new recombinant factor replacement products with an extended plasma half-life were approved by the Food and Drug Administration for use in the United States for prophylaxis use in adults with hemophilia A; in 2017, they were approved for the pediatric population. These extended half-life products (EHLs) were developed to reduce the burden of frequent factor replacement injections because conventional FVIII replacement therapy requires injections 3 times a week for severe hemophilia A prophylaxis.

There are currently 4 established strategies used to develop EHLs: (1) covalent attachment of polyethylene glycol (PEG) to the coagulation factor (ie, PEGylation) to reduce clearance, (2) integration of the coagulation factor with a fragmented crystallizable (ie, Fc) portion of IgG1 molecule to avoid lysosomal degradation, (3) combining the coagulation factor with a recombinant albumin to rescue endocytosed proteins from the intracellular degradation pathway, and (4) single-chain technology for augmenting the stability of the recombinant molecule. A list of available EHL factor replacement products is displayed in Table 1.

In terms of efficacy, EHL FIX replacement therapy has been more successful than its FVIII counterpart mainly due to its considerable increase in factor half-life compared with standard half-life preparations. EHL FIX options have decreased injection frequency from twice a week on average to weekly or even biweekly [36], whereas EHL FVIII options have decreased injection

Table 1
Available extended half-life factor replacement products [35]

	Factor VIII	Factor XI
Albumin Products		Idelvion (half-life: 104 h)
Fc Fusion Products	Eloctate (half-life: 13–20 h)	Alprolix (half-life: 54–90 h)
PEGylated Products	Adynovate (half-life: 13–16 h) Jivi (half-life: 17–21 h) Espercot (half-life: 17–22 h)	Rebinyn (half-life: 103–115 h)
Single Chain Products	Afstyla (half-life: 10–14 h)	

Data from National Hemophilia Foundation. Products Licensed in the US. Accessed August 2, 2021. https://www.hemophilia.org/healthcare-professionals/guidelines-on-care/products-licensed-in-the-us#IIA.

frequency from thrice a week to twice a week [37]. The difference in half-life extension is mainly due to the additional clearance of FVIII by vWF because FVIII binds to vWF for stabilization. Therefore, vWF half-life limits the extension that can be made to the half-life of FVIII to 15 to 19 hours.

There is recent progress in developing longer half-life FVIII products with the goal of bypassing vWF dependence of FVIII. New phase 1-2a investigational studies of a recombinant FVIII product that is fused to the vWF D'D3-domain (the factor VIII binding site; BIVV001) shows promising pharmacokinetic results, with a 3-fold to 4-fold increase in factor half-life [38].

Inhibitors

The mainstay of preventive care for children with hemophilia A is prophylactic infusion of FVIII to avoid bleeding and resultant joint destruction [10]. Although replacement therapy with CFCs is considered to be generally safe and effective, up to 30% of patients receiving CFCs develop "inhibitors." These neutralizing anti-FVIII autoantibodies render replacement therapy ineffective [8] and result in significant complications including increased morbidity and mortality, and reduced health-related quality of life [39,40]. Typically, inhibitors develop early in treatment, within 50 exposure days to FVIII therapy [41].

Inhibitor levels are measured by the Bethesda assay or the Nijmegen-modified Bethesda assay [42]. The laboratory definition of a positive inhibitor in hemophilia A is a titer of more than 0.6 Bethesda units (BU) for FVIII [8]. They are divided into 2 classes: a high-responding inhibitor (≥5 BU) and a low-responding inhibitor (<5 BU) [8]. Low-responding inhibitors are likely transient, usually dropping less than the definition threshold within 6 months of initial detection if there is no change in treatment regimen, despite antigenic challenge with CFCs. High-responding inhibitors are likely to persist. Although they may decrease and become undetectable after long periods without CFC exposure, they tend to increase 3 to 5 days after reexposure to CFCs [43].

Inhibitors need to be detected early to ensure appropriate management [10]. More than half of inhibitor cases are found in routine screening after initial exposures to CFCs. Therefore, patients with newly diagnosed hemophilia A should undergo screening at least every 6 to 12 months after the initiation of

CFC therapy, when the risk of developing inhibitors is greatest, and then annually [10]. Indications for inhibitor testing include the following [10]:

- After initial factor exposures
- After intensive (ie, more than 5 consecutive days) factor exposure
- For recurrent bleeding or target joint (ie, any joint where 3 or more spontaneous bleeding have occurred within consecutive 6 months) bleeding despite adequate CFC therapy
- For lack of response to CFC therapy
- For factor recovery or half-life less than the expectation after CFC therapy
- For inadequate clinical or laboratory response to CFC therapy
- Before surgery
- For inadequate postoperative response to CFC therapy

Therapeutic options for patients with hemophilia A and inhibitors

Treatment of patients with hemophilia A and inhibitors revolves around 2 principles: eradication of inhibitors and management of acute bleeds [44]. Eradication is the goal, given the marked contrast in prognosis and social burden between children who receive regular effective FVIII prophylaxis, and those who do not respond due to inhibitors [45]. Eradication requires immune tolerance induction (ITI) therapy, which usually consists of daily factor injections for months to years (Table 2). However, these intensive regimens do not guarantee eradication, with ITI being ineffective in 20% to 30% of patients with severe hemophilia A [10]. Response to ITI is even less favorable in patients with mild-to-moderate hemophilia A [10].

Management of acute bleeds in hemophilia A patients with inhibitors depends on whether the inhibitor is low-responding or high-responding [10].

Table 2
Immune tolerance induction protocols in hemophilia A [10,46]

Bonn protocol/high-dose protocol	100–150 IU FVIII/kg twice daily; concomitant treatment with FEIBA 50 U/kg or rFVIIa twice daily in accordance with bleeding tendency
High-dose protocol	200 IU FVIII/kg daily
Intermediate-dose protocol	100 IU FVIII/kg daily
van Creveld/low-dose protocol	25(-50) IU FVIII/kg every other day
Malmo protocol	Extracorporeal immune adsorption with protein A columns on 2 consecutive days, immunosuppression (cyclophosphamide), immunomodulation (IVIG), administration of FVIII concentrate at 8–12 h intervals
Protocols including immunosuppressive agents	Rituximab, mycophenolate mofetil, dexamethasone, IVIG and FVIII, respectively. FIX in hemophilia B

Abbreviation: FEIBA, factor eight inhibitor bypassing activity; IU, international units; IVIG, intravenous immunoglobulin; MASAC, Medical and Scientific Advisory Council.

Data from Srivastava A, Santagostino E, Dougall A, et al. WFH Guidelines for the Management of Hemophilia, 3rd edition. Haemophilia. Aug 2020;26 Suppl 6:1-158. https://doi.org/10.1111/hae.14046; and Valentino LA, Kempton CL, Kruse-Jarres R, et al. US Guidelines for immune tolerance induction in patients with haemophilia a and inhibitors. Haemophilia. Sep 2015;21(5):559-67. https://doi.org/10.1111/hae.12730.

As summarized in Table 3, standard replacement therapy with FVIII is recommended for patients with low-responding inhibitors, although at higher doses to overcome the effect of inhibitors. For those with high-responding inhibitors, bypass agents such as activated prothrombin complex concentrates (aPCC) and recombinant activated factor VII (rFVIIa) are recommended [48,49]. These agents essentially circumvent inhibitors and generate thrombin via alternate routes; however, they are less effective than CFC for bleed prevention in patients without inhibitors [44].

Due to suboptimal efficacy and substantial burden of conventional bypass agents for preventing bleeding episodes among patients with hemophilia A and inhibitors, efforts have been made to develop new therapies. Emicizumab is a bispecific monoclonal antibody that bridges activated FIX and FX, thereby restoring the function of activated FVIII (FVIIIa) [50]. Although emicizumab mimics the role of FVIIIa in the coagulation cascade, it is different from FVIIIa in that it has much lower affinity, does not require activation, and is not deactivated by protein C/s pathway (Fig. 1) [51,52]. Multiple clinical trials have shown that this novel therapy is effective prophylaxis among patients with hemophilia A and inhibitors [53–56]. Furthermore, the burden of prophylaxis is far less than with bypass agents because emicizumab is administered subcutaneously every 1, 2, or 4 weeks [10]. Thus, emicizumab is recommended for pre-ITI patients with high-responding inhibitors, patients on low-dose ITI, and patients who failed ITI [44]. It is also approved for hemophilia patients without inhibitors [10,51].

Emicizumab prevents, but does not treat, acute bleeds in patients with hemophilia A and inhibitors. Therefore, therapy with FVIII or bypass agents is required for the management of bleeding episodes [10]. rFVIIa is the preferred bypass agent versus aPCC due to the potential risk of thrombotic

Table 3
Treatment of acute bleeds in patients with hemophilia A and inhibitors [47]

	Low-responding inhibitors	High-responding inhibitors
Agent	FVIII[a]	rFVIIa or aPCC[b] or FVIII[c]
Monitoring	FVIII activity (FVIII:C) assay	Thromboelastography or thrombin generation assay

Abbreviations: aPCC, activated prothrombin complex concentrate; rFVIIa, recombinant activated factor VIIa.

[a]If half-life is shortened, will require higher, more frequent dosing.

[b]In patients receiving emicizumab prophylaxis, aPCC should be avoided or carefully used with lower doses due to the thrombotic microangiopathy risk (black box warning). rFVIIa should also be used with cautions in patients on emicizumab who have risk factors for thrombosis given increased risk of myocardial infarction or pulmonary embolism.

[c]In patients with high-responding inhibitors who currently have the low inhibitor titer, FVIII can be considered with close monitoring for the anamnestic response.

Data from Kempton CL, White GC, 2nd. How we treat a hemophilia A patient with a factor VIII inhibitor. Blood. Jan 1 2009;113(1):11-7. doi:10.1182/blood-2008-06-160432.

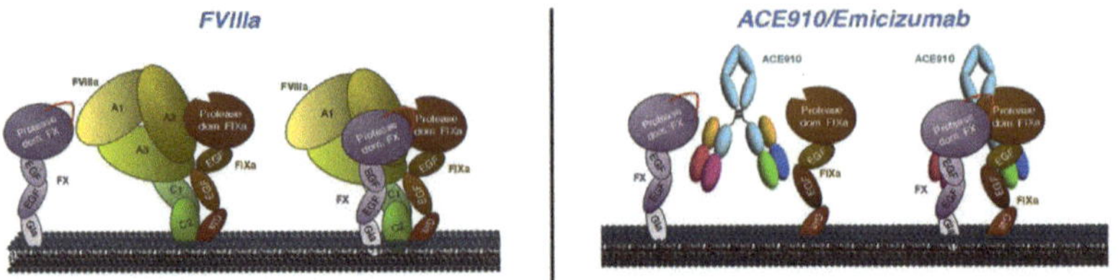

Multiple sites of interaction	Single sites of interaction
High affinity for enzyme & substrate *(low to high nanomolar range)*	Low affinity for enzyme & substrate *(micromolar range)*
Specific for FIXa and FX *(no binding to FIX and FXa)*	No distinction between zymogen and enzyme *(FIX vs FIXa and FX vs FXa)*
Full cofactor activity - *promotes phospholipid binding* - *stabilizes FIXa active site* - *bridges FIXa to FX*	Partial cofactor activity - *bridges FIXa to FX*
Enzyme and substrate are in excess over cofactor	Antibody is in excess over enzyme and substrate
FVIIIa has on/off mechanism	Emicizumab has no on/off mechanism
High level of self-regulation	Low level of self-regulation

Fig. 1. Differences between activated Factor VIII and emicizumab. (*Data from* National Hemophilia Foundation. MASAC Document 258 - Recommendation on the Use and Management of Emicizumab-kxwh (Hemlibra®) for Hemophilia A with and without Inhibitors. Updated March 16, 2020. Accessed August 20, 2021. https://www.hemophilia.org/healthcare-professionals/guidelines-on-care/masac-documents/masac-document-258-recommendation-on-the-use-and-management-of-emicizumab-kxwh-hemlibrar-for-hemophilia-a-with-and-without-inhibitors; and Lenting PJ, Denis CV, Christophe OD. Emicizumab, a bispecific antibody recognizing coagulation factors IX and X: how does it actually compare to factor VIII? Blood. 2017;130(23):2463-2468. https://doi.org/10.1182/blood-2017-08-801662.)

microangiopathy [51,53]. In addition, rFVIIa should be used cautiously in patients on emicizumab who have risk factors for thrombosis (eg, history of venous thromboembolism, smoking, obesity, chronic infection, and inflammation) due to risk of pulmonary embolism and acute non-STEMI [ST-elevation myocardial infarction (STEMI)] [57]. Close clinical monitoring for thrombosis and laboratory monitoring for inhibitor titers with bovine chromogenic Bethesda assay are advised [10].

Preoperative management of patients with hemophilia A and inhibitors

As discussed above, inhibitor testing is recommended for all patients with hemophilia A before surgery or invasive procedures. For patients with low-responding inhibitors, FVIII therapy with higher and more frequent doses than usual is recommended due to the short half-life of FVIII. Patients with high-responding inhibitors may also require escalated therapy with bypass agents. When response to a single agent is poor, sequential treatment (ie, alternating rFVIIa and aPCC every 3 hours) can be beneficial [58]. Once hemostasis is achieved for 3 to 5 days with a selected regimen, these agents can be tapered over 1 to 3 weeks [10].

For patients on emicizumab undergoing surgery or invasive procedures, the identical regimens are recommended: FVIII for those with low-responding inhibitors, and rFVIIa for those with high-responding inhibitors. Further evidence is needed to determine specific recommendations for dose, frequency, and duration [59]. Close clinical monitoring for thrombosis along with consideration for laboratory monitoring is recommended [10].

Gene therapy

Gene therapy is emerging as a novel treatment of hemophilia. Compared with the conventional treatment consisting of prophylactic factor infusion, gene therapy establishes continuous endogenous expression of FVIII or FIX after one treatment, essentially curing patients with hemophilia or transforming them to a milder phenotype. This treatment has the potential to significantly change the way we approach the treatment of hemophilia [60,61].

Many clinical trials of gene therapy for hemophilia A are currently ongoing. The gene therapy protocol varies slightly among trials because there may be variations in virus serotype, transgene modifications, manufacturing, dosing, and administration [62]. The overall process is shown in Fig. 2 [62]. The most commonly used vector is adeno-associated virus (AAV). This vector is ideal because it is not associated with human disease and can target specific cells [63]. All viral coding is removed, and the gene for FVIII or FIX is inserted into the viral vector [60]. The FIX gene is smaller than the FVIII gene; therefore, it is more easily packaged [64]. This size differential is the primary obstacle in the development of trials for hemophilia A. Once the package is

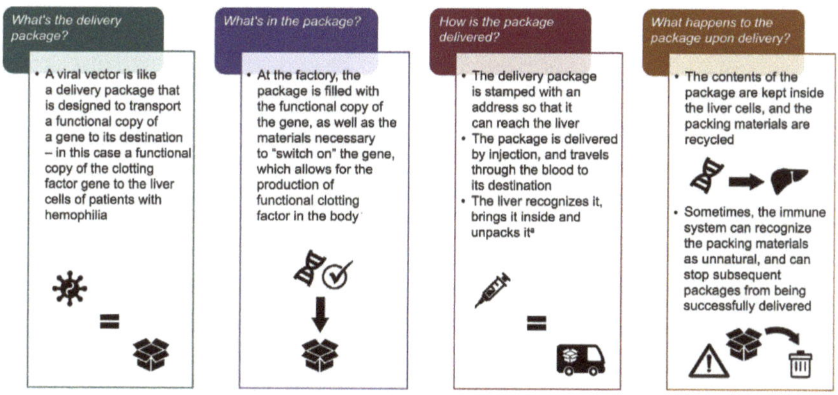

Fig. 2. Patient friendly figure of the process of gene therapy. [a]While the package is delivered at a high rate to the liver, it will also arrive at, and be unpacked by, many other cell types in the body. However, the gene encoding the functional protein will only be expressed in the liver, because liver-specific promoters are used to drive gene expression. (*From* Sidonio RF, Jr., Pipe SW, Callaghan MU, et al. Discussing investigational AAV gene therapy with hemophilia patients: A guide. Blood Rev. May 2021;47:100759. https://doi.org/10.1016/j.blre.2020.100759.)

created, it is administered to the patient, typically as a single, intravenous outpatient infusion over approximately 1 hour [65]. Once in the blood stream, the vector travels to liver cells, where it is internalized and the transgene is released into hepatocytes. The gene is transcribed and translated, and the liver produces functional clotting factor proteins [63]. Hemophilia is well suited for this type of therapy because it is responsive to a wide range of factor levels and precise regulation is not necessary [61]. In the recent clinical trials, gene therapy for hemophilia A was associated with reduction in bleeding and resultant decreased use or complete cessation of FVIII prophylaxis [66–68].

Gene therapy is considered a safe treatment option overall. Most trials have included only adult men with moderate-to-severe hemophilia B. Additionally, patients with HIV, hepatitis C, factor inhibitors, and antibodies to the viral vector were often excluded [62]. Therefore, understanding of the safety and efficacy of this treatment in some groups of individuals, including pediatric populations, is limited, warranting further research. The primary adverse reaction is elevated liver transaminases. Patients were monitored closely following treatment, particularly in the first month. Elevated transaminases were typically transient, asymptomatic, and resolved without treatment. In some studies, such transaminitis was defined as twice or more than baseline, which can be still within normal limits among some participants [69]. However, they often preceded or coincided with the loss of transgene expression and efficacy, which typically occurred within 12 weeks of infusion [70]. In some trials, corticosteroids were administered when transaminases were elevated, in an attempt to prevent loss of transgene expression. In other studies, corticosteroids were administered prophylactically. The efficacy of these strategies was mixed [66]. Despite early loss in some cases, a study in hemophilia B patients showed stable expression with no late toxicity up to 8 years after administration [71]. In studies with hemophilia A patients, the durability of transgenes expression was more limited, and some patients showed a late decline in clotting factor levels up to one to 2 years postadministration in the absence of transaminitis [66]. In mouse models, there has been increased risk of hepatocellular carcinoma [72]. Long-term data are required to better assess durability, efficacy, and safety of gene therapy, particularly in hemophilia A. Fortunately, in the event of unsuccessful gene therapy or loss of efficacy, patients can return to standard treatments of hemophilia [62].

One limitation of gene therapy is the upfront cost. Overall, gene therapy may be less expensive than recurrent prophylactic factor administration, yielding significant savings for the health-care system and society. However, the single treatment cost may not be feasible for many patients. Another barrier is patients with preexisting neutralizing antibodies or factor inhibitors because these would limit the efficacy of gene therapy. Large-scale production of clinical grade AAV vectors may be a limitation [60,61]. Finally, efficacy of gene therapy might be limited in pediatric populations due to a growing liver with significant hepatocyte turnover that can result in a dilutional effect [69]. However, overall, initial studies have been promising. Further studies on nonviral vectors and gene editing may provide solutions to some of these barriers [69].

CLINICS CARE POINTS

- Once the diagnosis of hemophilia A is made, comprehensive care in the hemophilia treatment center should be initiated to improve physical and psychosocial fitness and decrease morbidity, mortality, and hospitalization. Prophylaxis to prevent bleeding and its long-term complications including chronic arthropathy is essential in management of hemophilia A. Regular replacement therapy with clotting factor concentrates has been playing a pivotal role in prophylaxis, although there are some new modalities including extended half-life products and emicizumab, a biphasic monoclonal antibody mimicking activated Factor VIII.
- Patients with hemophilia A may develop "inhibitors" to clotting factor concentrates, which are anti-Factor VIII autoantibodies that dampen the efficacy of replacement therapies. Therefore, regular screening for inhibitors is required every 6-12 months after the initiation of replacement therapy.
- Treatment options for patients with hemophilia A and inhibitors include immune tolerance induction to eliminate inhibitors as well as bypassing agents and emicizumab to control acute bleeding episodes.

SUMMARY

Management of hemophilia A has evolved during the past few years. It is best offered in a setting of comprehensive care, ideally hemophilia treatment centers. Prophylaxis with regular factor replacement is now the gold standard management for people with moderate-to-severe hemophilia A. Novel EHLs reduce the burden of frequent factor replacement injections. For people with hemophilia A and inhibitors, therapeutic options include ITI, bypassing agents, and emicizumab. There are ongoing clinical trials on gene therapy for hemophilia A, which can be a great alternative to the current treatment options.

Acknowledgments

The authors would like to thank Jane Carver, PhD for assistance in writing and editing.

Disclosure

The authors have nothing to disclose.

References

[1] Peyvandi F, Garagiola I, Young G. The past and future of haemophilia: diagnosis, treatments, and its complications. Lancet 2016;388(10040):187–97.

[2] Chavin SI. Factor VIII: structure and function in blood clotting. Am J Hematol 1984;16(3):297–306.

[3] Schieve LA, Byams VR, Dupervil B, et al. Evaluation of CDC's hemophilia surveillance program - universal data collection (1998-2011) and community counts (2011-2019), United States. MMWR Surveill Summ 2020;69(5):1–18.

[4] Soucie JM, Evatt B, Jackson D. Occurrence of hemophilia in the United States. the hemophilia surveillance system project investigators. Am J Hematol 1998;59(4):288–94.

[5] Plug I, Mauser-Bunschoten EP, Brocker-Vriends AH, et al. Bleeding in carriers of hemophilia. Blood 2006;108(1):52–6.
[6] Bryant P, Boukouvala A, McDaniel J, et al. Hemophilia A in females: considerations for clinical management. Acta Haematol 2020;143(3):289–94, d.
[7] National Hemophilia Foundation. MASAC document 264 - MASAC recommendations regarding diagnosis and management of inherited bleeding disorders in girls and women with personal and family history of bleeding. 2021. Available at: https://www.hemophilia.org/healthcare-professionals/guidelines-on-care/masac-documents/masac-document-264-masac-recommendations-regarding-diagnosis-and-management-of-inherited-bleeding-disorders-in-girls-and-women-with-personal-and-family-history-of-bleeding. Accessed September 15, 2021.
[8] Blanchette VS, Key NS, Ljung LR, et al. Definitions in hemophilia: communication from the SSC of the ISTH. J Thromb Haemost 2014;12(11):1935–9.
[9] Israels S, Schwetz N, Boyar R, et al. Bleeding disorders: characterization, dental considerations and management. J Can Dent Assoc 2006;72(9):827.
[10] Srivastava A, Santagostino E, Dougall A, et al. WFH guidelines for the management of hemophilia, 3rd edition. Haemophilia 2020;26(Suppl 6):1–158.
[11] Manco-Johnson MJ, Abshire TC, Shapiro AD, et al. Prophylaxis versus episodic treatment to prevent joint disease in boys with severe hemophilia. N Engl J Med 2007;357(6):535–44.
[12] Bolton-Maggs PH. Optimal haemophilia care versus the reality. Br J Haematol 2006;132(6):671–82.
[13] Berntorp E, Boulyjenkov V, Brettler D, et al. Modern treatment of haemophilia. Bull World Health Organ 1995;73(5):691–701.
[14] Dunkley S, Lam JCM, John MJ, et al. Principles of haemophilia care: the Asia-Pacific perspective. Haemophilia 2018;24(3):366–75.
[15] Soucie JM, Nuss R, Evatt B, et al. Mortality among males with hemophilia: relations with source of medical care. the hemophilia surveillance system project investigators. Blood 2000;96(2):437–42.
[16] Moorehead PC, Chan AKC, Lemyre B, et al. A practical guide to the management of the fetus and newborn with hemophilia. Clin Appl Thromb Hemost 2018;24(9_suppl): 29S–41S.
[17] National Hemophilia Foundation. MASAC document 221 - recommendations on administration of vaccines to individuals with bleeding disorders. 2013. Available at. https://www.hemophilia.org/healthcare-professionals/guidelines-on-care/masac-documents/masac-document-221-recommendations-on-administration-of-vaccines-to-individuals-with-bleeding-disorders. Accessed September 17, 2021.
[18] Passeri EV, Martinelli M, Gatteri V, et al. Standard and water rehabilitation: An analysis of over 14 years' experience in patients with haemophilia or other clotting factor disorders after orthopaedic surgery. Haemophilia 2019;25(4):699–707.
[19] Kargarfard M, Dehghadani M, Ghias R. The effect of aquatic exercise therapy on muscle strength and joint's range of motion in hemophilia patients. Int J Prev Med 2013;4(1):50–6.
[20] Scully C, Diz Dios P, Giangrande P. Oral care for people with hemophilia or a hereditary bleeding tendency. 2nd edition. World Federation of Hemophilia; 2008. Available at: https://www1.wfh.org/publication/files/pdf-1164.pdf. Accessed September 18, 2021.
[21] Kalsi H, Nanayakkara L, Pasi KJ, et al. Access to primary dental care for patients with inherited bleeding disorders. Haemophilia 2012;18(4):510–5.
[22] Anderson JA, Brewer A, Creagh D, et al. Guidance on the dental management of patients with haemophilia and congenital bleeding disorders. Br Dent J 2013;215(10):497–504.
[23] Eyster ME, Asaad SM, Gold BD, et al. Upper gastrointestinal bleeding in haemophiliacs: incidence and relation to use of non-steroidal anti-inflammatory drugs. Haemophilia 2007;13(3):279–86.
[24] Rattray B, Nugent DJ, Young G. Celecoxib in the treatment of haemophilic synovitis, target joints, and pain in adults and children with haemophilia. Haemophilia 2006;12(5):514–7.

[25] Tsoukas C, Eyster ME, Shingo S, et al. Evaluation of the efficacy and safety of etoricoxib in the treatment of hemophilic arthropathy. Blood 2006;107(5):1785–90.
[26] Escobar MA, Brewer A, Caviglia H, et al. Recommendations on multidisciplinary management of elective surgery in people with haemophilia. Haemophilia 2018;24(5):693–702.
[27] Mannucci PM. Desmopressin (DDAVP) in the treatment of bleeding disorders: the first 20 years. Blood 1997;90(7):2515–21.
[28] Batty P, Austin SK, Khair K, et al. Treatment burden, haemostatic strategies and real world inhibitor screening practice in non-severe haemophilia A. Br J Haematol 2017;176(5): 796–804.
[29] Oldenburg J. Optimal treatment strategies for hemophilia: achievements and limitations of current prophylactic regimens. Blood 2015;125(13):2038–44.
[30] Astermark J, Petrini P, Tengborn L, et al. Primary prophylaxis in severe haemophilia should be started at an early age but can be individualized. Br J Haematol 1999;105(4): 1109–13.
[31] Warren BB, Thornhill D, Stein J, et al. Young adult outcomes of childhood prophylaxis for severe hemophilia a: results of the joint outcome continuation study. Blood Adv 2020;4(11):2451–9.
[32] Kurnik K, Bidlingmaier C, Engl W, et al. New early prophylaxis regimen that avoids immunological danger signals can reduce FVIII inhibitor development. Haemophilia 2010;16(2):256–62.
[33] Gouw SC, van der Bom JG, Marijke van den Berg H. Treatment-related risk factors of inhibitor development in previously untreated patients with hemophilia a: the CANAL cohort study. Blood 2007;109(11):4648–54.
[34] Gouw SC, van den Berg HM, Fischer K, et al. Intensity of factor VIII treatment and inhibitor development in children with severe hemophilia a: the RODIN study. Blood 2013;121(20): 4046–55.
[35] National Hemophilia Foundation. Products licensed in the US. Available at. https://www.hemophilia.org/healthcare-professionals/guidelines-on-care/products-licensed-in-the-us#IIA. Accessed August 2, 2021.
[36] Graf L. Extended half-life factor VIII and factor IX preparations. Transfus Med Hemother 2018;45(2):86–91.
[37] Berntorp E, Negrier C, Gozzi P, et al. Dosing regimens, FVIII levels and estimated haemostatic protection with special focus on rFVIIIFc. Haemophilia 2016;22(3):389–96.
[38] Konkle BA, Shapiro AD, Quon DV, et al. BIVV001 fusion protein as factor VIII replacement therapy for hemophilia A. N Engl J Med 2020;383(11):1018–27.
[39] Walsh CE, Soucie JM, Miller CH, et al. Impact of inhibitors on hemophilia A mortality in the United States. Am J Hematol 2015;90(5):400–5.
[40] D'Angiolella LS, Cortesi PA, Rocino A, et al. The socioeconomic burden of patients affected by hemophilia with inhibitors. Eur J Haematol 2018;101(4):435–56.
[41] Wight J, Paisley S. The epidemiology of inhibitors in haemophilia A: a systematic review. Haemophilia 2003;9(4):418–35.
[42] Verbruggen B, van Heerde WL, Laros-van Gorkom BA. Improvements in factor VIII inhibitor detection: from bethesda to nijmegen. Semin Thromb Hemost 2009;35(8):752–9.
[43] de Moerloose P, Fischer K, Lambert T, et al. Recommendations for assessment, monitoring and follow-up of patients with haemophilia. Haemophilia 2012;18(3):319–25.
[44] Young G. How I treat children with haemophilia and inhibitors. Br J Haematol 2019;186(3): 400–8.
[45] Brackmann HH, White GC 2nd, Berntorp E, et al. Immune tolerance induction: what have we learned over time? Haemophilia 2018;24(Suppl 3):3–14.
[46] Valentino LA, Kempton CL, Kruse-Jarres R, et al. US Guidelines for immune tolerance induction in patients with haemophilia a and inhibitors. Haemophilia 2015;21(5):559–67.
[47] Kempton CL, White GC 2nd. How we treat a hemophilia A patient with a factor VIII inhibitor. Blood 2009;113(1):11–7.

[48] Astermark J, Donfield SM, DiMichele DM, et al. A randomized comparison of bypassing agents in hemophilia complicated by an inhibitor: the FEIBA NovoSeven Comparative (FENOC) Study. Blood 2007;109(2):546–51.
[49] Leissinger C, Gringeri A, Antmen B, et al. Anti-inhibitor coagulant complex prophylaxis in hemophilia with inhibitors. N Engl J Med 2011;365(18):1684–92.
[50] Kitazawa T, Igawa T, Sampei Z, et al. A bispecific antibody to factors IXa and X restores factor VIII hemostatic activity in a hemophilia A model. Nat Med 2012;18(10):1570–4; https://doi.org/10.1038/nm.2942.
[51] National Hemophilia Foundation. MASAC document 258 - Recommendation on the use and management of emicizumab-kxwh (hemlibra®) for hemophilia A with and without inhibitors. Available at. https://www.hemophilia.org/healthcare-professionals/guidelines-on-care/masac-documents/masac-document-258-recommendation-on-the-use-and-management-of-emicizumab-kxwh-hemlibrar-for-hemophilia-a-with-and-without-inhibitors. Accessed August 20, 2021.
[52] Lenting PJ, Denis CV, Christophe OD. Emicizumab, a bispecific antibody recognizing coagulation factors IX and X: how does it actually compare to factor VIII? Blood 2017;130(23): 2463–8.
[53] Oldenburg J, Mahlangu JN, Kim B, et al. Emicizumab Prophylaxis in Hemophilia A with Inhibitors. N Engl J Med 2017;377(9):809–18.
[54] Oldenburg J, Mahlangu JN, Bujan W, et al. The effect of emicizumab prophylaxis on health-related outcomes in persons with haemophilia A with inhibitors: HAVEN 1 Study. Haemophilia 2019;25(1):33–44.
[55] Pipe SW, Shima M, Lehle M, et al. Efficacy, safety, and pharmacokinetics of emicizumab prophylaxis given every 4 weeks in people with haemophilia A (HAVEN 4): a multicentre, open-label, non-randomised phase 3 study. Lancet Haematol 2019;6(6):e295–305.
[56] Young G, Liesner R, Chang T, et al. A multicenter, open-label phase 3 study of emicizumab prophylaxis in children with hemophilia A with inhibitors. Blood 2019;134(24):2127–38.
[57] Gundabolu K, Goldsweig A, Bhatt VR, et al. ST-segment elevation myocardial infarction (STEMI) and pulmonary embolism in a hemophilia A patient receiving emicizumab and recombinant activated factor VII. Haemophilia 2020;26(1):e5–8.
[58] Seaman CD, Ragni MV. Sequential bypassing agents during major orthopedic surgery: a new approach to hemostasis. Blood Adv 2017;1(17):1309–11.
[59] Le Quellec S, Negrier C. Emicizumab should be prescribed independent of immune tolerance induction. Blood Adv 2018;2(20):2783–6.
[60] Nathwani AC. Gene therapy for hemophilia. Hematology Am Soc Hematol Educ Program 2019;2019(1):1–8.
[61] Perrin GQ, Herzog RW, Markusic DM. Update on clinical gene therapy for hemophilia. Blood 2019;133(5):407–14.
[62] Sidonio RF Jr, Pipe SW, Callaghan MU, et al. Discussing investigational AAV gene therapy with hemophilia patients: a guide. Blood Rev 2021;47:100759.
[63] Anguela XM, High KA. Entering the modern era of gene therapy. Annu Rev Med 2019;70: 273–88.
[64] Brunetti-Pierri N, Ng P. Adenoviral vectors for hemophilia gene therapy. J Genet Syndr Gene Ther 2013;2(Suppl 1):017.
[65] High KA, Roncarolo MG. Gene Therapy. N Engl J Med 2019;381(5):455–64.
[66] Rangarajan S, Walsh L, Lester W, et al. AAV5-factor VIII gene transfer in severe hemophilia A. N Engl J Med 2017;377(26):2519–30.
[67] Pasi KJ, Rangarajan S, Mitchell N, et al. Multiyear follow-up of AAV5-hFVIII-SQ gene therapy for hemophilia A. N Engl J Med 2020;382(1):29–40.
[68] George LA, Monahan PE, Eyster ME, et al. Phase I/II trial of SPK-8011: stable and durable FVIII expression after AAV gene transfer for hemophilia A [abstract]. Res Pract Thromb Haemost 2021;5(Suppl 2). Available at. https://abstracts.isth.org/abstract/phase-i-ii-trial-of-spk-8011-stable-and-durable-fviii-expression-after-aav-gene-transfer-for-hemophilia-a/.

[69] von Drygalski A, Young G. Recent advances in gene therapy for hemophilia clinical trials. Available at. https://genetherapy.isth.org/education/2020-virtual-learning-sessions/nhf-virtual-2021. Accessed November 15, 2021.
[70] Manno CS, Pierce GF, Arruda VR, et al. Successful transduction of liver in hemophilia by AAV-Factor IX and limitations imposed by the host immune response. Nat Med 2006;12(3):342–7.
[71] Nathwani AC, Reiss U, Tuddenham E, et al. Adeno-associated mediated gene transfer for hemophilia B:8 year follow up and impact of removing "empty viral particles" on safety and efficacy of gene transfer. Blood 2018;132(Supplement 1):491.
[72] Donsante A, Miller DG, Li Y, et al. AAV vector integration sites in mouse hepatocellular carcinoma. Science 2007;317(5837):477.

Advances in Pediatrics 69 (2022) 149–162

ADVANCES IN PEDIATRICS

Genital Herpes Simplex Virus—An Updated Review

Saida Omarova, MD*, Aileen Cannon, MD, Wendy Weiss, DO, Adrienne Bruccoleri, DNP, Joseph Puccio, MD

Department of Pediatrics, USF Morsani College of Medicine, 4202 East Fowler Avenue, SHS 100, Tampa, FL 33620, USA

Keywords

• Genital herpes • HSV-1 • HSV-2 • Emotional aspects of HSV • Valacyclovir

Key points

- Genital herpes is a common STI in the United States that is often unrecognized.
- The prevalence of both herpes simplex virus-1 (HSV-1) and HSV-2 has decreased in recent years.
- Increasingly, new genital herpes infections are caused by HSV-1.
- Primary genital herpes infection in pregnant women is responsible for most of the neonatal transmission.
- Treatment with nucleoside analogs reduces the frequency and severity of primary and episodic HSV infection.

INTRODUCTION

The herpes virus was named by the Greek physician Hippocrates who called it herpes because the lesions appeared near each other and were vesicular. Herpes is derived from the Greek word *herpein*, which means reptile, or to creep. Alphaherpesvirinae, Betaherpesvirinae and Gammaherpesvirinae are subfamilies of the human herpesvirus family. The Alphaherpesvirinae subfamily includes the simplex viruses-HSV-1 and 2 and Varicellovirus-varicella zoster virus (VZV). There are more than 200 members of the Herpesviridae family, which are capable of infecting different species, 8 of which are known to cause disease in humans [1]. The simplex viruses can cause lifelong genital infections and despite the prevalence of HSV-1 and HSV-2 infections in the United States

No authors have anv commercial or financial conflicts of interest.

*Corresponding author. *E-mail address:* somarova@usf.edu

https://doi.org/10.1016/j.yapd.2022.03.010

decreasing in the past 20 years, infections with these viruses continue to contribute to significant clinical and psychological morbidities.

EPIDEMIOLOGY/STATISTICS

The WHO estimates that approximately 45% of the US population is infected with HSV-1 and 14.4% with HSV-2 [2]. It is estimated that 48 million Americans have genital HSV-2; however, rates are likely higher because it is not a reportable disease. Most people infected with the virus may lack classic clinical symptoms, that is, vesicles and ulcers, which can delay diagnosis by months or even years. According to a 2016 NHANES survey, Mexican-American adults have the highest prevalence of HSV-1 (~71%) and non-Hispanic blacks have the highest prevalence of HSV-2 (~34%) [3,4]. Since 1999, the prevalence of both HSV-1 and HSV-2 in the United States has decreased among persons aged 14 to 49 years regardless of sex and gender. HSV-1 prevalence decreased from 59.4% in 1999 to 2000 to 48.1% in 2015 to 2016. HSV-2 prevalence decreased from 18.0% in 1999 to 2000 to 12.1% in 2015 to 2016 [4], likely due to safer sex practices and education about human immunodeficiency virus (HIV) [5]. Despite this decline, approximately one million new genital herpes infections are reported each year.

Genital herpes is primarily associated with HSV-2 and typically studied in HSV-2 positive people. In 18 to 49-year-old Americans, women accounted for 2/3 of the genital herpes infections in 2018 [6]. Table 1 [7] shows the estimated incidence and prevalence of HSV-2 among men and women in 2018.

As childhood exposure to orolabial HSV-1 decreases, the overall prevalence of HSV-1 is decreasing. However, as increasing adolescent sexual experiences involve oral-genital contact, genital HSV-1 infection rates have increased, accounting for greater than half of all new genital HSV infections in a 2016 report [8]. In a 9-year retrospective study of college students, genital HSV-1 infections as a percent of genital ulcer disease has increased by 40% since 1993 [9]. The use of condoms for vaginal sex among college students increased by 46% between 1985 and 2000, which may help explain decreased HSV-2 infections in this group. The use of condoms and other barrier methods for oral sex was reportedly as low as 5% in one study of college students [10].

Table 1
Estimated incidence and prevalence of herpes simplex virus-2 among US men and women in 2018

	HSV-2 incidence	HSV-2 prevalence
15–24 yo women	152,000	918,000
15–24 yo men	242,000	398,000
15–49 yo men	300,000	6.4 M
15–49 yo women	260,000	12.2 M

Data from Kreisel KM, Spicknall IH, Gargano JW, et al. Sexually Transmitted Infections Among US Women and Men: Prevalence and Incidence Estimates, 2018. Sexually transmitted diseases. 2021;48(4). https://doi.org/10.1097/OLQ.0000000000001355.

Genital HSV-1 is more common among younger women than younger men. In a study of young adult women, HSV-1 infections were 3 times more likely to be genital than oral. This study also concluded that in young adults, most HSV-1 infections are likely acquired as genital versus oral infections, which are more likely acquired in childhood [11]. Further studies are needed to better estimate the prevalence and incidence of genital herpes, HSV-1 and HSV-2 in all age groups. In 2008, the direct medical costs of genital herpes were $540 million, not accounting for indirect costs of mental health and wellness care [6].

HERPES CLINICAL COURSE

Infection with HSV is lifelong, characterized by primary infection followed by latent infection with episodic reactivation. HSV-1 and HSV-2 are enveloped dsDNA viruses known for their short replicative cycles and ability to infect a variety of host tissues resulting in a wide range of clinical presentations. HSV-2 usually results in genital infections, whereas HSV-1 can cause genital infections as well as other mucocutaneous infections such as orolabial herpes, herpetic gladiatorum, herpetic sycosis (HSV folliculitis), herpetic whitlow, eczema herpeticum, and ocular infections (herpetic keratitis). HSV can also cause more serious infections such as herpetic encephalitis, meningitis, hepatitis, and neonatal herpes [12].

HSV transmission occurs when a mucosal surface or abraded skin comes in contact with infected secretions or mucosa from someone actively shedding virus. Viral replication occurs in the infected cells causing cellular ballooning, nuclear degeneration, and eventual cell lysis resulting in the characteristic blistering or vesicles seen with HSV infection. The virus travels up a sensory nerve to a dorsal root ganglion (usually the sacral ganglion in genital herpes) where additional viral replication occurs and latency is established [13].

Most primary genital HSV infections are asymptomatic or subclinical during which patients are unaware of their infection. When symptomatic primary infection does occur, symptoms tend to be more severe with HSV-2 versus HSV-1 [14]. Systemic symptoms in primary infection occur more often in women (70%) versus men (40%) and can include headache, fever, myalgia, and anorexia. Prodromal symptoms of itching or lower back pain often occur 1 to 2 days before the appearance of lesions. Vesicular lesions usually erupt 4 to 7 days following sexual contact and can continue to erupt for up to 8 days. These painful lesions may evolve from vesicles to pustules to ulcers taking up to 3 weeks to fully resolve. Tender inguinal lymphadenopathy usually appears during the second to third week of the illness and is generally the last symptom to resolve [14].

Lesions of primary genital HSV infections in women usually involve the groin, vulva, vagina, and cervix. In men, lesions are usually found on the glans penis, prepuce, or penile shaft [15]. Perianal infections and proctitis can occur depending on sexual practices. Dysuria is common in both women (80%) and men (40%) and can last for 7 to 10 days [14]. During primary infection, the virus may also spread through peripheral sensory nerves resulting in lesions extending beyond the genital area [14]. Aseptic meningitis can occur in 36% of women and 13% of men with primary genital HSV-2 infections but is rarely a complication of primary HSV-1 genital infection [16].

Reactivation of HSV occurs more commonly than previously thought, often without symptoms. Multiple studies have documented asymptomatic shedding of HSV-2, even in patients without previous symptomatic infection. Genital shedding of HSV-1 is much less frequent than that of HSV-2 [17]. When symptomatic recurrences occur, they may begin with a prodrome of localized tingling, burning, or itching followed by the development of unilateral localized genital lesions [14]. Symptomatic versus primary recurrences tend to be more mild, lack systemic symptoms, and typically resolve within 7 to 10 days. Recurrence rates vary but are more common the first year following primary infection with HSV-2 with an average of 5 recurrences the first year versus HSV-1, which averages 1 recurrence per year. Recurrence rates for HSV-2 decrease after the first year to about 2 recurrences per year [17].

HSV-2 infections are associated with an increased risk for acquiring HIV infection. HIV shedding from genital ulcers has been demonstrated in HIV/HSV-2 infected individuals increasing the risk of HIV transmission [17]. HSV-2 shedding is also increased among HIV infected individuals [18].

DIAGNOSTIC TESTING FOR HERPES SIMPLEX VIRUS

The clinical diagnosis of genital herpes should be confirmed by laboratory testing using either a virologic (direct) testing method to detect viral presence or serologic (indirect) testing for HSV viral antibodies. In addition, serotype-specific testing to distinguish HSV-1 and HSV-2 should always be completed because this will affect clinical prognosis and aid in patient counseling [18].

The most commonly performed virologic testing methods used today include viral culture and nuclear acid amplification testing (NAAT) [18]. Historically, bright field microscopy was used to detect cytopathic changes on specimen samples collected from active lesions. This method, known as the Tzanck smear, is quick and inexpensive but requires expertise in the slide preparation and cytologic interpretation. The Tzanck smear should not be used for clinical diagnosis alone because it fails to distinguish between HSV-1, HSV-2, and VZV and has an overall low sensitivity (84%), necessitating the need to complete confirmatory testing with viral culture or NAAT [19]. Direct immunofluorescence assays (DFA) use fluorescein-labeled monoclonal antibodies to detect HSV antigens from infected specimens. The DFA assays have high specificity (90%–100%) but low sensitivity (61%), limiting their use in the clinical setting [18,19].

When genital lesions are present, a direct testing method with a serotype-specific viral culture or NAAT is preferred [18]. Viral cultures traditionally have been the reference standard for the diagnosis of herpes [20]. Viral cultures are widely available, and in many areas, they may be the only accessible HSV test [18]. The specificity of serotype-specific HSV viral culture approaches 100% for HSV-1 and HSV-2, whereas the sensitivity varies from 50% to

75% and is highly dependent on the stage of the lesion at the time of specimen collection [21]. Herpes virus can be isolated from culture for more than 90% of vesicular or pustular lesions, 70% of ulcerated lesions, and only 27% of crusted lesions [20]. Ideally, specimens for culture should come from vesicular or pustular lesions that are swabbed within the first 3 days of appearance. Samples from several lesions should be obtained–vesicles should be unroofed and then firmly swabbed at the bases. If only ulcerative lesions are present, the bases can similarly be firmly swabbed. Swabs should be immediately placed in viral transport media and specimens held at 4oC until processed by the laboratory [21]. The incubation time for viral cultures depends on the viral concentration in the sample and can vary from 48 hours to 4 to 6 days [20]. A positive culture result confirms HSV infection but a negative culture does not exclude infection. If the clinician is concerned about a possible false-negative culture result, serologic testing may be considered [18].

Multiple NAAT assays to detect HSV-1 and HSV-2 DNA are now commercially available. Polymerase chain reaction (PCR) testing has been the gold standard for the diagnosis of systemic and central nervous system HSV infections and is becoming the preferred testing method for genital infections [22]. Specimen collection from genital lesions for HSV PCR testing is similar to that for viral culture. The specificity of HSV NAAT assays ranges from 90% to 100% with sensitivity of 93% to 100% [19]. HSV NAAT assays also have several other advantages over viral cultures: DNA samples needed for PCR testing are more stable during transport compared with the whole virus sample needed for viral culture; viral cultures can take days to get results, whereas PCR testing can be completed within hours; PCR testing is better able to detect HSV in older lesions that have already ulcerated; HSV PCR testing of anogenital specimens has been found to be more sensitive than viral culture for detecting both HSV-1 and HSV-2 [20].

Serologic testing can detect serotype-specific selective antibodies to HSV-1 and HSV-2. Following primary infection, IgG antibodies to HSV can be detected as early as 2 to 3 weeks but can take up to 6 months to develop. The envelope protein, glycoprotein G, is unique to each virus type (gG1 for HSV-1 and gG2 for HSV-2). Serotype-specific selective testing detects antibodies to these proteins, thereby differentiating HSV-1 from HSV-2 infections. Western blot testing has been the reference standard in herpes serologic testing but is not widely available, limiting its use to mainly research [19]. The most commonly available serologic testing method is enzyme-linked immunosorbent assay (ELISA). Several ELISA tests, both laboratory based assays and point-of-care tests, are currently Food and Drug Administration (FDA) approved and commercially available but sensitivity (80%–98%) and specificity (92%–100%) vary greatly depending on the immunoassay used. False-negative results can occur with recent infection and repeat testing should be considered in 12 weeks if indicated. Similarly, false-positive results are common. In patients with minimal risk factors or who lack symptoms, confirmatory testing using a different method (eg, Western blot) should be considered [22].

The Centers for Disease Control and Prevention (CDC) has several recommendations for the use of HSV-2 type-specific serologic testing. Serologic testing may be useful in patients with atypical or recurrent genital symptoms whose HSV direct viral testing was negative and in patients with a clinical HSV genital infection who did not have confirmatory testing completed using a direct viral testing method. The CDC also recommends HSV-2 serologic testing be considered in specific high-risk patients such as those with greater than 10 lifetime sex partners, prior HIV infection, or men who have sex with men (MSM). These patients should be screened for a history of prior genital lesions or symptoms, and serologic testing for HSV-2 should be offered to those who report lesions or symptoms [18].

SCREENING FOR ASYMPTOMATIC HERPES SIMPLEX VIRUS INFECTION

HSV is a lifelong infection for which there is no cure. Antiviral medications are recommended to treat active lesions and as suppressive therapy to help reduce outbreaks in those with prior symptoms. Early detection and treatment of asymptomatic HSV infection does not alter the clinical prognosis and the CDC currently does not recommend episodic or suppressive antiviral medication in HSV serologic-positive patients without prior symptomatic infection [18]. Direct viral testing methods have poor sensitivity in diagnosing genital HSV infection in the absence of active lesions and the testing of random or blind genital swabs should be avoided [23]. Completing serologic screening of asymptomatic persons could result in a large number of false-positive results and there is currently limited access to confirmatory testing with Western blot. There are potential social and emotional implications associated with false-positive HSV diagnosis. In addition, false-positive HSV diagnoses may lead to unnecessary prescription of antiviral medication. For these reasons, the US Preventive Service Task Force and the CDC recommend against routine serologic screening for genital HSV infection in asymptomatic adolescents and adults, including those who are pregnant [24].

HSV-2 serologic testing may be useful in a select group of asymptomatic patients. The CDC recommends that asymptomatic individuals whose sex partners are diagnosed with genital herpes be screened for a history of genital lesions/symptoms and be offered HSV-2 serologic testing. Screening with HSV-2 serologic testing should also be considered in patients presenting for the initial HIV evaluation [18].

EMOTIONAL/PSYCHOSOCIAL IMPLICATIONS AND COUNSELING

The diagnosis of genital herpes can have a negative impact on both psychological and psychosexual wellbeing. Patients may experience a wide range of emotional responses including feelings of depression, anger, or distress, and a reduction in one's self-esteem and confidence. Some may feel hostility toward the person believed to be the source of their infection [25]. Patients also report being surprised, sad, disappointed, or confused at the diagnosis, whereas others may feel relief to finally know the cause of their symptoms. Patients may feel socially stigmatized and have concerns about transmitting the infection to a sex partner or newborn [26]. Patients can also experience a high level of anxiety because they anticipate disclosing their herpes diagnosis to a sex partner [27].

Being diagnosed with an STI can have a negative impact on relationships leading to challenges in developing and achieving intimacy. Those diagnosed with genital herpes have reported feeling sexually undesirable and some may purposely avoid sexual contact to prevent spreading the infections to others. Psychosexual morbidity from genital herpes can also include a change in libido, pain with sex, and erectile dysfunction [26].

Every effort should be made to make a rapid and reliable diagnosis. Patients should be educated regarding HSV infection and advised on available antiviral treatments [26]. For those with symptoms, psychological distress increases with each recurrence. In patients with recurrent genital herpes, studies have shown the use of antiviral suppressive therapy with acyclovir or valacyclovir can dramatically reduce psychological morbidity and improve quality of life [26]. The improvement in quality of life is due in part to the reduction of symptoms [27]. Patients should also be educated on effective HSV prevention and safer sex practice, so they can protect themselves from other STIs and reduce the risk of infecting others with HSV [27].

In addition to suppressive antiviral medications, psychotherapy focusing on cognitive coping strategies has been shown to decrease psychological and psychosexual morbidity [26]. Coping strategies should focus on helping an individual deal with further outbreaks, informing new partners or significant others of their diagnosis, and reducing anxiety and stress in daily life [26]. Patients taking daily suppressive antiviral medications, for example, acyclovir, may lower the risk of transmission to seronegative partners by 70% [28]. Daily or episodic antiviral medication reduces the risk of lesion recurrence and asymptomatic viral shedding. The psychological effects of HSV diagnosis may often be incongruent with disease severity [18].

According to the CDC, counseling patients with genital HSV should include the following:

- Awareness of prodromal symptoms and potential risk of transmission during asymptomatic shedding, which is more common in the first 12 months.
- The effectiveness of suppressive antiviral medication in preventing symptomatic recurrences and in reducing transmission of HSV-2.
- The importance of informing partners about genital HSV before starting a sexual relationship.
- The higher risk of vertical transmission to the neonate during primary genital HSV infection or active outbreak during delivery.
- The increased risk of HIV acquisition in those infected with HSV-2.
- The benefit of suppressive therapy to prevent transmission among asymptomatic genital HSV patients is unknown.

- The rate of recurrences and viral shedding are lower in HSV-1 than HSV-2 infection.
- Patients with frequent genital HSV-1 recurrences may be offered suppressive therapy.
- Patients with genital HSV should inform the providers who will be caring for them during pregnancy.
- Suppressive therapy may be offered to patients with significant psychological trauma from genital HSV diagnosis [18].

PREVENTION

Due to the often diverse presentation of genital HSV, counseling and education are key to prevention and management [18]. Sexual abstinence is the only method of complete prevention [29]. Consistent condom use greatly reduces the risk of genital HSV transmission from men to women but is less effective in the transmission from women to men [18]. Latex condom use is highly recommended in serodiscordant HSV couples to prevent transmission to the uninfected partner because asymptomatic shedding is common. Increased education and awareness of other methods of protection such as dental dams and female condoms may be important in lowering transmission because there have been increased rates of genital HSV-1 from oral sex. Because most HSV infections are asymptomatic, there is a need for better education, counseling, and discussion about the benefits of monogamous partnership. HSV is not a reportable disease; therefore, patients should be encouraged to learn about HSV and to discuss the condition before starting a sexual relationship. Factors that help prevent HIV transmission can also be effective for HSV. For example, rates of transmission to women are lower if the male partner is circumcised, and medical male circumcision in adulthood also decreases the rate of HSV transmission. Several studies have found decreased risk of HSV-2 acquisition among men over the age of 15 who received medical male circumcision, with subsequent lower risk of transmission to female partners [30]. Research has shown that preexposure prophylaxis (PrEP) for HIV lowers the risk of genital HSV-2 by 30% in heterosexual couples due to anti-HSV-2 activity of the antiviral drug tenofovir [31].

There is a 51% decreased incidence of HSV-2 with pericoital use of 1% tenofovir vaginal gel and tenofovir, and detectable intravaginal levels are associated with protection against HSV-1 and HSV-2 [32]. Ongoing studies are investigating the role of PrEP and tenofovir in the prevention of HSV-1 and HSV-2 in all populations. Despite various preventive HSV vaccine trials, results have failed to show significant efficacy in preventing genital HSV disease in both men and women [33].

TREATMENT

There are currently 3 FDA-approved antiviral medications for the treatment of genital herpes: acyclovir, valacyclovir, and famciclovir [34]. These drugs are nucleoside analogs that inhibit HSV replication via thymidine kinase activity

[34]. According to the CDC, patients with a first episode of symptomatic genital herpes should be treated with an antiviral agent for 7 to 10 days or until resolution of lesions occurs [18,35]. The treatment is aimed at reducing days with symptoms because there is no permanent cure. Table 2 [18] outlines the current treatment guidelines for genital herpes. Table 3 [18] lists the guidelines for the treatment of genital herpes in persons living with HIV infection.

There are ongoing clinical trials of a therapeutic HSV-2 vaccine that has shown decreased viral shedding and 50% reduction in recurrence rates in HSV-2-infected participants [3].

Table 2
2021 Centers for Disease Control and Prevention genital herpes treatment guidelines

Indication	Acyclovir	Valacyclovir	Famciclovir
First-episode infection (treatment can be extended if healing is incomplete after 10 d of therapy)	400 mg orally 3 times daily for 7–10 d or (acyclovir 200 mg orally 5 times daily is also effective but not recommended due to frequency of dosing)	1 g orally twice daily for 7–10 d	250 mg orally 3 times daily for 7–10 d
Suppressive therapy for HSV-2	400 mg orally 2 times daily	500 mg orally once daily or 1g orally once daily (higher dose may be needed for persons with recurrences >10/y)	250 mg orally twice daily
Episodic recurrent HSV-2	800 mg orally twice daily for 5 d or 800 mg orally 3 times daily for 2 d, (400 mg orally 3 times daily for 5 d is effective but not recommended due to frequency of dosing)	500 mg orally twice daily for 3 d or 1 g orally daily for 5 d	500 mg orally once, followed by 250 mg twice daily for 2 d or 125 mg orally twice daily for 5 d
Severe or disseminated disease	5–10 mg/kg intravenously every 8 h until clinical improvement, then oral therapy to complete 10 d		

Data from Workowski KA, Bachmann LH, Chan PA, et al. Sexually Transmitted Infections Treatment Guidelines, 2021. MMWR Recommendations and reports: Morbidity and mortality weekly report Recommendations and reports. 2021;70(4).

Table 3
2021 Centers for Disease Control and Prevention genital herpes treatment guidelines among persons with human immunodeficiency virus infection

Indication	Acyclovir	Valacyclovir	Famciclovir
First-episode infection (treatment can be extended if healing is incomplete after 10 d of therapy)	400 mg orally 3 times daily for 7–10 d or (acyclovir 200 mg orally 5 times daily is also effective but not recommended due to frequency of dosing)	1 g orally twice daily for 7–10 d	250 mg orally 3 times daily for 7–10 d
Suppressive therapy for HSV-2	400–800 mg orally 2–3 times daily	500 mg orally twice daily	500 mg orally twice daily
Episodic recurrent HSV-2	400 mg orally 3 times daily for 5–10 d	1 g orally twice daily for 5–10 d	500 mg orally twice daily for 5–10 d

Data from Workowski KA, Bachmann LH, Chan PA, et al. Sexually Transmitted Infections Treatment Guidelines, 2021. MMWR Recommendations and reports: Morbidity and mortality weekly report Recommendations and reports. 2021;70(4).

PREGNANCY AND HERPES SIMPLEX VIRUS

Vertical transmission to the neonate of an infected mother represents the greatest genital HSV concern related to pregnancy. HSV neonatal infection occurs through direct contact with virus shed from the cervix, vagina, vulva, or perianal area. Neonatal HSV infection has a high risk of mortality, and those that survive are often burdened with permanent disability. Most neonatal infections are acquired perinatally [36]. Most mothers of newborns with perinatally acquired HSV infection are asymptomatic and lack a history of clinically evident genital herpes at the time of delivery [37].

Primary genital HSV infection is defined as first occurrence of HSV infection in a previously seronegative mother. Primary infections acquired near the time of delivery present the highest risk of neonatal infection. Nonprimary first episode of HSV infections is defined as first occurrence of HSV infection in a mother who has preexisting antibody for a different HSV type. The risk of mothers developing a nonprimary first episode versus a primary infection is slightly lower, and the risk of vertical transmission is slightly lower. The differences in rates of neonatal infection for each class of infection (primary, nonprimary, and recurrent) seem to be related to the presence/absence of type-specific HSV antibodies and amount of viral exposure (both concentration and duration of viral shedding) in the mother [38]. Genital HSV infections acquired in the first half of pregnancy pose a lower risk of vertical transmission. Type-specific antibodies develop within 12 weeks after maternal infection and may play a protective role in lowering the frequency of neonatal infections in women with recurrent HSV [39]. The likelihood of transmission is largely dependent on the maternal HSV classification (primary vs recurrent), maternal HSV antibody status, duration of ruptured membranes, use of fetal scalp monitors, use of forceps or vacuum, and mode of delivery (cesarean vs vaginal) [40].

In women with previously confirmed HSV, there is no indication for repeat testing during pregnancy. Testing should be completed in women without a known history of HSV who present with suspicious lesions. Swabs from lesions should be collected for HSV type-specific testing such as viral culture or PCR. PCR testing is preferred due to the low sensitivity of viral cultures, particularly for recurrent or healing lesions. A negative PCR or viral culture result does not exclude the presence of infection. The American College of Obstetricians and Gynecologists (ACOG) does not recommend routine HSV screening of pregnant women and does not recommend antepartum genital HSV cultures in asymptomatic patients with recurrent disease [41].

Women who have no history of genital HSV and present with new genital ulcers during pregnancy should be treated empirically with acyclovir until healing is complete and culture results are known. Women with a history of recurrent genital HSV should be placed on suppressive therapy starting at 36 weeks gestation, which has been shown to decrease recurrences at term, thereby reducing the frequency of cesarean delivery [18] (Table 4). Although suppressive therapy may reduce maternal symptoms and shedding, reduction of neonatal infection has not been shown [42]. Women with recurrent HSV and no active lesions or prodromal symptoms do not need cesarean delivery because the neonatal risk is low, estimated to be 2/10,000 births [43]. In women who have a primary or nonprimary first episode infection in their third trimester, cesarean delivery is preferred but suppressive therapy may mitigate risk enough to allow for vaginal delivery. In women with active genital lesions or prodromal symptoms such as vulvar pain or burning, the CDC and ACOG recommend cesarean delivery as soon as possible after rupture of membranes or onset of labor.

Table 4
2021 Centers for Disease Control and Prevention genital herpes treatment guidelines in pregnancy

Indication	Acyclovir	Valacyclovir
First-episode infection	400 mg orally 3 times daily for 7–10 d	
Daily suppressive therapy (starting at 36 wk gestation)	400 mg orally 3 times daily	500 mg orally twice daily

Data from Workowski KA, Bachmann LH, Chan PA, et al. Sexually Transmitted Infections Treatment Guidelines, 2021. MMWR Recommendations and reports: Morbidity and mortality weekly report Recommendations and reports. 2021;70(4).

SUMMARY

HSV are endemic worldwide. In the alpha Herpesviridae family there are 2 major viruses, HSV-1 and HSV-2 [1]. Previously, HSV-1 was primarily associated with oral lesions and HSV-2 with genital lesions. Although the prevalence of HSV-1 genital infection from oral-to-genital contact has increased, the episodic recurrences are less frequent than for HSV-2. Often, genital HSV infection may be asymptomatic or it may result in painful ulcers [1]. HSV infection can be transmitted to neonates through infected mothers during birth and from oral contact with caregivers postnatally. Although neonatal infection is rare, it can be fatal or disabling. Those who have acquired HSV-2 infections are at increased risk for infection with the HIV. Symptomatic and asymptomatic viral shedding are common for both HSV-1 and HSV-2. Infected individuals can be asymptomatic yet contagious, which contributes to the infective burden of HSV [7].

CLINICS CARE POINTS

- Most new HSV-1 infections are genital versus oral in young adults.
- Most primary genital HSV infections are asymptomatic or subclinical and systemic symptoms with primary infection occur more commonly in women.
- Reactivation of HSV occurs more commonly than previously thought, often asymptomatically.
- IgG antibodies to HSV may take up to 6 months to be detected in serum of infected people.
- Genital HSV infections acquired in the first half of pregnancy pose a lower risk of vertical transmission to the fetus.

References

[1] Rechenchoski DZ, Faccin-Galhardi LC, Linhares REC, et al. Herpesvirus: an underestimated virus. Folia Microbiologica 2017;62(2); https://doi.org/10.1007/s12223-016-0482-7.

[2] Harris KD. Herpes Simplex Virus Keratitis. Home Healthc Now 2019;37(5); https://doi.org/10.1097/NHH.0000000000000791.

[3] Bernstein DI, Flechtner JB, McNeil LK, et al. Therapeutic HSV-2 vaccine decreases recurrent virus shedding and recurrent genital herpes disease. Vaccine 2019;37(26); https://doi.org/10.1016/j.vaccine.2019.05.009.

[4] McQuillan G, Kruszon-Moran D, Flagg EW, et al. Prevalence of Herpes Simplex Virus Type 1 and Type 2 in Persons Aged 14-49: United States, 2015-2016. NCHS data brief 2018;(304):1–8.

[5] Chemaitelly H, Nagelkerke N, Omori R, et al. Characterizing herpes simplex virus type 1 and type 2 seroprevalence declines and epidemiological association in the United States. PLoS One 2019;14(6); https://doi.org/10.1371/journal.pone.0214151.

[6] Spicknall IH, Flagg EW, Torrone EA. Estimates of the Prevalence and Incidence of Genital Herpes, United States, 2018. Sex Transm Dis 2021;48(4); https://doi.org/10.1097/OLQ.0000000000001375.

[7] Kreisel KM, Spicknall IH, Gargano JW, et al. Sexually Transmitted Infections Among US Women and Men: Prevalence and Incidence Estimates, 2018. Sex Transm Dis 2021;48(4); https://doi.org/10.1097/OLQ.0000000000001355.

[8] Groves MJ. Genital herpes: A review. Am Fam Physician 2016;93(11):928–34.
[9] Roberts CM, Pfister JR, Spear SJ. Increasing proportion of herpes simplex virus type 1 as a cause of genital herpes infection in college students. Sex Transm Dis 2003;30(10); https://doi.org/10.1097/01.OLQ.0000092387.58746.C7.
[10] American College Health Association. American College Health Association-National College Health Assessment. Reference Group Executive Summary.; 2020.
[11] Bernstein DI, Bellamy AR, Hook EW, et al. Epidemiology, clinical presentation, and antibody response to primary infection with herpes simplex virus type 1 and type 2 in young women. Clin Infect Dis 2013;56(3); https://doi.org/10.1093/cid/cis891.
[12] Mustafa M, Illzam EM, Muniandy RK, et al. Herpes simplex virus infections, Pathophysiology and Management. IOSR J Dental Med Sci 2016;15(07):85–91.
[13] Whitley R, Kimberlin DW, Prober CG. Pathogenesis and disease. In: Arvin A, Campadelli-Fiume G, Mocarski E, et al., editors. Human Herpesviruses: Biology, Therapy, and Immunoprophylaxis. Cambridge: Cambridge University Press; 2007. Chapter 32.
[14] Sauerbrei A. Herpes Genitalis: Diagnosis, Treatment and Prevention. Geburtshilfe Frauenheilkd 2016;76(12):1310–7.
[15] Whitley RJ. Herpesviruses. In: Baron S, editor. Medical microbiology. 4th edition. Galveston (TX): University of Texas Medical Branch at Galveston; 1996. p. 1996, *Chapter 68. Available From.*
[16] Berger JR, Houff S. Neurological Complications of Herpes Simplex Virus Type 2 Infection. Arch Neurol 2008;65(5); https://doi.org/10.1001/archneur.65.5.596.
[17] Johnston C, Corey L. Current concepts for genital herpes simplex virus infection: Diagnostics and pathogenesis of genital tract shedding. Clin Microbiol Rev 2015;29(1):149–61.
[18] Workowski KA, Bachmann LH, Chan PA, et al. Sexually Transmitted Infections Treatment Guidelines, 2021. MMWR Recommendations and reports : Morbidity and mortality weekly report Recommendations and reports 2021;70(4); https://doi.org/10.15585/mmwr.rr7004a1.
[19] Nath P, Kabir MA, Doust SK, et al. Diagnosis of herpes simplex virus: Laboratory and point-of-care techniques. Infect Dis Rep 2021;13(2):518–39.
[20] van Wagoner NJ, Hook EW. Herpes diagnostic tests and their use. Curr Infect Dis Rep 2012;14(2):175–84.
[21] Singh A, Preiksaitis J, Frcpc MD, Romanowski B. The Laboratory Diagnosis of Herpes Simplex Virus Infections. Vol 16.
[22] Strick LB, Wald A. Diagnostics for Herpes Simplex Virus Is PCR the New Gold Standard? Vol 10.; 2006.
[23] Morbidity and Mortality Weekly Report. MMWR Surveill Summ 2021;70(8); https://doi.org/10.15585/mmwr.mm7008a4.
[24] Bibbins-Domingo K, Grossman DC, Curry SJ, et al. Serologic screening for genital herpes infection: US preventive services task force recommendation statement. JAMA 2016;316(23):2525–30.
[25] Mindel A. Psychological and psychosexual implications of herpes simplex virus infections. Scand J Infect Dis Suppl 1996;100:27–32.
[26] Mindel A, Marks C. Psychological Symptoms Associated with Genital Herpes Virus Infections Epidemiology and Approaches to Management. Vol 19.; 2005.
[27] Merin A, Pachankis JE. The psychological impact of genital herpes stigma. J Health Psychol 2011;16(1):80–90.
[28] Leone P. Chapter 14. Genital Herpes. In: Klausner JD, Hook EW, editors. CURRENT diagnosis & treatment of sexually transmitted diseases. New York: The McGraw-Hill Companies; 2007. p. 84–90. Available at: http://accessmedicine.mhmedical.com/content.aspx?aid=3025329.
[29] Nath AK, Thappa DM. Newer trends in the management of genital herpes. Indian J Dermatol Venereol Leprol 2009;75(6); https://doi.org/10.4103/0378-6323.57716.

[30] Grund JM, Bryant TS, Jackson I, et al. Association between male circumcision and women's biomedical health outcomes: a systematic review. Lancet Glob Health 2017;5(11); https://doi.org/10.1016/S2214-109X(17)30369-8.
[31] Celum C, Morrow RA, Donnell D, et al. Daily oral tenofovir and emtricitabine-tenofovir pre-exposure prophylaxis reduces herpes simplex virus type 2 acquisition among heterosexual HIV-1-uninfected men and women: A subgroup analysis of a randomized trial. Ann Intern Med 2014;161(1); https://doi.org/10.7326/M13-2471.
[32] Karim SSA, Kashuba AD, Werner L, et al. Drug concentrations after topical and oral antiretroviral pre-exposure prophylaxis: Implications for HIV prevention in women. Lancet 2011;378(9787); https://doi.org/10.1016/S0140-6736(11)60878-7.
[33] Belshe RB, Leone PA, Bernstein DI, et al. Efficacy Results of a Trial of a Herpes Simplex Vaccine. N Engl J Med 2012;366(1); https://doi.org/10.1056/nejmoa1103151.
[34] Sauerbrei A. Optimal management of genital herpes: Current perspectives. Infect Drug Resist 2016;9; https://doi.org/10.2147/IDR.S96164.
[35] Parks G. Genital Herpes. In: Nelson AL, Woodward J, Wysocki S, editors. Sexually transmitted diseases: a practical guide for primary care. Totowa(NJ): Humana Press; 2006. p. 47–70; https://doi.org/10.1007/978-1-59745-040-9_3.
[36] Kimberlin DW. Herpes Simplex Virus Infections of the Newborn. Semin Perinatol 2007;31(1); https://doi.org/10.1053/j.semperi.2007.01.003.
[37] Pinninti SG, Kimberlin DW. Maternal and neonatal herpes simplex virus infections. Am J Perinatol 2013;30(2); https://doi.org/10.1055/s-0032-1332802.
[38] Brown ZA. Neonatal herpes simplex virus infection in relation to asymptomatic maternal infection at the time of labor. Pediatr Infect Dis J 1991;10(8); https://doi.org/10.1097/00006454-199108000-00028.
[39] Johnston C, Magaret A, Selke S, et al. Herpes simplex virus viremia during primary genital infection. J Infect Dis 2008;198(1); https://doi.org/10.1086/588676.
[40] Corey L, Wald A. Maternal and Neonatal Herpes Simplex Virus Infections. N Engl J Med 2009;361(14); https://doi.org/10.1056/nejmra0807633.
[41] ACOG. PB 220: Management of Genital Herpes in Pregnancy. Obstet Gynecol 2020;133(76).
[42] Hollier LM, Wendel GD. Third trimester antiviral prophylaxis for preventing maternal genital herpes simplex virus (HSV) recurrences and neonatal infection. Cochrane Database Syst Rev 2008;1; https://doi.org/10.1002/14651858.CD004946.pub2.
[43] Vontver LA, Hickok DE, Brown Z, et al. Recurrent genital herpes simplex virus infection in pregnancy: Infant outcome and frequency of asymptomatic recurrences. Am J Obstet Gynecol 1982;143(1); https://doi.org/10.1016/0002-9378(82)90686-X.

Advances in Pediatrics 69 (2022) 163–176

ADVANCES IN PEDIATRICS

Vaccine Hesitancy in Pediatrics

Andrea Lafnitzegger, DO[a],
Claudia Gaviria-Agudelo, MD[b,*]

[a]Pediatrics, University of South Florida Morsani College of Medicine, 2 Tampa General Circle, Tampa, FL 33606, USA; [b]Pediatric Infectious Diseases, University of South Florida Morsani College of Medicine, 2 Tampa General Circle, Tampa, FL 33606, USA

Keywords

• Vaccine hesitancy • Vaccine refusal • Vaccinations • Immunizations • Pediatrics • Children

Key points

- The term "vaccine hesitancy" encompasses a wide spectrum of vaccine attitudes and beliefs, which vary from cautious acceptance to complete refusal of vaccinations.
- Parents' opinions about vaccines are influenced by a multitude of individual and contextual factors that need to be acknowledged and understood by providers.
- Health care providers remain the most trusted source about vaccines for the general public.
- Motivational interviewing is an effective communication tool that can be used to address vaccine hesitancy among parents.

INTRODUCTION

For decades, vaccinations have decreased the burden of infectious diseases and have been described as one of the top 10 greatest public health achievements worldwide [1]. Vaccines have allowed for the eradication of smallpox, the near eradication of polio, and the prevention of over 21 million hospitalizations and 732,000 deaths among children born in the last two decades [2]. Despite these remarkable achievements, there continues to be a spectrum of parental concerns regarding childhood vaccinations. Unfortunately, this is an increasing trend [3], and parents consider human papillomavirus and influenza vaccines to

*Corresponding author. *E-mail address:* claudiag13@usf.edu

https://doi.org/10.1016/j.yapd.2022.03.011
0065-3101/22/Published by Elsevier Inc.

be particularly problematic [4,5]. SARS-CoV-2 vaccination in children is also a controversial topic at this time, which will not be covered in this review.

Parents' confidence in vaccines is critical to the success of national immunization programs [6]. However, vaccines can be a victim of their own success as the visibility of vaccine-preventable diseases (VPDs) is dramatically reduced [7–9]. Children who are not vaccinated due to parental refusal remain at increased risk of acquiring VPDs which can subsequently contribute to outbreaks [10], as has been noted with measles and pertussis over the last several years [11].

Additionally, parents are more often requesting exemptions to school entry requirements for vaccination, and providers perceive parental vaccine refusal as being more common [6]. It has been estimated that 13% to 27% of parents of young children delay recommended vaccinations and 6% to 16% decline recommended vaccinations in the United States [12].

The term "vaccine hesitancy" helps identify and define individual's concerns surrounding vaccination [11,13]. In this review, we discuss important aspects about general vaccine hesitancy regarding routine pediatric immunizations. We also provide strategies that health care professionals can use to address it in pediatric clinical practice.

DEFINING VACCINE HESITANCY

In 2012, the World Health Organization's (WHO) Strategic Advisory Group of Experts (SAGE) on Immunizations developed a working group to address vaccine hesitancy due to the growing concerns of its effects on vaccine uptake. The SAGE working group defines vaccine hesitancy as "delay in acceptance or refusal of vaccines despite availability of vaccination services" [14]. Although there are many barriers and identified factors that prevent parents from vaccinating their children, vaccine hesitancy focuses more on those who choose not to vaccinate despite elimination of these barriers [15].

Parents' vaccine attitudes influence their decision regarding child vaccination [16]. The WHO further explains that vaccine hesitancy is "complex and context specific, varying across time, place, and vaccines and is influenced by complacency, convenience, and confidence" [14]. Dube and colleagues reflect on the challenge of defining and categorizing vaccine attitudes while also providing a very comprehensive conceptual model of vaccine hesitancy (Fig. 1) [13].

The spectrum of vaccine acceptance

Before the use of the term "vaccine hesitancy," a more polarizing view of vaccine beliefs divided people into either "pro-vaccinators" or "anti-vaccinators" [17]. It is increasingly recognized that a spectrum or a continuum of vaccine acceptance exists [14]. This continuum ranges from individuals that accept all vaccines with no doubts, to those who completely refuse with no doubts, with vaccine-hesitant individuals between these two extremes (Fig. 2). It is important to note that a parent could have one or multiple concerns related to vaccines and still decide to vaccinate their child [18]. Leask and colleagues further defined five distinct parental groups, including the "unquestioning acceptor," the "cautious acceptor," the "hesitant," the "late or selective vaccinator," and the "refuser" of all vaccines [19]. Dividing vaccine hesitancy into these five groups not only helps providers understand the wide scope of vaccine attitudes but also helps them tailor their interventions.

MAJOR REASONS FOR VACCINE HESITANCY

Vaccine hesitancy is related to a range of both psychological and demographic determinants, such as attitudes toward vaccinations, social norms, and trust in science [20]. Two dominant themes emerged in the literature: understanding the parental decision-making framework and the individual factors that lead to vaccine hesitancy.

Of note, there have been inconsistencies in the descriptions of the demographic factors that predict vaccine hesitancy (age, gender, ethnicity, level of education, income, location, religiosity, political views, specific vaccine, etc.) [21]. Future research should continue to explore these factors and additional attitudinal predictors.

PARENTAL DECISION-MAKING

Several studies have described the complexity of parental decision-making regarding vaccinations [20,22–25]. Vaccine decision-making involves emotional, cultural, social, spiritual, and political factors in addition to cognitive factors [13]. Fig. 3 presents a conceptual model of parental vaccine decision-making.

The most common health model used to examine parental attitudes and beliefs toward vaccinations is the Health Belief Model [26]. This theoretic framework examines patient motivations for adopting a health-related behavior [6]. Other studies have used interviews through focus groups to identify patterns in parents' thoughts and attitudes toward vaccination. Blaisdell and colleagues reported that when parents perceived ambiguity related to vaccine-associated risks, they created their own subjective risk judgments. Predominantly, these judgments yielded three main approaches to parental vaccination risk assessments: "(1) maximizing perceived risk of harm from vaccines, (2) minimizing perceived risk of contracting VPDs, and (3) maximizing their perceived control over VPDs risk" [27].

Common reasons for vaccine refusal

Fear and mistrust in vaccines, which have existed since inoculation was introduced, are increasing among parents [16]. In a systematic review, Gidengil and colleagues identified seven themes for childhood vaccination in the United States, including adverse effects, mistrust, perceived lack of necessity, provaccine opinions, skepticism about effectiveness, desire for autonomy, and morality concerns [28].

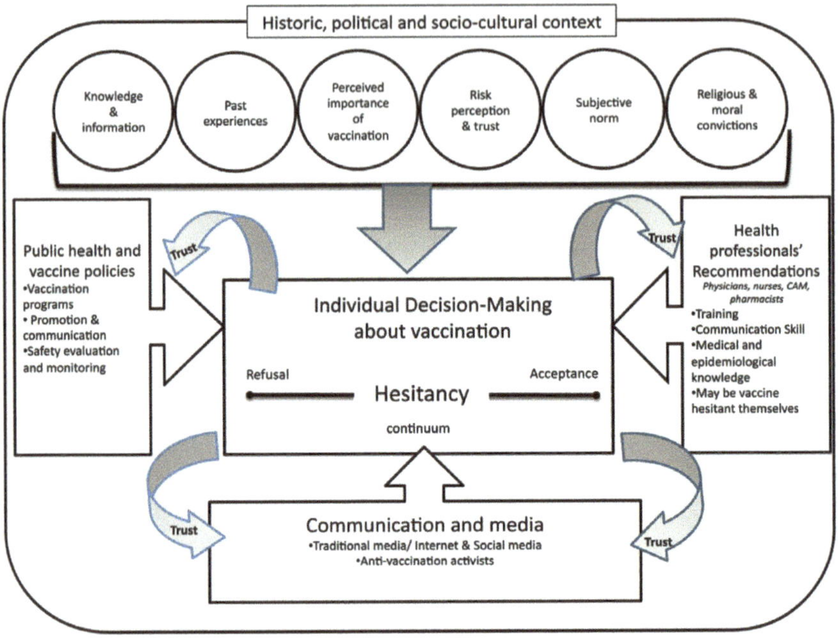

Fig. 1. Conceptual model of general vaccine hesitancy. (*From* [Dubé, E., Laberge, C., Guay, M., et al. (2013). Vaccine hesitancy: an overview. Human vaccines & immunotherapeutics, 9(8), 1763-1773.] with permission.)

Vaccine-hesitant parents often mention vaccine safety and vaccine effectiveness as their principal concerns [11,29]. Some are unsure why their children still need to be vaccinated "against diseases that are now rare" [7]. Protection from perceived risk of vaccines conflicts with protection from disease, as many parents today have never experienced VPDs and may underestimate the diseases' severity [24,29,30]. One study described how, for some parents, regrets can originate more from action than inaction regarding vaccines and risk perception [25].

Parents become concerned about possible negative consequences of vaccines including potential long-term effects. Surveys have found that the most common vaccine attitudes and beliefs were "vaccines cause illness," "too many vaccines overwhelm a child's immune system," "vaccines contain harmful ingredients," "natural immunity is better," "adverse events are more likely in younger children," and "the alternative motive that vaccination is done for business and profit" [30].

Additionally, some parents choose to customize the immunization schedule, with 34% believing children "get too many vaccines" during their first 2 years of life and 92% preferring that 3 or fewer vaccines be given at one time [30]. However, infants today actually receive fewer vaccine antigens than in the past [11,29]. Medical providers face the challenge of allowing accommodations

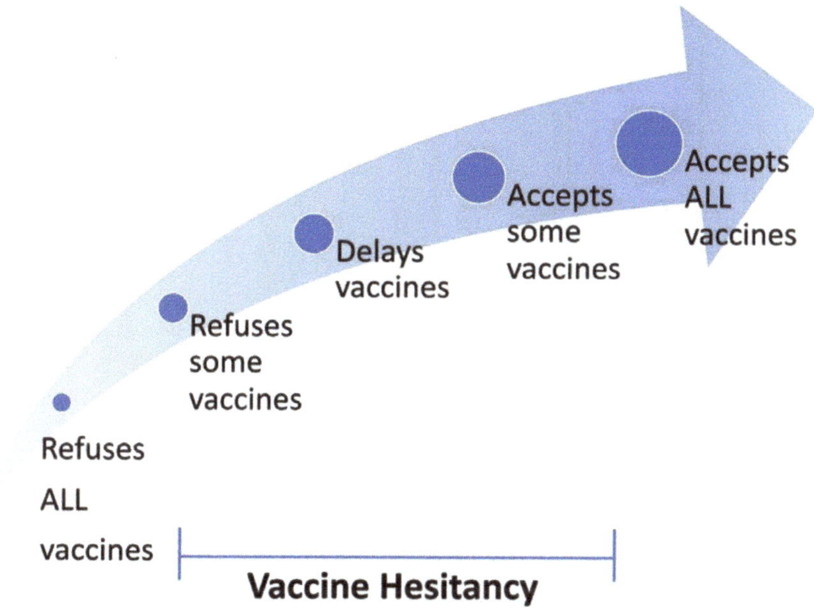

Fig. 2. Continuum of vaccine acceptance. (*Data from* [SAGE Working. (2014). Report of the SAGE working group on vaccine hesitancy. Geneva: World Health Organization].)

for parental preferences by creating alternative vaccine schedules with the goal of still providing all recommended immunizations [11].

At the same time, the "naturalistic view," which considers exposure to the disease itself to be often preferable to vaccinations, is growing in popularity among parents [4]. This approach seems to be common in parents who make choices they consider to be healthier and safer, for example, eating organic food and taking alternative approaches to health care and education [11,24]. It has been estimated that parents of unvaccinated children can be four times more likely to use services of alternative medicine providers such as a chiropractor for primary care [31].

Regarding vaccines and concerns about autism spectrum disorder, an article published by Andrew Wakefield in 1998 claimed that the measles, mumps, and rubella (MMR) vaccine caused an intestinal inflammation cascade ultimately leading to autism spectrum disorder [32]. The study was small ($n = 12$), uncontrolled, and the investigator had undisclosed financial interests. The article was eventually retracted, and the investigator was charged with ethical and scientific misconduct. Since the initial publication of this, multiple well-designed studies have debunked the claims that vaccinations increase the risk of autism spectrum disorder [11]. However, concerns and mistrust of the MMR vaccine and vaccines, in general, continue with parents fearing a link between the vaccination and development of autism.

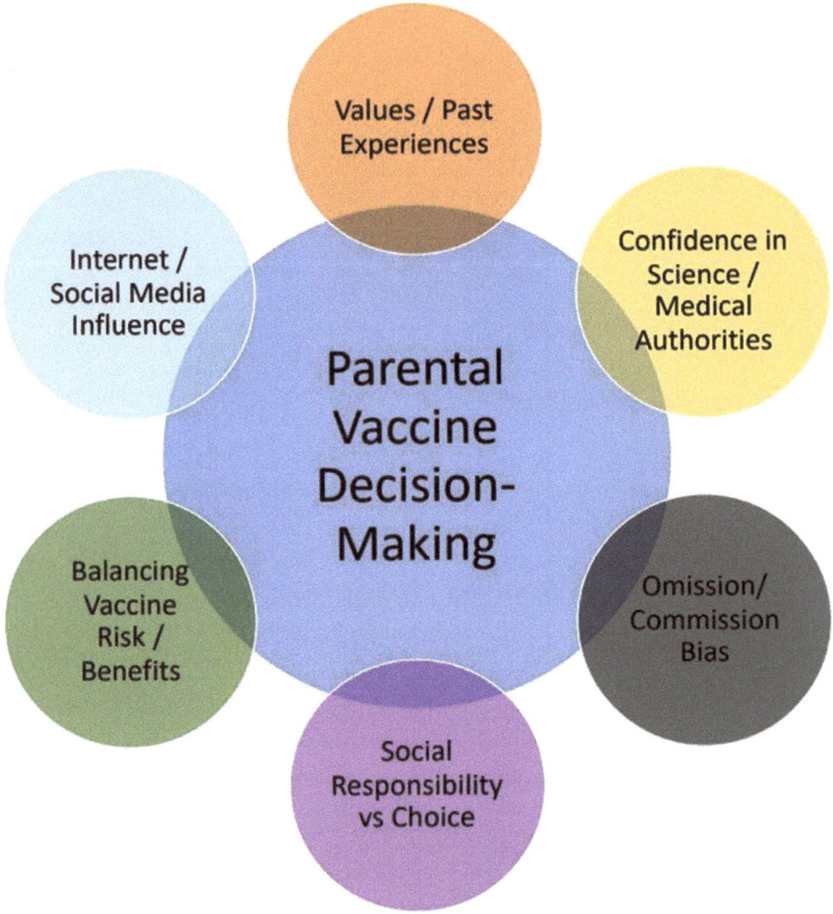

Fig. 3. Conceptual model of parental vaccine decision-making.

INDIVIDUAL FACTORS

Conspiracy theory

The effectiveness of educational interventions is limited by individuals' trust in the sources that provide risk and benefit information; this trust is influenced by ideology [33]. Several empirical studies indicate that people's ideologies strongly influence their perception and acceptance of risk; distrust in the medical establishment or other authoritative bodies coincides with distrust in the government and the pharmaceutical industry [24,34,35]. The pharmaceutical industry, in particular, is often considered untrustworthy, with its influence on research, medical professionals, and government being perceived negatively [24,36].

Widespread conspiracy beliefs that impact vaccination decisions can be mediated by feelings of powerlessness, disillusionment, and mistrust in authorities [23]. Vaccine conspiracy beliefs were among multiple significant predictors of parents' willingness to vaccinate [16], and the odds that parents who distrust the government have seen a complementary/alternative medicine provider were 2.1 times greater than those of parents who trust the government [37]. Parents who distrust the government also had increased odds of distrusting vaccine information acquired at their health care providers' offices [16].

Medical providers are frustrated that misinformation tends to be resistant to correction [23]. For some parents, providing evidence about the safety of vaccines may not be sufficient. There is ample evidence that most science deniers are not going to be convinced by even the most carefully presented information [9]. Parents choose "what" or "whom" they view as the expert system and, while placing trust in that system, they make the decision to vaccinate or not [24].

Contextual influences/social pressure

Parents feel a social pressure with vaccine decision-making [3] and deciding to vaccinate can be perceived as "a socially forced choice" [20]. This social pressure might lead to parents overemphasizing the potential side effects related to vaccines, rather than focusing on the benefits [20]. The biased focus on the potential risks is especially relevant for families that practice intensive parenting (child-centered, time-intensive, and self-sacrificing parenting)–one of the most dominant parenting styles today [20]. Additionally, parents who received vaccine information from friends, family, or books were more likely to have specific immunization concerns than parents who received it from physicians [38].

Pain perception

Fear of needles and vaccination-related pain are barriers to vaccination for 5% to 10% of parents [11,13,39]. Although techniques for minimizing pain including applying pressure, distraction, administration of local anesthetics, and breastfeeding can be used, childhood experiences of vaccine related pain are disturbing to caregivers and can contribute to needle phobia. Vaccine acceptance can be improved if the vaccination services acknowledge and address the discomfort, pain, and fear associated with vaccination [39].

ROLE OF SOCIAL MEDIA AND THE INTERNET

The use, popularity, and perceived importance of the Internet to get health information are impactful factors in parental attitudes and decisions about vaccines [3,40]. Online, parents have access to more resources on vaccinations than ever before, but the Internet can be a harmful tool when it is difficult to discern which information is reliable [36]. Parents often obtain medical information from a wide variety of sources without considering their credibility.

Misinformation (including deliberate misinformation) and myths can appear alongside accurate information, and parents often find it difficult to discern which information is trustworthy [3,36]. The use of the Internet for "research" to support decision-making is concerning as non-validated information from nonmedical sources includes inaccuracies, rumors, and myths which contribute to fear and hesitancy and unintentionally misinformed vaccine decisions [29,41].

Questioning the legitimacy of science and the expertise of medical authorities is increasingly common [13]. Vaccine safety issues are predominantly highlighted in print, broadcast, social media, and on the Internet [42]. Unfortunately, people may consider the Internet sources of information that oppose vaccinations to be highly reliable. Some of the top searches for vaccine-related search terms are websites that propagate anti-vaccine conspiracy theories [23]; a search on the word "vaccination" produced more anti-than pro-vaccination Web sites [3]. Reports of vaccine adverse events can be distorted and amplified through sensational media coverage [43]. Emotional appeals focused on the risks of vaccinating have also increased vaccine hesitancy [21].

Additionally, the Web 2.0 functions allow any user to create and share content using social networks (eg, Facebook, YouTube, Twitter), often without undergoing scrutiny to verify that their sources of information are reliable; the expressed viewpoints are usually not based on any official data [13].

At the same time, communication strategies have been developed to address vaccine hesitancy on the Internet [4,9,40]. Daley and colleagues recently developed an internet-based intervention (Web site with vaccine information and social media components), which improved attitudes about vaccines among vaccine-hesitant parents recruited during pregnancy [10]. More research is needed on these important interventions.

INTERVENTIONS: INCREASING VACCINATION AND DECREASING HESITANCY AND REFUSAL

The power of a multimodal and tailored approach

Data indicate that an individualized approach tailored to a specific community versus one targeting the general population is more effective [44]. In addition, passive educational interventions (eg, an informational handout or video) may improve parental attitudes toward vaccines but are not strong enough to create behavior change [45].

Educational interventions may be effective for some parents depending on their reasons for vaccine hesitancy [46]. Navin and colleagues reported that one-on-one educational sessions with parents were most effective with parents who had chosen an alternative vaccine schedule (39.2%) but were less effective among parents who believed that vaccines provide little benefit (10.5%), had concerns about the risks of vaccines (8.1%), or refused for religious reasons (4.4%) [46].

While it is recommended that providers discuss the benefits to others and herd immunity with vaccine-hesitant parents, there is limited evidence that it helps change vaccine attitudes and uptake [47]. Parents can experience a clash between individual freedom and collective responsibility with highly individualistic societies displaying less communal attitudes [48]. A systematic review showed that while parents considered the concept of "vaccines being beneficial to others" to be important, their decision was ultimately based on the perceived benefit to their own child [47]. Nevertheless, providers should still make the effort to review with parents the collective benefits of immunizations.[11].

The power of the medical provider

For all parents, health care providers are among the top-three trusted sources of vaccine information [49], and a strong provider commitment to vaccinations can influence vaccine-hesitant or resistant parents [11,29,50].

In a 2013 study, pediatricians reported that they were able to convince 30% of vaccine-hesitant parents who initially refused a vaccine for their child [11]. Trust is a recurring and predominant theme in the literature and a critical component of a strong provider-patient relationship [34,50]. This is especially important when some parents feel that information provided by their children's doctors is biased toward promoting vaccine benefits, while the side effects can be inadequately presented [51]. As pediatric providers, we need to bring unbiased and accurate scientific information to these conversations, so that parents can make informed decisions about immunizations.

The growing trend toward vaccine hesitancy poses a dilemma for pediatricians. Establishing a partnership that includes shared decision-making is the key [52], as parents who distrust their health care providers are more likely to have received vaccine information from an anti-vaccine organization [37]. Additionally, the rapid development of vaccinology makes it difficult for providers to keep up to date, causing potential confusion and mistrust when discussing vaccinations. It is particularly important to convey to parents that vaccines undergo comprehensive evaluation before being licensed [11].

The opinion of other health care professionals (eg, nurses, medical assistants) who interact with parents can serve as a source of advice, particularly for those who manifest concerns about vaccines [11]. However, provider attitudes toward immunizations vary [8], with up to 6% of pediatric medical providers labeling themselves as vaccine hesitant [35]. Additionally, recently graduated health care providers were 15% less likely to believe vaccines are efficacious, less likely to believe that many commonly used childhood vaccines were safe, and 3.7% believed that "immunizations do more harm than good" [8]. Curricula for health care professionals should emphasize the importance of vaccines to enhance their ability to respond to legitimate parental concerns.

Communication tools

The rise of patient-centered care has transitioned the traditional power from providers as sole directors of patient care to shared decision-making between the health professionals and patients [9]. Many parents no longer want to be passive, but instead they prefer to be active participants in the decisions concerning their children' health [43]. This is a main limitation for "presumptive delivery strategy" recommended in the literature.

At the same time, parents seek to be well informed and usually ask for more medical details [3,13]. The information provided should be transparent in presenting both the risks and benefits of vaccinations while providing assurance that vaccines are safe and effective [41]. Potential side effects should be fully disclosed; it should be emphasized that most side effects are mild (eg, fever or tenderness and swelling at the site of immunization), and the severe side effects are rare but can occur, with most of those being transient [11]. A clear language should be used to present the benefits and risks of VPDs fairly and accurately [4]. Providers should also communicate that there are not effective treatments for many VPDs [51].

A big challenge that providers face today is that some parents subscribe to an entirely different set of beliefs about health and illness [13], in contrast with the evidence-based medicine model used by most medical providers [24]. However, science-based statements about probabilities and risk are not as impactful for families as the anecdotes and emotional appeals often used in anti-vaccination claims [13].

Providers need to keep an open and respectful dialogue to build trust and guide parents to choose wisely about vaccinations [36], recognizing that parents' informational needs vary according to the extent of their vaccine-related concerns [6]. Medical providers are more effective when they share the evidence in a nonjudgmental/nonconfrontational way and acknowledge parents' concerns with empathy [52,53].

Motivational interviewing is an evidence-based communication tool recommended for parents determined to be "hesitant," "late or selective vaccinators," or "refusers" [9]. This "guiding style of communication" uses an empathetic approach to explore a person's existing motivations and concerns about a behavior (like vaccination) to elicit behavior change [19]; the intent is to empower the patient/caregiver to change by using a supportive and nonconfrontational approach [53]. This interviewing technique can enable pediatric providers to address parents' individual concerns more effectively [53].

Physicians often underestimate or overestimate parental concerns regarding vaccines [42] and should be cautious about using dramatic and fear-provoking narratives surrounding VPDs [9,53]. Paradoxically, an online-based intervention promoting MMR vaccination intent produced worsening vaccine attitudes

Table 1
Recommendations for addressing parental vaccine hesitancy

DON'T	DO
Overestimate parental vaccine hesitancy	Listen and ask open-ended questions Recognize that each parent has a unique opinion about vaccines
Use judgmental language	Show empathy and interest while stating the facts
Use scare tactics	Provide concise information and focus on the benefits of vaccines
Simply provide information about vaccines	Validate parents' emotions and use affirmations to empower parents
Allow misinformation to go unchallenged	Be clear, honest, and transparent while debunking misinformation
Simply tell parents what they need to do	Use motivational interviewing to target parents' concerns while tailoring the information provided

among some parents [54], and a recent research suggests that communicating that vaccination entails no risk may lead patients to view vaccines as riskier [5].

In summary, a willingness to listen respectfully to parents, encourage questions, acknowledge parental concerns, and provide accurate information about vaccines' risks and benefits is essential for developing rapport and trust [51,53]. Table 1 summarizes some recommendations that can be used by providers when addressing vaccine hesitancy with parents.

SUMMARY

Vaccine hesitancy is a complex and multifaceted phenomenon. It has been described as a spectrum of doubt among people that ranges from hesitant acceptance to complete refusal of vaccinations. This phenomenon exists even when barriers to vaccination are removed. Available literature about the topic has expanded to enable us to more fully understand this term, its driving factors, and the interventions that can help alleviate this evolving public health concern.

Reasons for vaccine hesitancy center around perceptions of vaccine safety and efficacy, individual characteristics, and social context. Unfortunately, one cannot apply a "one-size-fits-all" approach to addressing vaccine-hesitant parents. There is still much to learn regarding what drives parents' decision-making and, more importantly, how to address it. No single solution to this issue exists but interventions that are multimodal and tailored to specific populations are likely to be most successful. The COVID-19 pandemic and the hesitancy surrounding SARS-CoV-2 vaccines further confirm the urgent need for effective communication strategies.

The starting point is establishing a strong foundation of trust and respect between the providers and their patients and families. This will allow providers to create a safe space for parents to discuss their concerns and openly ask questions about vaccinations and, subsequently, follow their guidance. Providers should not underestimate the power of their knowledge and recommendations when addressing vaccine-hesitant parents.

CLINICS CARE POINTS

- Providers should approach vaccine-hesitant parents with a nonconfrontational and open dialogue to provide accurate and clear information about vaccine-preventable diseases and vaccinations while addressing parental concerns.
- Taking time to build rapport with parents allows providers to build trust and make meaningful recommendations to families. Many vaccine-hesitant parents are simply looking for a trusted source to address their questions and concerns.
- Motivational interviewing is an evidence-based communication tool that providers can use to target parental concerns and tailor information while discussing vaccines.

- Providers should continue to work at the clinical practice and advocacy level to approach vaccine hesitancy from multiple angles with a tailored approach specific to their communities.

FUTURE DIRECTIONS

- More research on demographic predictors of vaccine hesitancy
- Further examination of the usefulness of a variety of communication techniques
- Research into new and more effective strategies for delivering pro-vaccine messages
- Development of evidence-based interventions to reduce vaccine hesitancy at the individual and public health level

Disclosure

The authors have nothing to disclose.

References

[1] Centers for Disease Control and Prevention (CDC. Ten great public health achievements–United States, 2001-2010. MMWR Morbidity Mortality Weekly Report 2011;60(19):619–23.
[2] Whitney CG, Zhou F, Singleton J, et al. Benefits from immunization during the vaccines for children program era—United States, 1994–2013. MMWR Morbidity Mortality Weekly Report 2014;63(16):352.
[3] Harmsen IA, Mollema L, Ruiter RA, et al. Why parents refuse childhood vaccination: a qualitative study using online focus groups. BMC public health 2013;13(1):1–8.
[4] Cataldi JR, Kerns ME, O'Leary ST. Evidence-based strategies to increase vaccination uptake: a review. Curr Opin Pediatr 2020;32(1):151–9.
[5] Zimet GD, Rosberger Z, Fisher WA, et al. Beliefs, behaviors and HPV vaccine: correcting the myths and the misinformation. Prev Med 2013;57(5):414–8.
[6] Gilkey MB, McRee AL, Magnus BE, et al. Vaccination confidence and parental refusal/delay of early childhood vaccines. PloS one 2016;11(7):e0159087.
[7] Janko M. Vaccination: a victim of its own success. AMA J Ethics 2012;14(1):3–4.
[8] Mergler MJ, Omer SB, Pan WK, et al. Are recent medical graduates more skeptical of vaccines? Vaccines 2013;1(2):154–66.
[9] McClure CC, Cataldi JR, O'Leary ST. Vaccine hesitancy: where we are and where we are going. Clin Ther 2017;39(8):1550–62.
[10] Daley MF, Narwaney KJ, Shoup JA, et al. Addressing Parents' Vaccine Concerns: A Randomized Trial of a Social Media Intervention. Am J Prev Med 2018;55(1):44–54.
[11] Edwards KM, Hackell JM. Countering vaccine hesitancy. Pediatrics 2016;138(3).
[12] Nowak GJ, Cacciatore MA. Parents' confidence in recommended childhood vaccinations: Extending the assessment, expanding the context. Hum Vaccin Immunother 2017;13(3):687–700.
[13] Dubé E, Laberge C, Guay M, et al. Vaccine hesitancy: an overview. Hum Vaccin Immunother 2013;9(8):1763–73.
[14] SAGE Working. Report of the SAGE working group on vaccine hesitancy. Geneva: World Health Organization; 2014.
[15] MacDonald NE. Vaccine hesitancy: Definition, scope and determinants. Vaccine 2015;33(34):4161–4.
[16] Shapiro GK, Holding A, Perez S, et al. Validation of the vaccine conspiracy beliefs scale. Papillomavirus Res 2016;2:167–72.
[17] Manfredi P, Della Posta P, d'Onofrio A, et al. Optimal vaccination choice, vaccination games, and rational exemption: an appraisal. Vaccine 2009;28(1):98–109.

[18] Eby AZ. Impacting Parental Vaccine Decision-Making. Pediatr Nurs 2017;43(1):22–9, 34.
[19] Leask J, Kinnersley P, Jackson C, et al. Communicating with parents about vaccination: a framework for health professionals. BMC Pediatr 2012;12:154.
[20] Damnjanović K, Graeber J, Ilic S, et al. Parental Decision-Making on Childhood Vaccination. Front Psychol 2018;9:735.
[21] Reuben R, Aitken D, Freedman JL, et al. Mistrust of the medical profession and higher disgust sensitivity predict parental vaccine hesitancy. PLoS One 2020;15(9):e0237755.
[22] Aharon AA, Nehama H, Rishpon S, et al. Parents with high levels of communicative and critical health literacy are less likely to vaccinate their children. Patient Educ Couns 2017;100(4):768–75.
[23] Jolley D, Douglas KM. The effects of anti-vaccine conspiracy theories on vaccination intentions. PLoS One 2014;9(2):e89177.
[24] Attwell K, Leask J, Meyer SB, et al. Vaccine rejecting parents' engagement with expert systems that inform vaccination programs. J Bioethical Inq 2017;14(1):65–76.
[25] Lagoe C, Farrar KM. Are you willing to risk it? The relationship between risk, regret, and vaccination intent. Psychol Health Med 2015;20(1):18–24.
[26] Dyda A, King C, Dey A, et al. A systematic review of studies that measure parental vaccine attitudes and beliefs in childhood vaccination. BMC Public Health 2020;20(1):1253.
[27] Blaisdell, L.L., Gutheil, C., Hotsmans, N.A., et al., Unknown Risks: Parental Hesitation about Vaccination. *Med Decis Making.* **36** (4), 2016, 479-489.
[28] Gidengil C, Chen C, Parker A, et al. Beliefs around childhood vaccines in the United States: A systematic review. Vaccine 2019;37(45):6793–802.
[29] Geoghegan S, O'Callaghan KP, Offit PA. Vaccine safety: myths and misinformation. Front Microbiol 2020;11:372.
[30] Hulsey E, Bland T. Immune overload: Parental attitudes toward combination and single antigen vaccines. Vaccine 2015;33(22):2546–50.
[31] Carrion ML. An ounce of prevention: identifying cues to (in) action for maternal vaccine refusal. Qual Health Res 2018;28(14):2183–94.
[32] Wakefield, A. J., Murch, S. H., Anthony, A., et al., RETRACTED: Ileal-lymphoid-nodular hyperplasia, non-specific colitis, and pervasive developmental disorder in children. *Lancet.* **28**; 351 (9103), 1998, 637-641.
[33] Baumgaertner B, Carlisle JE, Justwan F. The influence of political ideology and trust on willingness to vaccinate. PLoS One 2018;13(1):e0191728.
[34] Eller NM, Henrikson NB, Opel DJ. Vaccine Information Sources and Parental Trust in Their Child's Health Care Provider. Health Educ Behav 2019;46(3):445–53.
[35] Suryadevara M, Handel A, Bonville CA, et al. Pediatric provider vaccine hesitancy: An under-recognized obstacle to immunizing children. Vaccine 2015;33(48):6629–34.
[36] Bianco A, Mascaro V, Zucco R, et al. Parent perspectives on childhood vaccination: How to deal with vaccine hesitancy and refusal? Vaccine 2019;37(7):984–90.
[37] Lee C, Whetten K, Omer S, et al. Hurdles to herd immunity: Distrust of government and vaccine refusal in the US, 2002–2003. Vaccine 2016;34(34):3972–8.
[38] Wheeler M, Buttenheim AM. Parental vaccine concerns, information source, and choice of alternative immunization schedules. Hum Vaccin Immunother 2013;9(8):1782–9.
[39] Noel M, Taddio A, McMurtry CM, et al. HELPinKids&Adults Knowledge Synthesis of the Management of Vaccination Pain and High Levels of Needle Fear: Limitations of the Evidence and Recommendations for Future Research. Clin J Pain 2015;31(10 Suppl): S124–31.
[40] Stahl JP, Cohen R, Gaudelus J, et al. The impact of the web and social networks on vaccination. New challenges and opportunities offered to fight against vaccine hesitancy. Med Mal Infect 2016;46(3):117–22.
[41] Ozawa S, Stack ML. Public trust and vaccine acceptance–international perspectives. Hum Vaccin Immunother 2013;9(8):1774–8.

[42] Healy CM, Montesinos DP, Middleman AB. Parent and provider perspectives on immunization: are providers overestimating parental concerns? Vaccine 2014;32(5):579–84.
[43] Siddiqui M, Salmon DA, Omer SB. Epidemiology of vaccine hesitancy in the United States. Hum Vaccin Immunother 2013;9(12):2643–8.
[44] Jarrett C, Wilson R, O'Leary M, et al. Strategies for addressing vaccine hesitancy–A systematic review. Vaccine 2015;33(34):4180–90.
[45] Williams SE, Rothman RL, Offit PA, et al. A randomized trial to increase acceptance of childhood vaccines by vaccine-hesitant parents: a pilot study. Acad Pediatr 2013;13(5): 475–80.
[46] Navin MC, Wasserman JA, Ahmad M, et al. Vaccine Education, Reasons for Refusal, and Vaccination Behavior. Am J Prev Med 2019;56(3):359–67.
[47] Quadri-Sheriff M, Hendrix KS, Downs SM, et al. The role of herd immunity in parents' decision to vaccinate children: a systematic review. Pediatrics 2012;130(3):522–30.
[48] Caplan A. Liberty has its responsibilities: holding non-vaccinators liable for the harm they do. Hum Vaccin Immunother 2013;9(12):2666–7.
[49] Chung Y, Schamel J, Fisher A, et al. Influences on immunization decision-making among US parents of young children. Matern child Health J 2017;21(12):2178–87.
[50] Connors JT, Slotwinski KL, Hodges EA. Provider-parent communication when discussing vaccines: a systematic review. J Pediatr Nurs 2017;33:10–5.
[51] Diekema DS. Provider dismissal of vaccine-hesitant families: misguided policy that fails to benefit children. Hum Vaccin Immunother 2013;9(12):2661–2.
[52] Alexander K, Lacy TA, Myers AM, et al. Should Pediatric Practices Have Policies to Not Care for Children With Vaccine-Hesitant Parents? Pediatrics 2016;138(4).
[53] Gagneur A. Motivational interviewing: A powerful tool to address vaccine hesitancy. Can Commun Dis Rep 2020;46(4):93–7.
[54] Nyhan B, Reifler J, Richey S, et al. Effective messages in vaccine promotion: a randomized trial. Pediatrics 2014;133(4):e835–42.

Advances in Pediatrics 69 (2022) 177–202

ADVANCES IN PEDIATRICS

Turner Syndrome: An Update

Margaret Steiner, MD*, Paul Saenger, MD

NYU Langone Health–Long Island, 101 Mineola Boulevard, Mineola, NY 11501, USA

Keywords

• Turner syndrome • Short stature • Long-acting growth hormone • Infertility

Key points

- Turner syndrome is the most common sex chromosome abnormality in women.
- Girls with Turner Syndrome almost all have short stature.
- Growth hormone is an effective treatment of girls with Turner syndrome.

The diagnosis of Turner syndrome is sometimes made at birth in the patient with classic physical features such as webbed neck and congenital lymphedema. Other patients are diagnosed later, when they present with either growth failure in childhood, failure to enter or complete puberty, or early ovarian failure.

INTRODUCTION

It has been more than 80 years since Henry Turner, an internist, reported in 1938 the clinical characteristics of the 7 patients whose phenotype now bears his name [1]. These women had short stature in association with sexual infantilism, webbing of the neck, low posterior hairline, and increased carrying angle of the elbows (cubitus valgus). In 1930, Ullrich described an 8-year-old girl with short stature; lymphedema of the neck, hands, and feet; subsequent neck webbing, cubitus valgus, and other phenotypic abnormalities (including a high arched palate, ptosis, low-set auricles, and small upwardly curved nails); and several other features that are now associated with Turner syndrome. This gave rise to the less common, but more appropriate eponym Ullrich–Turner syndrome.

Ullrich later recognized that his patients and those of Turner seemed to have the same condition [2]. He also called attention to the work of Bonnevie, who

*Corresponding author. *E-mail address:* Margaret.steiner@nyulangone.org

https://doi.org/10.1016/j.yapd.2022.03.004
0065-3101/22/

described a group of congenital anomalies in mice consisting of the distention of the neck and malformations of the ears, face, and limb buds-all secondary to the dissection of the subcutaneous tissues by fluid. This "bleb" mechanism for producing multiple anomalies was suggested by Ullrich as being responsible for the cervical lymphangiectasia noted in some human female abortuses that seemed to produce a scarred webbed neck (pterygium colli). Ullrich proposed the eponym status Bonnevie-Ullrich to describe the set of specific anomalies arising from a single mechanism (lymphangiectasia) and resulting in the phenotype of Turner syndrome.

The links among these phenotypic descriptions, the pathologic evidence of streak ovaries, and the abnormal X chromosomes came with the introduction of the technique for sex chromatin identification by Barr and the demonstration that most patients with Turner syndrome lacked sex chromatin material [3]. Initially, this absence of sex chromatin (or lack of a Barr body) was associated with "maleness" because a similar pattern was found in normal phenotypic men. Only after it was demonstrated that it was the second X chromosome that in the inactivated state constituted the Barr body was it clear that the 45,X karyotype would result in a chromatin pattern similar to the normal 46,XY karyotype.

It was not until 1961 that techniques became available for the analysis of the chromosomal constitution and the sex chromosome constitution was shown in a 14-year-old phenotypic female with Turner syndrome to be, indeed, 45,X[4]. Thus, patients with Turner syndrome were not XY males, but in most cases 45,X females. The original patient of Ullrich was studied in the 1960s and found to have a 45,X karyotype (D. Knorr, personal communication to the author). One of the original 7 patients Turner described was also reinvestigated and found to have a 45, X chromosomal karyotype [4].

INCIDENCE

Turner syndrome is the most common sex chromosome abnormality in women and occurs in approximately 1 in 2500 live births [5]. Turner syndrome is now more commonly diagnosed prenatally via amniocentesis and chorionic villous sampling. Gravholt and colleagues found that the prenatal prevalence of TS is 176 in 100,000 via amniocentesis and 392 in 100,000 via chorionic villous sampling [6]. The true prevalence, however, is uncertain as those with mild phenotypes may remain undiagnosed [7].

PATHOGENESIS

Molecular studies have shown that maternal X is retained in two-thirds of patients with Turner syndrome and paternal X in the remaining one-third [8]. More than one-half of all patients with Turner syndrome have a mosaic chromosomal complement (eg, 45,X/46,XX) detectable in peripheral blood leukocytes [9,10]. Mosaicism with a normal cell line in the fetal membranes may be necessary in all affected cases for adequate placental function and fetal survival [11].

The identification of mosaicism depends directly on the method of ascertainment. It varies from 34% with conventional cytogenetic techniques to 60% with fluorescence in situ hybridization (FISH) techniques to 74% in a study in which reverse transcriptase polymerase chain reaction (PCR) assays were used [12].

Some patients with Turner syndrome lack only part of one sex chromosome, and the Turner syndrome phenotype can be seen with a variety of structural abnormalities, such as isochromosomes, rings, or terminal deletions [13]. A rare but very informative class of Turner syndrome includes patients who have deletions of the Y chromosome that remove the testes-determining gene, SRY; these individuals develop as women. Based on this finding and the fact that men require only one X chromosome for normal development, Ferguson-Smith hypothesized that copies of Turner syndrome genes are also present on the Y chromosome.

Specific localization of Turner syndrome candidate genes proved elusive until one group successfully identified a pseudoautosomal deletion encompassing a novel homeobox gene, SHOX (short stature homeobox-containing gene on the X chromosome), which is associated with short stature not only in Turner syndrome but also in Leri–Weill dyschondrosteosis and in an estimated 2 to 15% of cases of idiopathic short stature [14–17].

The telomeres of the short arms of chromosome X and Y are logical sites for Turner syndrome genes, as sex chromosomes undergo meiotic recombination within the pseudoautosomal region and all genes in this region that have been examined escape X-inactivation. Characterization of XYp females provides additional support for the hypothesis of a distinct Turner syndrome stature locus: most of these patients have unbalanced X,Y translocations and, in the most fully documented patients with this karyotype, 2 intact copies of the pseudoautosomal region are present. It is not surprising that these patients attain normal stature, despite the presence of features consistent with Turner syndrome. As noted above, an absence of SHOX was identified as the genetic cause of the short stature phenotype in patients with Turner syndrome [14,16].

Studies that have examined the relationship between the chromosomal and karyotypic abnormalities and clinical findings in patients with Turner syndrome have been disappointing [18]. Short stature is the only clinical finding invariably associated with the 45,X karyotype; it also is the only phenotypic abnormality present in virtually 100% of patients. Specific karyotypic abnormalities may also correlate with the presence of hypothyroidism. The webbing of the neck, shield chest, and probably the ear malformations, renal anomalies, and cardiac defects may be a consequence of fetal lymphedema, which interferes with organ development [19–22].

Deletions of the long arm of the X chromosome have been reported in otherwise normal women (ie, normal stature) with secondary amenorrhea [23]. A 45,X/46,XY karyotype has been associated with a variety of phenotypes ranging from the typical phenotype of Turner syndrome to ovotesticular disorder of sexual development with genital ambiguity, to a normal male phenotype with infertility [24].

CLINICAL MANIFESTATIONS

Typical features- The most characteristic feature of girls and women with Turner syndrome is their short stature (Table 1). Other common features are a "shield" chest with widely spaced nipples, webbed neck, cubitus valgus, and Madelung deformity of the forearm. Neonates may have congenital lymphedema of the hands and feet and 2 or more of the following dysmorphic features: webbed neck, nail dysplasia, high-arched palate, and short fourth metacarpal [25]. The height of patients with Turner syndrome should be plotted on growth curves specific to this disorder [26,27].

Hearing loss, hypothyroidism, and liver function abnormalities can occur as these women get older [28,29]. Liver enzymes are mildly elevated in approximately 35 to 45% of adult patients [30,31], and improve with postmenopausal hormone therapy [30]. Intelligence is usually within the normal range, but patients may have specific neurocognitive deficits, for example, problems with visuo-spatial organization.

Other manifestations include autoimmune disease (including chronic autoimmune thyroiditis) [32] and specific morphologic defects of facial development and cardiovascular, urologic, and bone structure [28,33,34].

Ovarian failure- Although most affected women have no pubertal development and primary amenorrhea, some develop normally and then have secondary amenorrhea, while occasionally others have no morphologic defects and achieve normal stature. It should be noted that adrenarche is normal in Turner syndrome.

As an example, a retrospective study of 522 patients with Turner syndrome who were over the age of 12 years found that 84 (16%) had spontaneous menarche at an average age of 13.2 years; 30 of these women still had regular menses 9 years after menarche, and 3 became pregnant without medical assistance [35].

In a second retrospective study of 276 adults with cytogenetically proven Turner syndrome, 5 women had spontaneous puberty and spontaneous pregnancies, despite high-grade monosomy (45,X in $\geq$ 90% of a 50-cell karyotype) [36].

Manifestations in older patients include primary hypogonadism occurring either before or after puberty (gonadal dysgenesis). It is one of the most common causes of premature ovarian failure [37].

The ovaries in Turner syndrome characteristically consist of small amounts of connective tissue and no follicles or only a few atretic follicles ("streak gonads"). However, the degree of ovarian dysfunction and the extent of the defects are variable.

Careful histologic studies of the ovaries of 8 aborted 45,X fetuses many years ago are the basis of our understanding of the gonadal failure in Turner syndrome [38]. These ovaries contained apparently normal numbers of primordial germ cells for up to at least 6 weeks of gestation, but at later gestational ages, the numbers of germ cells were decreased and connective tissue was increased, as compared with age-matched normal fetuses. These results

Table 1
Clinical features in girls with Turner syndrome

Physical diagnosis		Percentage affected
Skeletal	Short stature	100
	Short neck	40
	↑ Upper: lower body ratio	97
	Cubitus valgus	47
	Short metacarpal	37
	Scoliosis	12.5
	Madelung deformity	7.5
	Micrognathia/high palate	60
Lymphatic obstruction	Neck Webbing	25
	Low posterior hairline	42
	Edema of hands/feet	22
	Nail dysplasia	13
Others	Strabismus	18
	Ptosis	11
	Multiple nevi	26
Screening Evaluation		
Cardiovascular anomaly	All	44
	Bicuspid aortic valve	30
	Aortic coarctation	12
	Dilated aorta	11
	Other*	12
Renal anomaly	All	18
	Horseshoe Kidney	11
	Duplicated collecting ducts	4
	Unilateral agenesis	3
Liver disorder	All	36
	Abnormal liver function tests(LFTs)	27
	Fatty infiltration	19
Hypertension	All	34
	Prehypertension	14
	Overt hypertension	20
Autoimmunity	All	51
	Hashimoto thyroiditis	51
	Graves' disease	1
	Type 1 diabetes	0
	Celiac	5
	Inflammatory bowel	3

"Physical Diagnosis" describes findings from physical examinations of more than 200 girls seen by Drs Barbara Lippe and paul Saenger between 1985 and 2000. Information on puberty development is not included because many girls were not old enough to assess. The "screening evaluation" data are from 100 girls aged 7 to 17 who underwent standardized imaging laboratory testing as a part of the NIH natural history study performed between 2001 and 2008. The cardiovascular evaluation included MRI and cardiac echo. Under the cardiovascular listing, the "other" category included partial anomalous pulmonary veins, aberrant right subclavian monitors. All patients also had renal and hepatic ultrasound studies. Abnormal liver function was defined as greater than 10% elevation of aminotransferase(s). Hashimoto's was defined by the history of clinical hypothyroidism or elevation of circulating thyroid antibodies.

indicate that the gonadal dysgenesis may be caused by accelerated apoptosis rather than abnormal germ cell formation.

Another study evaluated 104 girls aged 0.2 to 17.4 years with complete or partial X chromosome deletions using pelvic ultrasonography [39]. Approximately one-third have visible, nonstreak ovaries. The girls with visible ovaries had apparently normal ovarian growth and follicular development up to the time of puberty, and were more likely to have spontaneous breast development and uterine growth, indicating some ovarian function; many, but not all, of these girls had incomplete X chromosome deletions. These findings are consistent with several case reports of adult women with both 45,X and partial X deletions who have conceived and borne children before developing secondary amenorrhea [40,41].

Thus, the consequences of X chromosome deletions are highly variable, ranging (at the extremes) from intrauterine death to normal health with normal menarche and normal reproductive function for a few years thereafter. The incidence of 45,X and 45,X/46,XX mosaic karyotypes in women with normal fertility is unknown.

Only one X chromosome is active in somatic cells after the third week of gestation. As a result, deletion of any part of one X chromosome will affect fertility only if the normal copies of the missing gene or genes do one of the following:

- Imprint somatic cells before 3 weeks of gestation
- Escape inactivation so that 2 copies are normally required
- Are critical for oocyte development (as oocytes have 2 active X chromosomes).

Short stature– Short stature combined with a square appearance is the most common clinical feature of Turner syndrome. The adult height of untreated patients correlates significantly with midparental height (ie, the height corresponds to the average of the height percentiles of the mother and the father).Is this correct? I would have thought for the untreated patients, the height would be lower than that correlated with midparental height. Recombinant human growth hormone therapy is recommended to maximize final height (see later in discussion).

Renal anomalies–Renal anomalies are common in patients with Turner syndrome. Congenital malformations of the urinary system are present in approximately 30 to 40%. The most common abnormalities are collecting system malformations (20%) and horseshoe kidneys (10%), followed by malrotation and other positional abnormalities (5%) [5]. Patients should undergo renal ultrasonography at the time of diagnosis, and, if structural abnormalities are identified, the patient should be monitored yearly for urinary tract infection.

Anomalies associated with the obstruction of the ureteropelvic junction can produce clinically significant hydronephrosis or pyelonephritis. Idiopathic hypertension is common in Turner syndrome, even in the absence of recognizable renal or cardiac malformations. Blood pressure should, therefore, be monitored carefully, and hypertension treated vigorously.

Cardiovascular disease–There is an increased risk of cardiovascular morbidity in women with Turner syndrome, presumably due to their risk of cardiovascular malformations, renal abnormalities, and hypertension [42,43]. The malformations are associated with increased risks for aortic dissection and increased mortality rates. Neck webbing and increased thoracic anterior-to-posterior diameters are predictors for cardiovascular abnormalities [44].

In a series of 173 patients with Turner syndrome at a single center, the following rates of cardiac malformations were reported [43]: any malformation 44.5%; aortic valve abnormalities (primary bicuspid aortic valve) 34.1%; aortic arch abnormalities (primarily coarctation) 19.1%; systemic venous abnormalities 8.1%; ventricular septal defects 5.2%; pulmonary venous abnormalities 4%; hypoplastic left heart/single ventricle 3.5%, atrial septal defects 1.7%; coronary artery abnormalities 1.6%.

Coarctation/aortic valve disease–The prevalence of cardiovascular malformations in patients with Turner syndrome is variable across studies. Approximately 30% have aortic valve disease, while up to 30% have coarctation [42,43,45–47]. Patients with the relatively common anomaly of a bicuspid aortic valve are more likely to have other cardiovascular abnormalities, such as aortic arch defects [43,47]. The variability among estimates could be due to differences in the age group examined, the degree of mosaicism in the population, or a technical difficulty in visualizing the valvular defect using echocardiography. Usually, MRI will give better results than echocardiogram because shield chest phenotype in patients with Turner syndrome can cause challenges for reliable echocardiograms. The prevalence of cardiovascular malformations seems to be higher in those with 45,X compared with those with a mosaic chromosomal complement (45,X/46,XX) (38 vs 11%) [45]. Even when initial magnetic resonance imaging does not show aortic root dilation or coarctation, subsequent imaging may show the development of these abnormalities during the next 2 to 6 years [48].

Aortic dissection–Aortic dissection or rupture is an increasingly recognized cause of death in women with Turner syndrome [49,50]. In a study of 166 women with Turner syndrome and 26 healthy controls, one-third of the patients had aortic size index values (ascending aortic diameters normalized to body surface area) greater than the 95th percentile (2.0 cm/m^2) [50]. After 3 years of follow-up, aortic dissections occurred in 3 patients (all 3 had an aortic size index >2.5 cm/m^2), for an annualized rate of 618 cases/100,000 woman-years, approximately 100-fold higher than that seen in women of similar age without Turner syndrome. In a report of 20 women with Turner syndrome who had already experienced an aortic dissection, mean aortic size index as 2.7 ± 0.6 cm/m [2,51].

Pregnancy–Of greater concern is a possible increase in mortality due to aortic dissection or rupture that has been reported in women with Turner syndrome achieving pregnancy through in vitro fertilization (IVF) with oocyte donation [52]. Therefore, before attempting to become pregnant, women with Turner syndrome should undergo a complete medical evaluation, with particular attention paid to blood pressure, cardiovascular and renal function, as recommended by the American Society of Reproductive Medicine [53].

To minimize the risk of dissection, the authors suggest close cardiovascular monitoring in patients with Turner syndrome with a dilated ascending aorta [37].

Hypertension–Hypertension is more common in women with Turner syndrome compared with controls [54–56]. In a series of 62 patients (age range 5–22 years) with Turner syndrome, 30% were mildly hypertensive and 50% had an abnormal diurnal blood pressure profile as measured by 24-h ambulatory blood pressure monitoring [54], the physiologic nighttime dip in blood pressure did not occur. Neither the presence of renal or cardiac abnormalities nor treatment with growth hormone or estrogen had an effect on blood pressure.

Other–Other cardiovascular anomalies have been reported in patients with Turner syndrome. A prolonged QT interval has been reported in some series, including in young children with Turner syndrome [57–60]. In a study of 93 women with Turner syndrome, 11 with 46,XX primary amenorrhea, and 25 normal controls, mean carotid intima-media thickness was increased to a similar degree in the 2 hypogonadal groups, suggesting a primary role for estrogen deficiency [61]. However, the patients with Turner syndrome had additional abnormalities when compared with both the 46,XX primary amenorrhea and control groups, including increased common carotid, aortic root, and brachial artery diameters, suggesting additional genetic factor that contribute to their vasculopathy.

Osteoporosis–Osteoporosis and fractures have been reported to be common in women with Turner syndrome, thought to be due to both ovarian failure and possibly haploinsufficiency for bone-related X chromosome genes [62,63]. However, in some studies, patients who receive standard estrogen therapy seem to have normal bone density when compared with age-matched healthy women. As an example, in a study of 70 adult women with Turner syndrome who underwent bone mineral density testing (by dual-energy x-ray absorptiometry [DXA]), osteoporosis was diagnosed in 7 (10%), six of whom were more than 45 years [64]. None of the women with osteoporosis had ever received prolonged estrogen replacement. Fracture rates in the patients who had received estrogen therapy were no different from age-matched controls while in untreated patients, fracture rate was markedly elevated, radial fracture being the most common.

Some of the osteopenia reported in patients with Turner syndrome may be due to an underestimation of bone mineral density in short subjects. This was suggested in a study of 40 adult women with Turner syndrome, in which osteoporosis was overdiagnosed in patients less than 150 cm tall unless bone mineral density measurements were adjusted for body size (and therefore bone size). After adjustment for body size, the prevalence of osteoporosis and fractures in patients with Turner syndrome who had been treated with estrogen was the same as age-matched controls without Turner syndrome [65].

However, the ideal controls to which patients with Turner syndrome should be compared are women with ovarian failure and a normal karyotype, thereby controlling for the ovarian hormone deficiency. In a study comparing 41 women with Turner syndrome to a control group of 35 karyotypically normal women with premature ovarian failure, a selective reduction in cortical (forearm) bone mineral density was seen in patients with Turner syndrome [66]. This difference persisted after adjustment for height, age of puberty, lifetime estrogen exposure, and serum 25-hydroxyvitamin D concentrations.

Thus, there seems to be a selective reduction in bone mineral density in women with Turner syndrome that is independent of ovarian hormone exposure.

Risk of malignancy–Women with Turner syndrome whose karyotype includes a Y chromosome (such as 45,X/46,XY mosaicism), are at increased risk for gonadoblastoma, a neoplasm that occurs in dysgenetic gonads [67]. In a population-based study that included 3425 women with Turner syndrome followed for a mean of 17 years, 5 women, all with Y chromosome material, developed gonadoblastoma (cumulative risk of 7.9% by age 25 years) [68].

These patients may also be at increased risk for other tumors. In the population-based study noted above, the overall risk of cancer was not increased, but site-specific risks were increased for meningioma, childhood brain tumors, bladder, and uterine cancer (but not breast cancer), when compared with the general population. However, the clinical importance of this finding is unclear, as the number of cases was small.

The risk of breast cancer has been a concern in women with Turner syndrome who receive long-term postmenopausal hormone therapy, but no excess risk has been reported thus far.

Ocular abnormalities–Ocular abnormalities are common among patients with Turner syndrome [69]. Amblyopia, strabismus, ptosis, hypertelorism epicanthus, farsightedness, and red-green color blindness have been noted in small case series [70,71]. Keratoconus, glaucoma, anterior lenticonus, cataracts, retinal vascular changes, and retinal detachment have been noted in case reports [69,72].

Autoimmune disorders–Turner syndrome is associated with an increased risk of autoimmune disorders, most importantly hypothyroidism (Hashimoto's thyroiditis), celiac disease, and inflammatory bowel disease [32,73,74]. The best evidence comes from a prospective study of autoimmune diagnoses in women with Turner syndrome (n = 244) or karyotypically normal (46,XX) primary ovarian insufficiency (POI; ovarian failure) (n = 457), compared with normative data for the United States population of women [32]. Autoimmune hypothyroidism (Hashimoto's thyroiditis) occurred in 37% of women with Turner syndrome compared with 15% in women with POI; the prevalence in both groups was higher than that in normally cycling women (5.8%).

The prevalence of both inflammatory bowel disease and celiac disease was significantly increased in Turner syndrome (4 and 2.7%, respectively), but not in POI. No other autoimmune diagnosis, including type 1 diabetes or hyperthyroidism due to Grave's disease, was increased.

In the second study of 389 girls with Turner syndrome screened with IgA antigliadin antibodies and/or antiendomysial antibodies, 25 (6.4%) had celiac disease [75]. Of these, 10 had typical symptoms, 8 had atypical symptoms, and 7 had no symptoms. The prevalence of celiac disease in the general population is estimated to be 1 in 184 (0.54%) [37].

Metabolic issues–Patients with Turner syndrome are at risk for metabolic disorders. Insulin resistance, as measured by euglycemic clamp studies, is an early metabolic defect in girls with Turner syndrome [76]. Abdominal adiposity is lower and glucose tolerance better in growth hormone-treated girls with Turner syndrome compared with untreated girls [13]. In addition, an increased frequency of central obesity, insulin resistance, type 2 diabetes, and dyslipidemia has been reported in adult women with Turner syndrome when compared with women without Turner syndrome [29].

Skin–Girls with Turner syndrome may be more likely than others to develop pilomatricoma, an uncommon benign skin neoplasm thought to arise from cells of the hair follicle [77–81]. In one study, these asymptomatic papules or nodules that most typically develop as single lesions on the head or neck were identified in 8 of 331 patients (2.6%) with Turner syndrome; there was no association between prior growth hormone therapy and the presence of skin lesions [77]. Although the prevalence of pilomatricoma in the general population is not known, it is thought to be considerably lower than 2.6%.

An increased rate of pigmented nevi has been reported in Turner syndrome [80] especially after growth hormone treatment, but a higher rate of melanoma has not; in fact, a lower rate has been observed [81]. It was previously thought that the risk for keloid formation was increased in these patients, but that is no longer the case.

Otologic Disorders–Perhaps the most common medical problem experienced by girls with Turner syndrome is bilateral otitis media. Anderson and coworkers [82] first described medically significant middle ear pathology in girls with Turner syndrome, with many recurrent episodes, spontaneous perforations, frequent need for surgical treatment, and significant hearing loss in about 25%. Additional studies confirmed the problem of recurrent, often refractory, otitis in Turner syndrome, usually associated with conductive hearing loss and correlated with karyotypes demonstrating loss of the C chromosome short arm, XP [83–86].

The chronic and severe otitis does not seem to be related to a specific or generalized immunologic dysfunction. Other types of infections and disorders of the mucous membranes do not occur with increased frequency in Turner syndrome. It seems rather that the frequent otitis may be the consequence of abnormalities in the growth of the cranial base disturbing the relationship of the middle ear to the Eustachian tube, which coupled with abnormalities in the shape of the palate, create a predisposition to fluid collection and secondary infection.

Conductive hearing loss is most common and severe in children and is correlated with middle ear pathology [83], whereas sensorineural hearing loss is more common in adults. This sensory defect is generally bilateral and characterized by symmetric sensorineural dips in the audiogram in the midfrequency range. Thus, the sensorineural hearing deficit seems to progress over time and is not strictly a congenital abnormality. There remains a significant conductive component of hearing loss in adults with Turner syndrome that may signify ongoing middle ear pathology [83]. The assiduous treatment of ear, nose, and throat problems in childhood and avoiding potential injuries to the inner ear may reduce the risk of hearing loss.

Liver disease–Minor elevations of hepatic aminotransferases are common in girls and women with Turner syndrome, usually in the absence of signs or symptoms of liver disease. Approximately 20% to 25% of girls [87] and 40% of women [88] demonstrate abnormal liver function tests including aspartate-, alanine-, and gamma-glutamyl transferaseand, less commonly, alkaline phosphatase. In some cases, liver enzyme elevations may be associated with pharmacologic estrogen, progestin, or oxandrolone treatments [87,89], but over the long-term estrogen treatment is associated with the normalization of hepatic enzymes [88]. Among 100 girls from age 7 to 17 evaluated in the NIH natural history study between 2002% and 2007%, 27% had modest transaminase elevation that was not correlated with growth hormone (GH) or estrogen use, nor with fatty infiltration observed on liver ultrasound [90]. Aside from a rare case report, there does not seem to be any association between autoimmunity and hepatic abnormalities. Liver biopsies in adults with typical enzyme abnormalities have not consistently defined any unique or diagnostic pathology in women with Turner syndrome [91]. Roulot and coworkers have suggested hepatic disorder may be linked to intrinsic vascular disease. Gravholt and colleagues reported an increased frequency of cirrhosis in a Danish National Health registry study, but this has not been observed in clinical series on health in patients with Turner syndrome.

MANAGEMENT

Once the diagnosis of Turner syndrome has been established and a chromosomal confirmation established, additional diagnostic procedures are indicated. These diagnosis and management strategies have been published as recommendations from consensus workshops [92].

Initial and Follow-up Evaluation–Screening studies at the time of diagnosis and ongoing monitoring for age groups are summarized in Table 2. All newly diagnosed patients require a thorough cardiovascular evaluation. Blood pressure should be measured in all 4 extremities, and 24-h ambulatory monitoring may be helpful in detecting nocturnal hypertension in girls as disappearance of the night time dip in blood pressure is one of the earliest signs of beginning hypertension. Routine renal ultrasound may detect structural abnormalities in renal architecture or collecting system anatomy. If no abnormalities are present, follow-up studies are not routinely indicated. If significant abnormalities are detected, follow-up evaluation and therapy may be indicated and long-term screening for urinary tract infection may be necessary. Scoliosis and

Table 2
Recommendations for screening in Turner syndrome (excluding cardiac and neuropsychological screening recommendations)

	At diagnosis	After Diagnosis (Childhood)	After Diagnosis (adults)
Weight/BMI	Yes	Every visit	Every visit
Blood pressure	Yes	Every visit	Every visit
Thyroid function tests (TSH and T4 or free T4)	Yes	Annually beginning around 4 y of age	Annually
Lipids			Annually if at least 1 cardiovascular risk factor[a] or regional recommendation
Liver enzymes (ALT, AST, GGTP, and alkaline phosphate)		Annually after 10 years of age	Annually
HbA1c with or without fasting plasma glucose		Annually after 10 years of age	Annually
25-hydroxyvitamin D		Every 2–3 y after 9–11 y of age	Every 3–5 y
Celiac screen		Starting at 2 y; thereafter, every 2 y	With suggesting symptoms
Renal ultrasound	Yes		
Audiometric evaluation	Yes[b]	Every 3 y	Every 5 y
Ophthalmologic examination	Yes[c]	Every 3 y	
Dental evaluation	Yes, if no previous care has been established		
Clinical investigation for congenital hip dysplasia	Yes, in newborns		
Skin examination	Yes	Annually	Annually
Bone mineral density			Every 5 y and when discontinuing estrogen
Skeletal assessment		Spine radiographs at 5–6 y and at 12–14 y of age	

The recommendations are for screening only. A clinical suspicion of active disease should always lead to relevant investigations. For details, please refer to UpToDAte topic text, or to the guideline cited later in discussion.

Abbreviations: ALT, alanine aminotransferase; AST, Aspartate aminotransferase; BMI, body mass index; GGTP, Gamma-glutamyl transpeptidase; HbA1c, hemoglobin A1c; T4, thyroxine; TSH, Thyroid-stimulating hormone.

[a]Cardiovascular risk factor: hypertension, overweight, tobacco use, diabetes, and physical inactivity.

[b]When 9 to 12 month old.

[c]When 12 to 18 month old.

From Gravholt CH et, al; International Turner Syndrome Consensus Group. Clinical practice guidelines for the care of girls and women with Turner syndrome: proceedings from the 2016 Cincinnati International Turner Syndrome Meeting. Eur J Endocrinol. 2017 Sep;177(3):G1-G70. https://doi.org/10.1530/EJE-17-0430. PMID: 28705803.

kyphosis are evaluated at diagnosis and during growth. If noted, the degree and cause of scoliosis should be determined radiographically.

Otologic and ophthalmologic consultations should begin by age 2 to 3 years and continue as clinically indicated. Otitis media is extremely common and should be treated vigorously. Myringotomy and polyethylene tube placement are considered the primary modes of therapy for serous otitis media in Turner syndrome. The high prevalence of hearing loss, either primary or secondary to residual serous otitis media, mandates that regular ENT evaluation with audiometry is needed for most patients. In infancy, feeding measures such as specific bottles and nipples often used for patients with cleft palate may also be indicated. Because abnormalities in speech may be a consequence of palatal deformity, speech evaluation is needed for most girls by age 7, as the narrow palate and small jaw cause malocclusion and crowded dentition frequently requiring orthodontic treatment.

Screening for autoimmune thyroid and celiac diseases begins at age 4 and includes thyroxine, thyroid-stimulating hormone, antithyroid antibodies, and tissue transglutaminase antibodies. Subsequently, thyroxine and thyroid-stimulating hormone or thyroid-stimulating hormone alone should be determined at 1- to 2-year intervals. Celiac screen is usually repeated every few years or as indicated by signs or symptoms. Metabolic screening including liver function tests, renal function tests, fasting glucose, or hemoglobin A1c and lipids should commence at about age 10 or earlier in the context of excess adiposity.

Hypertension is common in Turner syndrome, and blood pressure should be measured at each visit. In addition, 24-h ambulatory monitoring is ideal for detecting nocturnal or stress-related hypertensive episodes that may support the introduction of antihypertensive treatment.

The decision to seek consultation for plastic surgery to correct the webbed neck deformity or the forwardly displaced ears is individual. It must be pointed out to the patient and family that in addition to the webbing, the neck may also be short. Therefore, cosmetic surgery may be somewhat disappointing. In some cases, however, satisfactory results are achieved. Potentially increased keloid formation after plastic surgery should be discussed with the patients.

If, or when, psychometric testing should be performed is an individual family decision. Nevertheless, a preschool evaluation to rule out major areas of cognitive dysfunction might be advisable. School performance should be monitored, and specific problems should be attended to with skilled cognitive specialists. Girls with hearing loss will benefit from preferential seating in the classroom, and those with attention deficit disorder (ADD) may benefit from untimed testing in school when appropriate. The Turner Syndrome Society of the United States (www.turnerysyndrome.org) is an excellent resource.

Growth hormone–In the 1990s, recombinant human growth hormone (GH) was shown to increase growth velocity and final adult height for girls with Turner syndrome. Rosenfeld and coworkers demonstrated a gain in height compared with historical controls [92] and Sas and colleagues showed a clear dose-response effect with increasing GH doses associated with increasing height [93]. The first randomized study with an untreated contemporaneous control group showed that adult height was increased by about 7.3 cm after an average duration of 5.7 years of treatment, at a dose of 0.3 mg/kg/wk [94], which is lower than the current recommended dose of 0.375 mg/kg/wk. Very young girls 9 months to 4 years of age treated with GH maintained a normal growth rate compared with untreated Turner controls [95]. The results of a randomized, double-blind, placebo-controlled study begun at the NI in the Netherlands in 1987 showed an average gain in adult height of 3 cm with GH alone, and 5 cm with GH combined with prepubertal treatment with ultra-low-dose ethinyl estradiol [96]. The ethinyl estradiol dose for girls younger than 12 in the NIH study was less than 1 μg/d, compared with 20 μg in the low-dose birth control pill. These findings are consistent with a growth promoting effect of low, nonfeminizing estradiol levels in the prepubertal years. The growth-enhancing effects of low-dose estradiol are in contrast to the growth-inhibiting effect of feminizing doses of estrogen used to induce pubertal development [97], which is associated with epiphyseal fusion. Ranke and colleagues analyzed height prediction for GH treatment in Turner syndrome [98]. Height at the start of treatment, GH dose, and duration of treatment are identified as important predictive factors.

GH treatment has been evaluated for safety in a group of approximately 5000 girls with Turner syndrome followed for 10 to 20 years in the Genetech National Cooperative Growth Study [99]. An increased frequency of intracranial hypertension (pseudotumor cerebri), scoliosis, and slipped epiphyses was noted, as well as an unexpected higher incidence in the diagnosis of type 1 diabetes. On the beneficial side, GH treatment tends to normalize body proportions, although foot size is disproportionally enlarged [100]. GH treatment has beneficial effects on body composition, as shown in a comparison of age-matched girls who have never received GH (n = 26) to girls treated with GH (n = 76) participating in the NIH natural history study. BMI and visceral adiposity were significantly greater and glucose tolerance significantly worse in the untreated group (off GH treatment of 2 weeks before and during the study), with effects apparent years after the discontinuation of therapy [101].

GH treatment seems to have no adverse effects on the cardiovascular system over short-term follow-up, with body size-adjusted ventricular and aortic dimensions similar in treated and untreated patients [102,103]. Moreover, systemic lipids and aortic compliance were relatively better in girls treated with high-dose GH. A comparison of cortical and trabecular bone in GH-treated and age-matched untreated controls with Turner syndrome reveals no apparent effect of GH treatment on bone mineral density [104].

Late diagnosis of Turner syndrome in girls age 10 and older is a common problem that compromises the attainment of optimal adult stature. In the past, such girls were treated with GH for several years and induction of puberty was delayed to age 15 or older. Such a delay in puberty is now viewed as detrimental to social and sexual development and may impair optimal bone mineralization. Statural growth in these girls may be increased by treatment with the nonaromatizable androgen oxandrolone at a dose of 0.05 mg/kg/d or less, in addition to GH, which may augment growth by up to 4 cm, usually without virilizing effects [105,106]. Oxandrolone is also used to enhance stature when GH is not available, but patients and families must be warned about potential adverse metabolic effects and diminution of breast development associated with androgen treatment.

GH treatment usually begins at the standard recommended dose of 0.05 mg/kg/d, with close monitoring for height velocity, IGF1 level, and potential adverse effects of intracranial hypertension, scoliosis, and slipped capital epiphyses. Treatment of 3 to 4 years is usually required to experience significant height gain and is discontinued when the target height is attained, when bone age is greater than 14 years, or when growth velocity is less than 1.5 cm per year. It is important to keep in mind that the safety data for GH in Turner syndrome represent intermediate-range follow-up of girls in whom treatment was typically initiated in mid-childhood and continued for several years at the preceding dosage. Although reaching an adult height of 5 feet or greater seems desirable from many points of view, there are as yet no proven medical or psychosocial benefits to this pharmacologic achievement, and hence safety should never be compromised to this end.

Extensive reviews of the emerging field of long-acting growth hormone (LAGH) have recently seen published, including by the author of this article [107–109]. The approaches taken for the development of LAGH preparations vary and can influence the pharmacokinetics and/or the pharmacodynamics of rhGH. To date, LAGH preparations have been developed using various approaches to prolong GH action, including forming emulsions (using gelatin and triglycerides), GH encapsulation (using degradable microspheres), GH pegylation, GH conjunction (to albumin or amino acid "tails"), and GH fusion proteins (by means of linking an inert peptide with rhGH at a region that does not interact with the growth hormone receptor) [107,109].

As the era of LAGH approaches, we need to consider whether there will be additional safety risks of LAGH compared with daily rhGH. In this regard, we need to consider issues related to the persistent elevation of GH and GH-related biomarkers, such as IGF1, as well as issues related to the mechanism of making GH long acting. Depending on the structure of LAGH, there may be off-target effects due to components of LAGH not present in rhGH. Treatment with daily rhGH given at bedtime attempts to mimic the normal daily profile of increased GH production overnight. However, daily rhGH is a single peak of GH action, which differs from the physiologic GH production of multiple GH pulses of different durations and intensities. Thus, our current daily rhGH treatment regimen does not provide a physiologic GH profile. LAGH products will likely have different pharmacokinetic profiles of GH release from the injection site into the bloodstream, to the target tissue, and to the GH receptor. The peak and trough levels of IGF1 during daily rhGH and LAGH therapy have been an area of intense debate. The goal of GH therapy has been to increase the IGF1 to promote growth. It remains to be determined whether LAGH will achieve similar or better growth than daily rhGH and whether individualizing LAGH therapy to target IGF1 to the upper part of the normal range would improve efficacy without decreasing safety. Due to the differing pharmacodynamics profile or different forms of LAGH, it will be important to determine the best time to measure IGF1 for safety and efficacy [110].

Puberty–As noted earlier, spontaneous puberty develops in 10% to 30% of girls with Turner syndrome. The higher rate applies mainly to girls with mosaicism for cells with more than one X chromosome, but a significant number of girls with less favorable chromosomal constitutions will also start puberty on their own. Aside from karyotype, the major indicators of potential natural pubertal onset are normal-range values for FSH and anti-Mullerian hormone (AMH). AMH may be particularly informative, because hormone levels directly reflect the presence of developing ovarian follicles and hence potential fertility [111]. Pelvic ultrasound may be helpful, although failure to visualize ovarian tissue does not preclude the presence of follicles. Patients and families are often very interested in potential fertility, and the clinician needs to have this information to provide counseling about reproductive options (discussed later). In most girls more than the age of 10, FSH will have elevated into the menopausal range, and AMH will be undetectable with pelvic ultrasound showing no evidence of ovaries and an immature uterus; these patients will need pubertal induction and maintenance estrogen/progestin treatment.

The aim of estrogen treatment in Turner syndrome is to mimic the beneficial effects of endogenous estrogen in breast and genital development, healthy fat distribution, and bone mineralization, while minimizing the risk for estrogen-associated gynecologic cancers and thrombogenic complications. In the past, the choice for estrogen treatment was limited to metabolized estrogens purified from pregnant mare urine (conjugated equine estrogens [CEE], "Premarin."), and the highly potent, synthetic ethinyl estradiol (EE2). In recent years, transdermal patches containing the natural ovarian product, 17-beta estradiol have become available and are now the preferred delivery method. In addition to replicating the molecular action of the ovary's natural hormone, this formulation is directly absorbed into the venous circulation, bypassing first-pass hepatic effects associated with excessive production of prothrombotic proteins. Moreover, the administration of transdermal estradiol allows the measurement of estradiol levels in the circulation, which may be helpful for monitoring adherence. Because estradiol levels vary widely throughout the monthly cycles in eugonadal females, target estradiol levels in pharmacologic treatment are not known. In sexually mature girls, the average daily ovarian estradiol production over the monthly cycle is 100 μg/d, which is approximated by transdermal patches delivering 100 μg/d. Physiologic estradiol repletion is not expected to normalize the FSH level, because FSH secretion is jointly regulated by estrogen and other ovarian products such as the inhibins. Thus, suppression of FSH is not a measure of adequate estrogen therapy.

Current recommendations for estrogen treatment of the induction of puberty suggest beginning the therapy at age 12 for most girls [112]. The aim of treatment is to initiate development with the lowest possible dose so that sexual maturation will begin on par with peers, while avoiding premature fusion of the epiphyses that would limit growth in stature. Thus, breast development and bone age are evaluated at 6-month intervals during estrogen treatment of pubertal induction. A sufficient phase of "unopposed" estrogen exposure is required for optimal breast development, and androgen or progesterone treatments may inhibit optimal development. Thus, oxandrolone should be discontinued before the initiation of estrogen treatment, and progestins should not be initiated until breast development is satisfactory. Some girls with prominent stigmata of fetal lymphedema may have damaged breast anlage and demonstrate minimal development in response to estrogen. These girls may benefit from breast implantation surgery, if so inclined.

Progestin treatment is necessary to suppress estrogen's proliferative effect on the uterine endometrium and should be introduced after 1 to 2 years of unopposed estrogen treatment, or sooner if breakthrough bleeding occurs. This recommendation is given because chronic exposure to estrogen treatment, in the absence of progestin effect, leads to endometrial hyperplasia and risk for hemorrhage and neoplasia. The most physiologic form of progestin is progesterone, which is available in a micronized form for oral administration and in cream and gel form. Regrettably, there have been no controlled studies to establish the most effective form of estrogen/progestin treatment of girls with Turner syndrome. The accepted dose of oral micronized progesterone proven to protect the uterus is 200 mg taken at bedtime for the last 10 to 12 days of a monthly cycle, or the last 20 to 30 days of a trimonthly cycle. Progesterone is soporific and hence the bedtime administration. The efficacy of topical progesterone in preventing uterine hyperplasia is unknown. More androgenic, synthetic progestins such as medroxyprogesterone or norethindrone may inhibit optimal breast and uterine development and have unfavorable metabolic effects in some individuals, although these agents are effective in endometrial protection.

Patients and families must be educated as to the importance of this physiologic hormone treatment regimen for healthy growth and development, especially with regard to building and maintaining strong bones. Discontinuation of hormone therapy during young adulthood is all too common and may result in irreversible loss of bone minerals especially in the spine, leading to height loss, kyphosis, and chronic pain and disability. Families may have legitimate concerns about the risks of heart disease and cancer associated with hormone replacement therapy, and it must be explained that these adverse effects were observed in postmenopausal women receiving less physiologic forms of treatment. It is also important to discuss "natural" hormones that are widely touted on women's health sites as an alternative to standard treatments underlining the fact that these products are not known to be effective or safe. Many older girls and young women may prefer taking oral or transdermal contraceptive formulations for reasons of convenience, tolerability, or financial concerns. Although these are not the most physiologic choices and have greater thrombogenic risk, estrogen/progestin contraceptive formulations are effective in maintaining bone mineralization and protecting the uterus.

It is important to point out that spontaneous puberty, even with menses that seem cyclic, does not always mean that normal ovulatory cycles are occurring or will continue to occur. Some girls have anovulatory cycles that do not achieve normal endometrial maturation and predispose them to endometrial hyperplasia, dysfunctional bleeding, or cancer. Irregular cycles may lead to the discontinuation of treatment in many cases. Every effort should be made to educate patients and parents as to the importance of continuing hormone replacement, with openness to consultation with experts in adolescent gynecology and adoption of alternative regimes such as oral contraceptive treatment that may ensure continued adherence. Girls with irregular cycles may still have an occasional ovulatory cycle and, if sexually active, are at risk for unplanned pregnancy. For these girls, contraceptive formulations may be the best choice for hormone therapy.

Hormone treatment requires regular breast examinations, and patients should be instructed about monthly self-examination. Girls who become sexually active need regular gynecologic follow-up with annual pelvic examinations and Pap tests. Regular discussion of issues of concern related to sexual maturation and counseling on the need for ongoing hormone treatment to maintain strong bones will be of paramount importance. There is no need to measure bone mineral density during childhood or adolescence unless there is an unusual clinical concern-for example, a low-impact or atraumatic fracture. Short stature is associated with the underestimation of bone mineral density obtained by DXA and results need to be normalized for bone size [113]. Size-adjusted vertebral bone mineral density is usually normal in adults with Turner syndrome that have received routine hormone replacement treatment, but it may decline dramatically with the discontinuation of treatment [114]. Bone mineral density of the hip and wrist is often lower than normal, reflecting a selective reduction in cortical bone that is not sensitive to estrogen [115] but may reflect the SHOX defect in bone.

Reproductive options–About 2% of women with Turner syndrome may have spontaneous pregnancies. Assisted reproduction using donor oocytes with in vitro fertilization has been successful when the uterus has been given adequate hormonal preparation before embryo transfer [116]. However, both spontaneous and assisted pregnancies are associated with a high risk for maternal complications, including catastrophic aortic dilatation, dissection, and rupture [117]. In most well-documented cases, the women had preexisting risk factors for dissection such as bicuspid aortic valve or aortic coarctation, although these problems were often not detected before pregnancy due to inadequate screening [118]. Patients known to have such defects should be counseled about alternatives to pregnancy such as adoption or surrogacy. If not already done, girls and young women with Turner syndrome should have a cardiovascular MRI before getting involved in counseling about reproductive options, because significant aortic malformations are often not detected on routine echocardiography and their presence would discourage planning for pregnancy. Girls with ovarian function may be candidates for the cryopreservation of recovered oocytes or ovarian tissue obtained by laparoscopy [116] given the very high probability of premature ovarian failure. This technology has been successful in preserving fertility for girls and women undergoing cancer treatment, although pregnancy resulting from this approach has not yet been reported in Turner syndrome. Girls and families interested in this possibility should be referred to reproductive endocrinology specialists associated with an academic medical center for consultation.

Psychological and educational issues–Psychologic assessment should be part of the initial evaluation and ongoing management plan for each child with Turner syndrome. Assessment of intellectual skills, learning skills, motor skills, and social maturity is recommended before enrollment in preschool programs [119]. Intelligence is usually normal, except in the rare patient with a tiny X-ring chromosome, who may have severe mental retardation because tiny X-ring chromosomes fail to undergo X inactivation [120,121].

Although most individuals with Turner syndrome have normal intelligence, there are increased risks for selective impairment in nonverbal skills [5,122]. This may include deficits in social cognition; difficulty with nonverbal problem-solving tasks such as mathematics; psychomotor deficits, such as clumsiness; and problems with visual-spatial organization, which may cause difficulty driving [18]. There is also an increased risk of attention deficit disorder. By contrast, verbal skills are often strong. These neurodevelopmental abnormalities may result from the X chromosome monosomy or from sex steroid deficiencies due to gonadal dysgenesis.

Imprinting by material from the paternal X chromosome was suggested in one report, implying that social functioning is influenced by an imprinted gene on the X chromosome that is switched off when this gene is inherited from the mother [123]. The existence of such a gene may partly explain the male–female differences in social cognition; it does not, however, provide an explanation for all psychological findings in Turner syndrome. Such an explanation would most likely involve an interplay between many genes and interacting environmental factors.

As these young women make the transition to independent living, counselors should stress that their learning difficulties do not disappear with age.

Family support–Information for caregivers and patients can be obtained from:

Turner Syndrome Society of the United States Tel: 1 to 800 to 365 to 9944
www.turnersyndrome.org
Turner Syndrome Society of Canada Tel: 1 to 800 to 465 to 6744
www.TurnerSyndrome.ca
Turner Syndrome Society of UK Tel: +44(0)1389 to 380385
www.tss.org.uk/

SUMMARY

- Turner syndrome, the most common sex chromosome abnormality (loss of part or all of an X chromosome), affects approximately 1 in every 2500 liveborn female newborns. It is a disorder of growth and development that is almost always associated with short stature and primary amenorrhea due to early ovarian failure.
- Girls/women with Turner syndrome whose karyotype includes a Y chromosome (such as 45,X/46,XY mosaicism) are at increased risk for gonadoblastoma, a neoplasm that occurs in dysgenetic gonads. These patients require gonadectomies.
- Patients with Turner syndrome are at increased risk for cardiovascular morbidity, presumably due to their risk of cardiovascular malformations, renal abnormalities, and hypertension. Abnormalities include aortic valvular disease, aortic arch anomalies (primarily coarctation), systemic venous abnormalities, ventricular septal defects, and hypoplastic left heart syndrome. Patients are at risk for aortic dissection, particularly during pregnancy.
- Osteoporosis and fractures are common in women with Turner syndrome, thought to be due to both ovarian failure and possibly haploinsufficiency for bone-related X chromosome genes.
- Girls with Turner syndrome are more likely than girls without Turner syndrome to develop abdominal obesity, insulin resistance, and type 2 diabetes; all may improve with growth hormone therapy. Patients with Turner syndrome are at increased risk for autoimmune endocrinopathies, most importantly, hypothyroidism.
- The diagnosis of Turner syndrome is sometimes made at birth in the patient with classic physical features such as webbed neck and congenital lymphedema. Other patients are diagnosed later, when they present with either growth failure in childhood, failure to enter or complete puberty, or early ovarian failure.

CLINICS CARE POINTS

- Turner syndrome, the most common sex chromosome abnormality (loss of part or all of an X chromosome), affects approximately 1 in every 2500 liveborn female newborns. It is a disorder of growth and development that is almost always associated with short stature and primary amenorrhea due to early ovarian failure.
- Girls/women with Turner syndrome whole karyotype includes a Y chromosome (such as 45,X/46,XY mosaicism) are at increased risk for gonadoblastoma, a neoplasm that occurs in dysgenetic gonads. These patients require gonadectomies.
- Patients with Turner syndrome are at increased risk for cardiovascular morbidity, presumably due to their risk of cardiovascular malformations, renal abnormalities, and hypertension. Abnormalities include aortic valvular disease, aortic arch anomalies (primary coarctation), systemic venous abnormalities, ventricular septal defects, and hypoplastic left heart syndrome. Patients are at risk for aortic dissection, particularly during pregnancy.

- Osteoporosis and fractures are common in women with Turner syndrome, thought to be due to both ovarian failure and possibly haploinsufficiency for bone-related X chromosome genes.
- Girls with Turner syndrome are more likely than girls without Turner syndrome to develop abdominal obesity, insulin resistance, and type 2 diabetes; all may improve with growth hormone therapy. Patients with Turner syndrome are at increased risk for autoimmune endocrinopathies, most importantly, hypothyroidism.

Disclosure

The authors have nothing to disclose.

References

[1] Turner HH. A syndrome of infantilism, congenital webbed neck and cubitus valgus. Endocrinology 1938;23:566.
[2] Ullrich O. Turner's syndrome and status Bonnevie-Ullrich. Am J Hum Genet 1949;1:179.
[3] Barr ML, Bertram EG. A morphological distinction between neurons of the male and female and the behavior of the nucleolar satellite during accelerated nucleo-protein synthesis. Nature 1949;163:676.
[4] Males JL, Seely JR. Turner's syndrome: Index case after 44 years (a tribute to Dr. Henry H. Turner). K Clin Endocrinol Metab 1978;46:163.
[5] Bondy CA, Turner Syndrome Study Group. Care of girls and women with Turner syndrome: a guideline of the Turner Syndrome Study Group. J Clin Endocrinol Metab 2007;92:10.
[6] Gravhold CH, Juul S, Naeraa RW, et al. Prenatal and postnatal prevalence of Turner's syndrome: a registry study. BMJ 1996;312(7022):16–21.
[7] Gunther DF, Eugster E, Zagar AJ, et al. Ascertainment bias in Turner syndrome: new insights from girls who were diagnosed incidentally in prenatal life. Pediatrics 2004;114:640.
[8] Mathur A, Stekol L, Schatz D, et al. The parental origin of the single X chromosome in Turner syndrome: lack of correlation with parental age or clinical phenotype. Am J Hum Genet 1991;48:682.
[9] Ferguson-Smith MA. Karyotype-Phenotype correlations in gonadal dysgenesis and their bearing on the pathogenesis of malformations. J Med Genet 1965;2:142.
[10] Simpson JL. Gonadal dysgenesis and abnormalities of the human sex chromosomes: current status of phenotypic-karyotypic correlations. Birth Defects Orig Artic Ser 1975;11:23.
[11] Held KR, Kerber S, Kaminsky E, et al. Mosaicism in 45,X Turner syndrome: does survival in early pregnancy depend on the presence of two sex chromosomes? Hum Genet 1992;88: 288.
[12] Binder G, Koch A, Wajs E, et al. Nested polymerase chain reaction study of 53 cases with Turner's syndrome: is cytogenetically undetected Y mosaicism common? J Clin Endocrinol Metab 2008;93:2109.
[13] Wooten N, Bakalov VK, Hill S, et al. Reduced abdominal adiposity and improved glucose tolerance in growth hormone-treated girls with Turner syndrome. J Clin Endocrinol Metab 2008;93:2109.
[14] Rao E, Weiss B, Fukami M, et al. Pseudoautosomal deletions encompassing a novel homeobox gene cause growth failure in idiopathic short stature and Turner syndrome. Nat Genet 1997;16:54.
[15] Ross JL, Scott C Jr, Marttila P, et al. Phenotypes Associated with SHOX Deficiency. J Clin Endocrinol Metab 2001;86:5674.

[16] Ross JL, Kowal K, Quigley CA, et al. The phenotype of short stature homeobox gene (SHOX) deficiency in childhood: contrasting children with Leri-Weill dyschondrosteosis and Turner syndrome. J Pediatr 2005;147:499.
[17] Huber C, Rosilio M, Munnich A, et al. High incidence of SHOX anomalies in individuals with short stature. J Med Genet 2006;43:735.
[18] Sybert VP, McCauley E. Turner's syndrome. N Engl J Med 2004;351:1227.
[19] Loscalzo ML, Van PL, Ho VB, et al. Association between fetal lymphedema and congenital cardiovascular defects in Turner syndrome. Pediatrics 2005;115:732.
[20] Clark EB. Neck web and congenital heart defects: a pathogenic association in 45 X-O Turner syndrome? Teratology 1984;29:355.
[21] Mazzanti L, Cacciari E. Congenital heart disease in patients with Turner's syndrome. Italian Study Group for Turner Syndrome (ISGTS). J Pediatr 1998;133:688.
[22] McCarthy K, Bondy CA. Turner syndrome in childhood and adolescence. Expert Rev Endocrinol Metab 2008;3:771.
[23] Wyss D, DeLozier CD, Daniell J, et al. Structural anomalies of the X chromosome: personal observation and review of non-mosaic cases. Clin Genet 1982;21:145.
[24] dos Santos AP, Andrade JG, Piveta CS, et al. Screening of Y chromosome microdeletions in 46, XY partial gonadal dysgenesis and in patients with a 45,X/46,XY karyotype or its variants. BMC Med Genet 2013;14:115.
[25] Sävendahl L, Davenport ML. Delayed diagnoses of Turner's syndrome: proposed guidelines for change. J Pediatr 2000;137:455.
[26] Ranke MB, Pflüger H, Rosendahl W, et al. Turner syndrome: spontaneous growth in 150 cases and review of the literature. Eur J Pediatr 1983;141:81.
[27] Brook CG, Mürset G, Zachmann M, et al. Growth in children with 45,XO Turner's syndrome. Arch Dis Child 1974;49:789.
[28] Sylvén L, Hagenfeldt K, Bröndum-Nielsen K, et al. Middle-aged women with Turner's syndrome. Medical status, hormonal treatment and social life. Acta Endocrinol (Copenh) 1991;125:359.
[29] Freriks K, Timmermans J, Beerendonk CC, et al. Standardized multidisciplinary evaluation yields significant previously undiagnosed morbidity in adult women with Turner syndrome. J Clin Endocrinol Metab 2011;96:E1517.
[30] Elsheikh M, Hodgson HJ, Wass JA, et al. Hormone replacement therapy may improve hepatic function in women with Turner's syndrome. Clin Endocrinol (Oxf) 2001;55:227.
[31] El-Mansoury M, Berntorp L, Byman I, et al. Elevated liver enzymes in Turner syndrome during a 5-year follow-up study. Clin Endocrinol (Oxf) 2008;68:568.
[32] Bakalov VK, Gutin L, Cheng CM, et al. Autoimmune disorders in women with turner syndrome and women with karyotypically normal primary ovarian insufficiency. J Autoimmun 2012;38:315.
[33] Chiovato L, Larizza D, Bendinelli G, et al. Autoimmune hypothyroidism and hyperthyroidism in patients with Turner's syndrome. Eur J Endocrinol 1996;134:568.
[34] Ostberg JE, Conway GS. Adulthood in women with Turner syndrome. Horm Res 2003;59:211.
[35] Pasquino AM, Passeri F, Pucarelli I, et al. Spontaneous pubertal development in Turner's syndrome. Italian Study Group for Turner's Syndrome. J Clin Endocrinol Metab 1997;82:1810.
[36] Hadnott TN, Gould HN, Gharib AM, et al. Outcomes of spontaneous and assisted pregnancies in Turner syndrome: the U.S. National Institutes of Health experience. Fertil Steril 2011;95:2251.
[37] Saenger P. Clinical manifestations and diagnosis of Turner syndrome (gonadal dysgenesis). UpToDate 2015.
[38] Singh RP, Carr DH. The anatomy and histology of XO human embryos and fetuses. Anat Rec 1966;155:369.

[39] Massarano AA, Adams JA, Preece MA, et al. Ovarian ultrasound appearances in Turner syndrome. J Pediatr 1989;114:568.
[40] King CR, Magenis E, Bennett S. Pregnancy and the Turner syndrome. Obstet Gynecol 1978;52:617.
[41] Reyes FL, Koh KS, Faiman C. Fertility in women with gonadal dysgenesis. Am J Obstet Gynecol 1976;126:668.
[42] Gravholt CH, Juul S, Naeraa RW, et al. Morbidity in Turner syndrome. J Clin Epidemiol 1998;51:147.
[43] Cramer JW, Bartz PJ, Simpson PM, et al. The spectrum of congenital heart disease and outcomes after surgical repair among children with Turner syndrome: a single-center review. Pediatr Cardiol 2014;35:253.
[44] Ho VB, Bakalov VK, Cooley M, et al. Major vascular anomalies in Turner syndrome: prevalence and magnetic resonance angiographic features. Circulation 2004;110:1694.
[45] Gøtzsche CO, Krag-Olsen B, Nielsen J, et al. Prevalence of cardiovascular malformations and association with karyotypes in Turner's syndrome. Arch Dis Child 1994;71:433.
[46] Elsheikh M, Casadei B, Conway GS, et al. Hypertension is a major risk factor for aortic root dilatation in women with Turner's syndrome. Clin Endocrinol (Oxf) 2001;54:69.
[47] Sachdev V, Matura LA, Sidenko S, et al. Aortic valve disease in Turner syndrome. J Am Coll Cardiol 2008;51:1904.
[48] Ilyas M, Chu C, Ettles D, et al. Evaluation by magnetic resonance imaging of aortic dilatation and coarctation in adult Turner syndrome patients. Clin Endocrinol (Oxf) 2006;65:154.
[49] Lin AE, Lippe B, Rosenfeld RG. Further delineation of aortic dilation, dissection, and rupture in patients with Turner syndrome. Pediatrics 1998;102:e12.
[50] Matura LA, Ho VB, Rosing DR, et al. Aortic dilatation and dissection in Turner syndrome. Circulation 2007;116:1663.
[51] Carlson M, Airhart N, Lopez L, et al. Moderate aortic enlargement and bicuspid aortic valve are associated with aortic dissection in Turner syndrome: report of the international turner syndrome aortic dissection registry. Circulation 2012;126:2220.
[52] Karnis MF, Zimon AE, Lalwani SI, et al. Risk of death in pregnancy achieved through oocyte donation in patients with Turner syndrome: a national survey. Fertil Steril 2003;80:498.
[53] Practice Committee of the American Society for Reproductive Medicine. Increased maternal cardiovascular mortality associated with pregnancy in women with Turner syndrome. Fertil Steril 2006;86:S127.
[54] Nathwani NC, Unwin R, Brook CG, et al. The influence of renal and cardiovascular abnormalities on blood pressure in Turner syndrome. Clin Endocrinol (Oxf) 2000;52:371.
[55] Landin-Wilhelmsen K, Bryman I, Wilhelmsen L. Cardiac malformations and hypertension, but not metabolic risk factors, are common in Turner syndrome. J Clin Endocrinol Metab 2001;86:4166.
[56] Fudge EB, Constantacos C, Fudge JC, et al. Improving detection of hypertension in girls with turner syndrome using ambulatory blood pressure monitoring. Horm Res Paediatr 2014;81:25.
[57] Bondy CA, Van PL, Bakalov VK, et al. Prolongation of the cardiac QTc interval in Turner syndrome. Medicine (Baltimore) 2006;85:75.
[58] Bondy CA, Bakalov VK. Investigation of cardiac status and bone mineral density in Turner syndrome. Growth Horm IGF Res 2006;16(Suppl A):S103.
[59] Bondy CA, Ceniceros I, Van PL, et al. Prolonged rate-corrected QT interval and other electrocardiogram abnormalities in girls with Turner syndrome. Pediatrics 2006;118:e1220.
[60] Dalla Pozza R, Bechtold S, Urschel S, et al. QTc interval prolongation in children with Turner syndrome: the results of exercise testing and 24-h ECG. Eur J Pediatr 2009;168:59.
[61] Ostberg JE, Donald AE, Halcox JP, et al. Vasculopathy in Turner syndrome: arterial dilatation and intimal thickening without endothelial dysfunction. J Clin Endocrinol Metab 2005;90:5161.

[62] Rubin K. Turner syndrome and osteoporosis: mechanisms and prognosis. Pediatrics 1998;102:481.
[63] Gravholt CH, Vestergaard P, Hermann AP, et al. Increased fracture rates in Turner's syndrome: a nationwide questionnaire survey. Clin Endocrinol (Oxf) 2003;59:89.
[64] Landin-Wilhelmsen K, Bryman I, Windh M, et al. Osteoporosis and fractures in Turner syndrome- importance of growth promoting and oestrogen therapy. Clin Endocrinol (Oxf) 1999;51:497.
[65] Bakalov VK, Chen ML, Baron J, et al. Bone mineral density and fractures in Turner syndrome. Am J Med 2003;115:259.
[66] Bakalov VK, Axelrod L, Baron J, et al. Selective reduction in cortical bone mineral density in turner syndrome independent of ovarian hormone deficiency. J Clin Endocrinol Metab 2003;88:5717.
[67] Gravholt CH, Fedder J, Naeraa RW, et al. Occurrence of gonadoblastoma in females with Turner syndrome and Y chromosome material: a population study. J Clin Endocrinol Metab 2000;85:3199.
[68] Schoemaker MJ, Swerdlow AJ, Higgins CD, et al. Cancer incidence in women with Turner syndrome in Great Britain: a national cohort study. Lancet Oncol 2008;9:239.
[69] Denniston A. Turner's syndrome. Lancet 2001;358:2169.
[70] Chrousos GA, Ross JL, Chrousos G, et al. Ocular findings in Turner syndrome. A prospective study. Ophthalmology 1984;91:926.
[71] Adhikary HP. Ocular manifestations of Turner's syndrome. Trans Ophthalmol Soc U K 1981;101(Pt 4):395.
[72] Mason JO 3rd, Tasman W. Turner's syndrome associated with bilateral retinal detachments. Am J Ophthalmol 1996;122:742.
[73] Elsheikh M, Wass JA, Conway GS. Autoimmune thyroid syndrome in women with Turner's syndrome—the association with karyotype. Clin Endocrinol (Oxf) 2001;55:223.
[74] El-Mansoury M, Bryman I, Berntorp K, et al. Hypothyroidism is common in turner syndrome: results of a five-year follow-up. J Clin Endocrinol Metab 2005;90:2131.
[75] Bonamico M, Pasquino AM, Mariani P, et al. Prevalence and clinical picture of celiac disease in Turner syndrome. J Clin Endocrinol Metab 1991;87:85495.
[76] Caprio S, Boulware S, Diamond M, et al. Insulin resistance: an early metabolic defect of Turner's syndrome. J Clin Endocrinol Metab 1991;72:832.
[77] Handler MZ, Derrick KM, Lutz RE, et al. Prevalence of pilomatricoma in Turner syndrome: findings from a multicenter study. JAMA Dermatol 2013;149:559.
[78] Wood S, Nguyen D, Hutton K, et al. Pilomatricomas in Turner syndrome. Pediatr Dermatol 2008;25:449.
[79] Bengtzen AR, Grossniklaus HE, Bernardino CR. Multiple pilomatrixoma in Turner syndrome. Ophthal Plast Reconstr Surg 2009;25:229.
[80] Brazzelli V, Larizza D, Martinetti M, et al. Halo nevus, rather than vitiligo, is a typical dermatologic finding of Turner 's syndrome: clinical, genetic, and immunogenetic study in 72 patients. J Am Acad Dermatol 2004;51:354.
[81] Lowenstein EJ, Kim KH, Glick SA. Turner's syndrome in dermatology. J Am Acad Dermatol 2004;50:767.
[82] Anderson H, Filipsson R, Fluur E, et al. Hearing impairment in Turner's syndrome. Acta Otolaryngol Suppl 1969;247:1.
[83] King KA, Makishima T, Zalewski CK, et al. Analysis of auditory phenotype and karyotype in 200 females with Turner syndrome. Ear Hear 2007;28:831–41.
[84] Barrenäs ML, Nylén O, Hanson C. The influence of karyotype on the auricle, otitis media and hearing in Turner syndrome. Hear Res 1999;138:163–70.
[85] Stenberg AE, Nylén O, Windh M, et al. Otological problems in children with Turner's syndrome. Hear Res 1998;124:85–90.
[86] Dhooge IJ, De Vel E, Verhoye C, et al. Otologic disease in Turner syndrome. Otol Neurotol 2005;26:145–50.

[87] Salerno M, Di Maio S, Gasparini N, et al. Liver abnormalities in Turner syndrome. Eur J Pediatr 1999;158:618–23.
[88] Koulouri O, Ostberg J, Conway G. Liver dysfunction in Turner's syndrome: prevalence, natural history, and effect of exogenous oestrogen. Clin Endocrinol 2008;69:306–10.
[89] Wemme H, Pohlenz J, Schönberger W. Effect of oestrogen/gestagen replacement therapy on liver enzymes in patients with Ullrich-Turner syndrome. Eur J Pediatr 1995;154: 807–10.
[90] McCarthy K, Bondy C. Turner syndrome in childhood and adolescence. Expert Rev Endocrinol Metab 2008;3:771–5.
[91] Roulot D. Liver involvement in Turner syndrome. Liver Int 2013;33:24–30.
[92] Rosenfeld RG, Attie KM, Frane J, et al. Growth hormone therapy of Turner's syndrome: beneficial effect on adult height. J Pediatr 1998;132:319–24.
[93] Sas TC, de Muinck Keizer-Schrama SM, Otten BJ, et al. Normalization of height in girls with Turner syndrome after long-term growth hormone treatment: results of a randomized dose-response trial. J Clin Endocrinol Metab 1999;84:4607–12.
[94] Stephure DK. Impact of growth hormone supplementation on adult height in turner syndrome: results of the Canadian randomized controlled trial. J Clin Endocrinol Metab 2005;90:3360–6.
[95] Davenport ML, Crowe BJ, Travers SH, et al. Growth hormone treatment of early growth failure in toddlers with Turner syndrome a randomized, controlled, multicenter trial. J Clin Endocrinol Metab 2007;92:3406–16.
[96] Ross JL, Quigley CA, Cao D, et al. Growth hormone plus childhood low-dose estrogen in Turner's syndrome. N Engl J Med 2011;364:1230–42.
[97] Chernausek SD, Attie KM, Cara JF, et al. Growth hormone therapy of Turner syndrome: the impact of age of estrogen replacement on final height. Genentech, Inc., Collaborative Study Group. J Clin Endocrinol Metab 2000;85:2439–45.
[98] Ranke MB, Lindberg A, Chatelain P, et al. Prediction of long-term response to recombinant human growth hormone in Turner syndrome: development and validation of mathematical models. KIGS International Board. Kabi international Growth Study. J Clin Endocrinol Metab 2000;85:4212–8.
[99] Bolar K, Hoffman AR, Maneatis T, et al. Long-term safety of recombinant human growth hormone in Turner syndrome. J Clin Endocrinol Metab 2008;93:344–51.
[100] Sas TC, Gerver WJ, de Bruin R, et al. Body proportions during long-term growth hormone treatment in girls with Turner syndrome participating in a randomized dose-response trial. J Clin Endocrinol Metab 1999;84:4622–8.
[101] Wooten N, Bakalov NK, Hill S, et al. Reduced abdominal adiposity and improved glucose tolerance in growth hormone-treated girls with Turner syndrome. J Clin Endocrinol Metab 2008;93:2109–14.
[102] Matura LA, Sachdev V, Bakalov VK, et al. Growth hormone treatment and left ventricular dimensions in Turner syndrome. J Pediatr 2007;150:587–91.
[103] Bondy CA, Van PL, Bakalov VK, et al. Growth hormone treatment and aortic dimensions in Turner syndrome. J Clin Endocrinol Metab 2006;91:1785–8.
[104] Ari M, Bakalov VK, Hill S, et al. The effects of growth hormone treatment on bone mineral density and body composition in girls with Turner syndrome. J Clin Endocrinol Metab 2006;91:4302–5.
[105] Zeger MP, Shah K, Kowal K, et al. Prospective study confirms oxandrolone-associated improvement in height in growth hormone-treated adolescent girls with Turner syndrome. Horm Res Paediatr 2011;75:38–46.
[106] Gault EJ, Perry RJ, Cole TJ, et al. Effect of oxandrolone and timing of pubertal induction on final height in Turner's syndrome: randomized, double blind, placebo controlled trial. BMJ 2011;342:d1980.
[107] Saenger PH, Mejia-Corletto J. Long-acting growth hormone: an update. Endocr Dev 2016;30:79–97.

[108] Yuen KCJ, Miller BS, Biller BMK. The current state of long-acting growth hormone preparations for growth hormone therapy. Curr Opin Endocrinol Diabetes Obes 2018;25(4):267–73.
[109] Christiansen JS, Backeljauw PF, Bidlingmaier M, et al. Growth Hormone Research Society perspective on the development of long-acting growth hormone preparations. Eur J Endocrinol 2016;174(6):C1–8.
[110] Collett-Solberg PF, Jorge AA, Boguszewski MC, et al. Growth hormone therapy in children; research and practice—A review. Growth Horm IGF Res 2019;44:20–32.
[111] Hagen CP, Aksglaede L, Sørensen K, et al. Serum levels of anti-Mullerian hormone as a marker of ovarian function in 926 healthy females from birth to adulthood and in 172 Turner syndrome patients. J Clin Endocrinol Metab 2010;95:5003–10.
[112] Bondy CA. Turner Syndrome Study Group. Care of girls and women with Turner syndrome: a guideline of the Turner Syndrome Study Group. J Clin Endocrinol Metab 2007;92:10–25.
[113] Bakalov VK, Chen ML, Baron J, et al. Bone mineral density and fractures in Turner syndrome. Am J Med 2003;115:257–62.
[114] Hanton L, Axelrod L, Bakalov VK, et al. The importance of estrogen replacement in young women with turner syndrome. J Women's Health (Larchmt) 2003;12:971–7.
[115] Bakalov VK, Axelrod L, Baron K, et al. Selective reduction in cortical bone mineral density in Turner syndrome independent of ovarian hormone deficiency. J Clin Endocrinol Metab 2003;88:5717–22.
[116] Hovatta O. Ovarian function and in vitro fertilization (IVF) in Turner syndrome. Pediatr Endocrinol Rev 2012;9(Suppl. 2):713–7.
[117] Hadnott TN, Bondy CA. Risks of pregnancy for women with Turner syndrome. Expert Rev Obstet Gynecol 2011;6:217–27.
[118] Boissonnas CC, Davy C, Bornes M, et al. Careful cardiovascular screening and follow-up of women with Turner syndrome before and during pregnancy is necessary to prevent maternal mortality. Fertil Steril 2009;91:929 e5–e7.
[119] Bender B, Puck M, Salbenblatt J, et al. Cognitive development of unselected girls with complete and partial X monosomy. Pediatrics 1984;73:175.
[120] Migeon BR, Luo S, Stasiowski BA, et al. Deficient transcription of XIST from tiny ring X chromosomes in females with severe phenotypes. Proc Natl Acad Sci U S A 1993;90:12025.
[121] Collins AL, Cockwell AE, Jacobs PA, et al. A comparison of the clinical and cytogenetic findings in nine patients with a ring (X) cell line and 16 45,X patients. J Med Genet 1994;31:528.
[122] McCauley E, Feuillan P, Kushner H, et al. Psychosocial development in adolescents with Turner syndrome. J Dev Behav Pediatr 2001;22:360.
[123] Skuse DH, James RS, Bishop DV, et al. Evidence from Turner's syndrome of an imprinted X-linked locus affecting cognitive function. Nature 1997;387:705.

Advances in Pediatrics 69 (2022) 203–217

ADVANCES IN PEDIATRICS

Clinical Indications for Growth Hormone Therapy

Melinda Danowitz, DO[a], Adda Grimberg, MD[b,c,*]

[a]CHOP Division of Pediatric Endocrinology, Abramson Building, Office 804F, 3401 Civic Center Boulevard, Philadelphia, PA 19104, USA; [b]Children's Hospital of Philadelphia, The Hub for Clinical Collaboration, Division of Endocrinology, 7th floor, 3500 Civic Center Boulevard, Philadelphia, PA 19104, USA; [c]Department of Pediatrics, Perelman School of Medicine, University of Pennsylvania, Philadelphia, PA, USA

Keywords

• Growth hormone • Growth • Short stature • Growth hormone deficiency • Prader–Willi syndrome • Turner syndrome • Idiopathic short stature

Key points

- Food and Drug Administration (FDA)-approved indications for pediatric GH therapy in the US include GH deficiency, Prader–Willi Syndrome, small for gestational age (SGA) without catch-up growth, idiopathic short stature, Turner syndrome, *SHOX* gene haploinsufficiency, Noonan Syndrome, and chronic renal insufficiency.
- Short stature may be secondary to an underlying genetic abnormality, malnutrition, or systemic condition, or can present in a healthy child; practitioners should evaluate for systemic causes of short stature and consider referral to a pediatric endocrinologist if workup is unrevealing.
- Rare but serious possible complications of GH treatment include intracranial hypertension, SCFE, worsening of scoliosis, obstructive sleep apnea, and pancreatitis.

Funding sources: A. Grimberg is supported by NIH grant 1 R01 HD097129 from the Eunice Kennedy Shriver National Institute of Child Health and Human Development. The NIH played no role in the writing of the article. The content of this article is solely the responsibility of the authors and does not necessarily represent the official views of NICHD or NIH.

*Corresponding author. CHOP Div Pediatric Endocrinology, The Hub for Clinical Collaboration, 7th floor, 3500 Civic Center Boulevard, Philadelphia, PA 19104. *E-mail address:* Grimberg@chop.edu

https://doi.org/10.1016/j.yapd.2022.03.005

Abbreviations

GH	growth hormone
GHD	growth hormone deficiency
SGA	small for gestational age
PWS	prader-Willi syndrome
FDA	food and Drug Administration
ISS	idiopathic short stature
IGF	insulin-like growth factor
SD	standard deviation
TS	turner syndrome
CRI	chronic renal insufficiency

INTRODUCTION

Recombinant human growth hormone (GH) first received approval from the United States Food and Drug Administration (FDA) for clinical treatment in 1985 for pediatric GH deficiency, and its indications subsequently have expanded. Short stature is one of the most common chief comlpaints for referral to a pediatric endocrinologist. Short stature may be secondary to an underlying genetic abnormality, malnutrition, or systemic condition, or can present in a healthy child. There are currently 8 FDA-approved indications for pediatric GH therapy in the United States. Of these, short stature in GH deficiency and Prader–Willi syndrome is due to a deficiency of GH. The other 6 indications do not involve GH deficiency; treatment aims to augment height by adding to the body's own endogenous GH production. We will describe the characteristic features for each of these indications, as well as summarize the use of GH, other endocrine manifestations of the conditions, and relevant diagnostic testing. We also will review patterns of growth that warrant referral to a pediatric endocrinologist as well as safety updates on the use of GH treatment.

FOOD AND DRUG ADMINISTRATION-APPROVED INDICATIONS FOR GROWTH HORMONE THERAPY

Growth hormone deficiency

Overview

Growth hormone deficiency (GHD) can be congenital or acquired. Congenital forms are due to gene differences or structural anomalies of the pituitary. GHD due to underlying pituitary anomaly may be accompanied by midline facial defects including cleft lip or palate, solitary median maxillary central incisor, or CHARGE syndrome, or associated with structural defects of the brain including septo-optic dysplasia, holoprosencephaly, hydrocephalus, or agenesis of the corpus callosum [1–3]. Acquired causes include central nervous system (CNS) tumors, the most common being craniopharyngioma, as well as CNS trauma, irradiation, infection, or inflammation. Many cases of GHD, however, are idiopathic. In the neonatal period, boys with GHD may present with micropenis, and neonates have an increased incidence of hypoglycemia and prolonged conjugated hyperbilirubinemia causing jaundice. Children with GHD may have midface hypoplasia, high-pitched voice, thin sparse hair, dental crowding, and acromicria (disproportionally small hands and feet). Typically children with GHD present with growth deceleration after a period of normal growth in infancy. A child should be evaluated for GHD if they have severe short stature (more than 2 standard deviations [SD] below the population mean for age and gender or below their midparental target height) and/or growth deceleration, or history of brain tumor or pituitary anomaly [4].

Growth hormone treatment in children with growth hormone deficiency

Dosing of GH is calculated based on the child's weight or body surface area, and titration to maintain normal levels of insulin-like growth factor (IGF)-I has been suggested [1,2]. In addition to its impact on growth, GH treatment can have positive effects on lipid profile, cardiac performance, body composition (muscle mass vs adiposity), and bone mineral density [1,5]. GH treatment can increase adult height, with a change in mean height SD scores between 1.8 and 3.5 [6].

Other endocrine-related problems

Neonates with GHD are at risk for hypoglycemia, and low blood glucose may be the first presenting symptom. Children can have isolated GHD or GHD associated with deficiency of other pituitary hormone(s). Sometimes those deficiencies may develop over time and in that case, GHD is typically the first deficiency to manifest.

Diagnostic testing

Testing GH levels is challenging because beyond the newborn period, GH secretion is pulsatile, especially during deep sleep. As a screening test, IGF-I and insulin-like growth factor binding protein-3 (IGFBP-3) concentrations are measured because their production is GH-dependent and their circulating levels are more consistent throughout the day [7]. IGF-I levels also are nutritionally dependent and can be low due to malnutrition independent of GH status [8]. Worrisome results on the screening test can be evaluated further by GH stimulation testing, whereby serial GH levels are measured in response to pharmacologic secretagogues. Agents used during this test can include arginine, clonidine, glucagon, insulin, and L-Dopa. To diagnose GHD, peak GH levels must be less than the diagnostic threshold in response to 2 separate pharmacologic agents [1,2,9]. Due to the complexities of diagnosis and testing, referral to a pediatric endocrinologist is warranted for the performance and interpretation of GH stimulation testing.

Prader–Willi syndrome

Overview

Prader–Willi syndrome (PWS) is a genetic disorder that leads to developmental differences, obesity, and short stature. Infants with PWS have hypotonia, poor reflexes, and poor suck leading to malnutrition and failure to thrive, often necessitating feeding tubes. Older children develop hyperphagia, typically starting around age 2 years, that is likely hypothalamic in origin and leads to central obesity [10]. Body composition is characterized by high body fat and low muscle mass. Dysmorphic facial features are seen, including almond-shaped palpebral fissures, narrow bifrontal diameter, thin upper vermillion, and down-turned corners of the mouth. Other characteristic phenotypic features are acromicria and straight ulnar borders. Children have developmental delay with delayed achievement of milestones, and children and adults often have mild intellectual disability with a tendency for perseveration and temper tantrums [11–13].

Growth hormone treatment in children with Prader–Willi syndrome

Without treatment, the average adult height for men with PWS is 155 cm, and for women is 148 cm [13]. Most children with PWS have low IGF-I levels, and 40% to 100% of children meet the criteria for GHD [14]. Treatment with GH leads to increased growth and adult height, as well as improved body composition including decreased fat and increased muscle mass [14]. GH treatment also has shown to improve motor development [15] and lipid profile [16]. Children with PWS treated with GH therapy earlier than age 2 years were found to have increased height, improved motor strength and cholesterol profile, and decreased body fat [17].

Other endocrine-related problems

Central hypothyroidism, central adrenal insufficiency, and hypogonadotropic hypogonadism occur at higher incidences than in the general population. Central adrenal insufficiency may place patients with PWS at higher risk of sudden death in times of infection or severe stress [18]. Hypogonadism can lead to genital hypoplasia in men (small phallus, hypoplastic scrotum, cryptorchidism), primary amenorrhea in women, and infertility in both sexes. There is a high incidence of comorbidities related to obesity, including impaired glucose tolerance or type 2 diabetes mellitus, dyslipidemia, NASH, and obstructive sleep apnea.

Diagnostic testing

PWS is due to the lack of expression of genes on the 15q11.2-q13 region of the paternally inherited chromosome, either due to imprinting defect, deletion, or uniparental disomy. Initial genetic testing for PWS includes DNA methylation analysis. If the methylation study is abnormal, FISH or chromosomal microarray should be performed to screen for deletions [19].

Small for gestational age without catch-up growth

Overview

Small for gestational age (SGA) is defined by having, for both sex and gestational age, a birth length at least 2 SD below the mean, or birth weight below 10th population centile. SGA can include infants who had intrauterine growth restriction (IUGR), infants small due to an underlying genetic change, as well as infants who are small but otherwise healthy [20]. Maternal risk factors for having an infant born SGA include short stature or personal history of being born SGA, cigarette or cocaine use during pregnancy, hypertension, renal disease, and nulliparity [21]. Infants born SGA are at higher risk for hypothermia, hypoglycemia, lung disease, low blood pressure, necrotizing enterocolitis, and polycythemia [22].

Growth hormone treatment in children with small for gestational age

Approximately 85% of infants born SGA experience catch-up growth within the first 2 years of life. The mean adult height for children born SGA with appropriate catch-up growth is 0.7 SD, whereas the mean adult height for children born SGA without catch-up growth is −1.7 SD [23]. Birth length is often more sensitive than birth weight in predicting catch-up growth for SGA infants born prematurely. SGA infants have a 7-fold increased risk of short stature as an adult [23]. GH treatment is approved for children born SGA who did not have catch-up growth in the first 2 years of life; the deferred initiation of treatment is designed to avoid unnecessarily treating all those children who will experience catch-up growth on their own. GH treatment increases adult height; one study cited an increase of 1.1 to 2 SD [24].

Other endocrine-related problems

In the newborn period, SGA infants are at higher risk for hypoglycemia, and blood glucose should be monitored for 48 hours after birth. Children and adults with a history of SGA are at increased risk for developing metabolic syndrome and type 2 diabetes mellitus, especially those with rapid catch-up weight gain in early life [22,25]. Treatment with GH does not alter the risk of developing metabolic syndrome [26].

Diagnostic testing

Diagnosis is made based on anthropometric criteria at birth.

Idiopathic short stature

Overview

Idiopathic short stature (ISS) is defined as having a height more than 2 SD below the mean for age and gender without evidence of systemic, genetic, or nutritional abnormality [27]. ISS is a diagnosis of exclusion, whereby other causes of short stature, including GHD, are ruled out.

Growth hormone treatment in children with idiopathic short stature

In 2003, the US FDA approved GH to treat children with ISS whose height is below −2.25 SD, whose height velocity is not expected to reach an adult height in the normal range, and who do not have evidence of other abnormality that should be observed or treated differently [1,2]. Height response to GH treatment in children with ISS is generally less than in patients with GHD and is highly variable, including some children with no response [1]. GH treatment of 6 years in children with ISS showed a mean adult height increase of 6 cm [28].

Other endocrine-related problems

None.

Diagnostic testing

As ISS is a diagnosis of exclusion, diagnostic testing should be obtained to rule out other genetic or systemic causes of short stature that are treated more appropriately by other means. Even if a child qualifies by anthropometric criteria for GH treatment under the ISS indication, it is still important to evaluate first for possible GHD. Diagnosing GHD informs both, the need for screening for other possibly associated problems such as pituitary lesions and/or deficiency of other pituitary hormones, and the expectations and management of GH treatment in these patients [1].

Turner syndrome

Overview

Turner syndrome (TS) is caused by partial or complete absence of the second X chromosome in girls, resulting in a 45,X genotype. There can be mosaicism, which leads to a variable phenotypic presentation. The only features that are universal are female and short stature. The average adult height of a woman with TS in the US is 143 cm, or 4 foot 8 inches [29]. Without GH treatment, adult heights of women with TS are typically 20 cm below target height based on calculated midparental height [29]. Approximately 1 in 2000 female live births have TS. Cardiovascular features include bicuspid aortic valve, coarctation of the aorta, and hypertension. Children with TS should have an echocardiogram at diagnosis, and subsequent cardiac management is determined by the presence or absence of congenital anomalies; even if no anomalies are seen, echocardiogram or cardiac MRI should be performed every 5 years in childhood due to increased risk of developing aortic dilation and dissection/rupture. [30]. There is an increased incidence of collecting system anomalies and horseshoe kidney, resulting in higher risk for hypertension and urinary tract infections. Girls should have a renal ultrasound at diagnosis. Children commonly have conductive or sensorineural hearing loss as well as frequent otitis media, possibly secondary to slow growth of the temporal bone. Hearing screen should be performed at diagnosis and every 2 to 3 years. There is an increased risk of congenital hip dislocation and scoliosis later in life. Other common physical features include nuchal fold, webbed neck, low-set ears, low posterior hairline, cubitus valgus, genu valgum, hyperconvex nails, shortened fourth metacarpals, high-arched palate, epicanthal folds, hypertelorism, and in infancy, edema of the hands and feet [31,32].

Growth hormone treatment in girls with Turner syndrome

Short stature in TS is due to haploinsufficiency of the short-stature homeobox-containing gene (*SHOX*), which is located on the pseudoautosomal region of the X chromosome (see later in discussion). Girls with TS who are treated with GH have a mean height gain of 5.7 cm compared with untreated girls with TS; however, this gain has ranged from 1 to 10 cm in various studies [29]. The incidence of scoliosis, slipped capital femoral epiphysis (SCFE), and intracranial hypertension is higher in patients with TS receiving GH compared with those receiving GH for other indications; however, it is believed to be secondary to a higher than baseline risk due to the underlying TS [33].

Other endocrine-related problems

Children with TS commonly have hypergonadotropic hypogonadism due to gonadal dysgenesis, which can cause absent or delayed puberty and typically requires sex steroid replacement therapy. There is also a higher incidence of premature ovarian failure [34]. This presents as primary or secondary amenorrhea and absent pubertal development with no pubertal growth spurt. The preferred route for estrogen replacement is transdermal. Hormone replacement therapy is needed for the induction of puberty and to optimize bone health and maintain secondary sex characteristics [35]. There is also a high incidence of autoimmune diseases including thyroiditis and celiac disease, as well as obesity and glucose intolerance. Thyroid function tests should be monitored annually.

Diagnostic testing

Diagnosis is made by karyotype [36]; if karyotype is normal and there is a high clinical suspicion, FISH studies can detect mosaicism.

SHOX gene haploinsufficiency

Overview

The short-stature homeobox-containing gene (*SHOX*) encodes a homeodomain transcription factor and is a gene implicated in short stature. *SHOX* gene is located on the short arm pseudoautosomal region 1 (PAR 1) of both the X and Y chromosomes. Men and women express 2 active copies of this gene; it does not become inactivated on the second X chromosome in women [37,38]. *SHOX* gene is expressed during skeletal development in the fetal period, as well as within the chondrocytes of the epiphyseal growth plate. *SHOX* mutations have variable phenotypes, including mild to severe short stature, and mesomelia (shortened forearms and lower legs). Children with *SHOX* mutations often have Madelung deformity of the wrist, which consists of bowing of the radial shaft, palmar and ulnar deviation of the carpals, and a prominent distal ulna due to premature fusion of the distal radial growth plate. Other clinical features include scoliosis, hypertrophy of leg musculature, high arched palate, shortened metacarpals, and micrognathia [38]. Mesomelic limb shortening leads to decreased arm span and increased sitting height/standing height ratio, which is one of the most predictive indicators of *SHOX* mutations [39]. One copy of *SHOX* can be missing by deletion or mutation, or as part of a larger chromosomal loss as is seen in TS. Conversely, expressing an extra copy of *SHOX* can cause tall stature, as is seen in Klinefelter syndrome (47, XXY) [38]. Haploinsufficiency of *SHOX* can cause Léri–Weill dyschondrosteosis, characterized by mesomelic shortening of the limbs and Madelung deformity, while loss of both copies causes Langer mesomelic dysplasia, with severe disproportionate short stature [37,40].

Growth hormone treatment in children with SHOX gene haploinsufficiency

Children with *SHOX* mutations have decreased prepubertal height velocity, with significantly decreased height velocity at puberty due to premature fusion of the epiphyseal growth plates [41]. The mean height of children with *SHOX* gene haploinsufficiency has been reported as −2.2 to −3 SD before the initiation of GH treatment [38,40,42]. GH treatment can result in height increase of 0.25 to 0.53 SD in 1 year, and an increase in height velocity [40,42]. The growth response to GH treatment in patients with *SHOX* gene haploinsufficiency is similar to that of girls with TS.

Other endocrine-related problems
None.

Diagnostic testing
SHOX mutations or deletions are identified using PCR amplification [43].

Noonan syndrome

Overview
Noonan syndrome is caused by germline mutations in the RAS/mitogen-activated protein kinase (MAPK) pathway, which encompasses many genes [44]. *PTPN11* is the most common gene mutation, implicated in approximately half of the patients with Noonan syndrome [45,46]. While the gene mutation is autosomal dominantly inherited, more than half the cases of Noonan syndrome are from de novo mutations. The incidence is 1/11,000 to 2500 live births, but may be closer to 1/100 for milder phenotypes. Noonan syndrome is characterized by dysmorphic facial features including hypertelorism, ptosis, low set ears, upturned lip, high arched palate, tall forehead, epicanthal folds, micrognathia, low posterior hairline, deep philtrum, broad nose, and triangle-shaped head [45–47]. The facial dysmorphisms are more prominent in infancy to midchildhood, and become more subtle as people with Noonan syndrome approach adulthood [48]. Other features of Noonan syndrome include short stature, congenital heart defects (most commonly pulmonary valve stenosis, stenosis of the peripheral pulmonary artery, atrial septal defect), skeletal malformations, learning difficulties, renal and lymphatic anomalies, cryptorchidism, webbed neck, cubitus valgus, genu valgum, and pectus deformities (pectus carinatum superiorly and pectus excavatum inferiorly) [48]. There is an increased risk of hearing loss, so children with Noonan syndrome should have annual hearing evaluation [45]. Due to the high incidence of cardiac malformations, children should have echocardiogram and electrocardiography performed at diagnosis, and if no heart disease is detected, examination should be performed with a cardiologist every 5 years. There is increased risk of hematologic abnormalities, particularly bleeding disorder, and children should get a coagulation profile at diagnosis or after 1 year of life. Due to increased incidence of renal anomalies, renal ultrasound should be obtained at the time of diagnosis [45].

Growth hormone treatment in children with Noonan syndrome
Short stature is prominent in both sexes and can be present in up to 70% of people with Noonan syndrome. Without treatment mean adult height is 150 to 155 cm in women and 160 to 168 cm in men, with height SDS around −2.1 [45]. Typically the birth length and weight are within normal limits, and height falls below the 3rd percentile closer to age 2 to 4 years [49]. The

severity of growth failure is variable and may relate to the specific gene mutation. There is conflicting research on mutation and response to GH; specifically with *PTPN11* mutations, there are reports that this mutation confers resistance to GH treatment, whereas other studies showed greater height gain with GH treatment [50–52]. Data from a GH registry showed that treatment with GH for approximately 5 to 6 years led to a gain of 1.2 to 1.3 height SDS [53]. Patients with Noonan syndrome are at increased risk of solid tumors and cancer, and therefore, treatment with GH should proceed with caution, as GH can promote tumor growth. The Pediatric Endocrine Society report on neoplasia risk with pediatric GH treatment pointed out the baseline malignancy risk in patients with *PTPN11* mutations, though whether GH treatment can further increase this risk was yet unknown [54].

Other endocrine-related problems

Delayed pubertal onset is common, with a mean onset of puberty for men at 13.5 to 14.5 years, and for women at 13 to 14 years. Children with Noonan syndrome grow for longer than their peers, with spontaneous height gains into the late teenage years in women and early 20s in men [49]. There is also an increased incidence of thyroid autoantibodies, but not of hypothyroidism [48]. Fertility is impaired in men, partially due to high incidence of cryptorchidism in infancy, while fertility is unaffected in women [55].

Diagnostic testing

Diagnosis is made based on the presence of characteristic clinical features, and can be confirmed with molecular genetic testing (*PTPN11*, *SOS1*, *RAF1*, and *KRAS*).

Chronic renal insufficiency

Overview

Chronic renal insufficiency (CRI) is defined by having reduced creatinine clearance. Renal insufficiency can be caused by structural defects including obstructive uropathy, intrinsic kidney disease including focal segmental glomerulosclerosis, aplastic kidney, polycystic kidney disease, or other systemic diseases affecting the kidney [56]. In adults with CRI, increased mortality is due to increased incidence of cardiovascular disease, especially left ventricular hypertrophy, and infections. There is also an increased risk of malignancies, with the most common being skin cancer [57]. Common problems in children with CRI include anemia and acidosis. Blood pressure control is crucial in children and adults with CRI, as chronic hypertension can lead to cardiac changes as well as the progression of kidney disease independent of other risk factors [58].

Growth hormone treatment in children with chronic renal insufficiency

Approximately 40% of children with CKD achieve adult heights below the 3rd percentile without GH treatment [59]. Height SDS ranges from −0.55 to −1.65 on various reports from cohorts in North America and Europe, with the greatest height deficit found in toddlers [56,60]. One early study showed an increase in height SDS from −2.6 to −0.7 after 5 years of GH treatment; another study showed an increase in height SDS from −3.4 to −0.8 after 8 years of treatment [61,62]. GH treatment does not seem to have a negative impact on underlying kidney disease. A recent consensus statement recommended the consideration of GH therapy in children with CKD stage 3 to 5 with a height below the 3rd percentile, or height velocity below the 25th percentile. GH therapy can be considered also in patients with renal transplant 1 year after transplantation if catch-up growth is not achieved [59]. In addition to GH treatment, optimizing nutrition can impact the growth of children with CRI; dietary goals include reducing protein, phosphorus, and salt intake [63]. Other comorbidities related to CKD also may impact growth, including longstanding hyponatremia, metabolic bone disease, anemia, and metabolic acidosis [59].

Other endocrine-related problems

Children with CRI have a higher incidence of hypocalcemia and hyperphosphatemia, often requiring calcium and/or calcitriol supplementation and phosphorus binders [56].

Diagnostic testing

Diagnosis of CRI is made using creatinine clearance, which is calculated using serum creatinine, sex, height, and age.

WHEN TO REFER TO A PEDIATRIC ENDOCRINOLOGIST?

Children should have regular measurements of height/length and weight with their primary provider, with height measurements obtained using a wall-mounted stadiometer when age-appropriate and length measured by the recumbent length board [64]. The following features indicate growth failure and should prompt further evaluation: height SDS below −2, height more than 2 SD below their midparental height SDS, abnormally slow height velocity, or significant decrease in height SDS on the growth chart [4,65]. Providers should consider malnutrition if linear growth failure is accompanied by poor weight gain, evidenced by low or dropping BMI or weight-for-length, or if slowing of weight gain precedes slowing of height gain. Nutritional deficiencies should be addressed, and when applicable, referral to a dietician should be considered. Providers should consider systemic causes of short stature or poor linear growth and may consider obtaining screening laboratory tests including complete blood count (CBC), comprehensive metabolic panel (CMP), celiac panel, thyroid function tests, inflammatory markers, and in girls, karyotype. If a cause of growth failure is identified, treatment of the underlying condition and/or subspecialty referral should occur accordingly. Initial evaluation also should include a bone age (AP radiograph of the left wrist and hand), to assess the degree of skeletal maturation. Detailed family history should be obtained, including the timing of puberty of parents and other relatives. If one or both parents had delayed pubertal growth spurt, constitutional delay of growth and puberty (CDGP) should be considered in the child; children with CDGP often have delayed bone ages.

Table 1
Potential benefits and complications of pediatric GH treatment

Benefits	Complications
Increased height velocity	Intracranial hypertension
Increased adult height	Worsening of scoliosis
Prevention of hypoglycemia[a]	Slipped capital femoral epiphysis
Favorable effects on lipid profile[b]	Worsening of obstructive sleep apnea
Increased muscle mass[b]	Pancreatitis
Decreased adiposity[b]	Increased insulin resistance
Increased bone mineral density[b]	
Improved motor control[c]	
Improved cardiovascular health[b]	

[a]GHD.
[b]GHD and PWS.
[c]PWS.

A practitioner should refer a patient to a pediatric endocrinologist for growth evaluation if the child has growth failure without an identifiable cause, or if they have any of the FDA-approved indications for GH treatment other than CRI. Referral to pediatric endocrinology should occur before pubertal onset when possible.

SIDE EFFECTS OF GROWTH HORMONE TREATMENT

The safety and efficacy of GH treatment in children have been studied extensively, although long-term effects and risks are still unknown as recombinant GH became commercially available in 1985 [66]. Many of these studies were industry-sponsored postmarketing surveillance studies and lack both, control populations for comparison and long-term follow-up after the discontinuation of treatment. Adverse effects that have been reported include limb pain, myalgias, arthralgias, peripheral edema, injection site pain, and injection site reaction [67].

Rare but serious possible complications of GH treatment include intracranial hypertension, worsening of scoliosis, SCFE, obstructive sleep apnea (OSA), and pancreatitis [1,65,68]. (Table 1). OSA is of particular concern in patients with PWS due to their higher baseline risk of OSA, and pancreatitis is included in the package insert although the causal relationship to GH treatment is unclear [68]. GH therapy affects glucose metabolism and can increase insulin resistance. Clinical evidence does not support an association between GH treatment and development of cancer in children without risk factors for malignancies. There is currently insufficient evidence to conclude whether GH treatment increases the risk of neoplasm in children who are already at higher risk of developing cancer [54].

SUMMARY

GH treatment involves nightly subcutaneous injections in attempt to mirror the pituitary's endogenous GH secretion. GH therapy is expensive, with median costs per child exceeding $25,000 annually [69]. Nonetheless, GH use in the US pediatric population almost tripled from 2001 to 2016 [69]. Over the past 35 years, pediatric GH treatment has expanded from its initial indication to correct GHD, to now using the medication to increase height in conditions whereby endogenous GH production is already adequate [70]. Treatment efficacy in such conditions is variable and generally less than in patients with GHD, and unresolved safety concerns require ongoing scrutiny [66].

CLINICAL CARE POINTS

- An extended pedigree can be helpful in distinguishing polygenic familial short stature from a dominantly inherited growth problem that had not been diagnosed previously.
- Girls with unexplained short stature should be screened for Turner syndrome even in the absence of other phenotypic features.
- Even if a child qualifies by anthropometric criteria for GH treatment under the ISS indication, it is still important to evaluate first for possible GHD.
- IGF-I levels can be lowered by malnutrition as well as by GHD, so growth curves should always be interpreted in the context of the weight and BMI (or weight-for-length) curves.

Disclosure

A. Grimberg received the 2020 Growth Hormone Research Competitive Grant Program Award from Pfizer. M. Danowitz has nothing to disclose.

References

[1] Grimberg A, DiVall SA, Polychronakos C, et al. Guidelines for growth hormone and insulin-like growth factor-1 treatment in children children and adolescents: growth hormone deficiency, idiopathic short stature, and primary insulin-like growth factor-1 deficiency. Horm Res Paediatr 2016;86(6):361–97.

[2] Collett-Solberg PF, Ambler G, Backeljauw PF, et al. Diagnosis, Genetics, and Therapy of Short Stature in Children: A Growth Hormone Research Society International Perspective. Horm Res Paediatr 2019;92:1–14.

[3] Bosch L, Katugampola H, Dattani MT. Congenital Hypopituitarism During the Neonatal Period: Epidemiology, Pathogenesis, Therapeutic Options, and Outcome. Front Pediatr 2021;8:1–17.

[4] Halas JG, Grimberg A. Dilemmas of Growth Hormone Treatment for GH Deficiency and Idiopathic Short Stature: Defining, Distinguishing, and Deciding. Minerva Pediatr 2020;72(3):206–25.

[5] Lanes R, Soros A, Gunczler P, et al. Growth hormone deficiency, low levels of adiponectin, and unfavorable plasma lipid and lipoproteins. J Pediatr 2006;149(3):324–9.

[6] Polak M, Blair J, Kotnik P, et al. Early growth hormone treatment start in childhood growth hormone deficiency improves near adult height: analysis from NordiNet® International Outcome Study. Eur J Endocrinol 2017;177(5):421–9.

[7] Hawkes CP, Grimberg A. Measuring Growth Hormone and Insulin-like Growth Factor-1 in Infants: What is Normal? Pediatr Endocrinol Rev 2013;11:126–46.

[8] Hawkes CP, Grimberg A. Insulin-like growth factor-1 is a marker for the nutritional state. Ped Endocrinol Rev 2015;13:499–511.
[9] Kamoun C, Hawkes CP, Grimberg A. Provocative growth hormone testing in children: how did we get here and where do we go now? J Pediatr Endocrinol Metab 2021;34(6): 679–96.
[10] Miller J, Lynn CH, Driscoll DC, et al. Nutritional phases in prader-willi syndrome. Am J Med Genet A 2011;155a:1040–9.
[11] Goldstone AP, Holland AJ, Hauffa BP, et al. Recommendations for the diagnosis and management of Prader-Willi Syndrome. J Clin Endocrinol Metab 2008;93(11):4183–97.
[12] Cassidy SB, Driscoll DJ. Prader-Willi syndrome. Eur J Hum Genet 2009;17:3–13.
[13] Cassidy SB, Schwartz S, Miller JL, et al. Prader-Willi syndrome. Gen Med 2012;14:10–26.
[14] Burman P, Ritzen EM, Lindgren AC. Endocrine Dysfunction in Prader-Willi Syndrome: A Review with Special Reference to GH. Endocr Rev 2001;22(6):787–99.
[15] Whitman B, Carrel A, Bekx T, et al. Growth Hormone Improves Body Composition and Motor Development in Infants with Prader-Willi Syndrome After Six Months. J Pediatr Endocrinol Met 2004;17:591–600.
[16] Colmenares A, Pinto G, Taupin P, et al. Effects on Growth and Metabolism of Growth Hormone Treatment for 3 years in 36 Children with Prader-Willi Syndrome. Horm Res Paediatr 2011;75:123–30.
[17] Carrel AL, Myers SE, Whitman BY, et al. Long-term growth hormone therapy changes the natural history of body composition and motor function in children with Prader-Willi Syndrome. J Clin Endocrinol Metab 2010;95(3):1131–6.
[18] de Lind van Winjgaarden RFA, Otten BJ, Festen DAM, et al. High Prevalence of Central Adrenal Insufficiency in Patients with Prader-Willi Syndrome. J Clin Endocrinol Metab 2008;93(5):1649–54.
[19] Angulo MA, Butler MG, Cataletto ME. Prader-Willi syndrome: a review of clinical, genetic, and endocrine findings. J Endocrinol Investig 2015;38:1249–63.
[20] Clausson B, Gardosi J, Francis A, et al. Perinatal outcome in SGA births defined by customized versus population-based birthweight standards. BJOG 2001;108:830–4.
[21] McCowan L, Horgan RP. Risk factors for small for gestational age infants. Best Pract Res Clin Obstet Gynaecol 2009;23:779–93.
[22] Zeve D, Regelmann MO, Holzman IR, et al. Small at Birth, but How Small? The Definition of SGA Revisited. Horm Res Paediatr 2016;86:357–60.
[23] Albertsson-Wikland K, Karlberg J. Natural growth in children born small for gestational age with and without catch-up growth. Acta Paediatr 1994;399:64–70.
[24] Lem AJ, van der Kaay DCM, de Ridder MAJ, et al. Adult height in short children born SGA treated with growth hormone and gonadotropin releasing hormone analog: results of a randomized, dose-response GH trial. JCEM 2012;97(11):4096–105.
[25] Arends NJT, Boonstra VH, Duivenvoorden J, et al. Reduced insulin sensitivity and the presence of cardiovascular risk factors in short prepubertal children born small for gestational age (SGA). Clin Endocrinol 2005;62(1):44–50.
[26] van Dijk M, Bannink EMN, van Pareren YK, et al. Risk Factors for Diabetes Mellitus Type 2 and Metabolic Syndrome are Comparable for Previously Growth Hormone-Treated Young Adults Born Small for Gestational Age (SGA) and Untreated Short SGA Controls. JCEM 2007;92(1):160–5.
[27] Cutfiled WS, Albert B. Growth Hormone Treatment for Idiopathic Short Stature. Pediatr Endocrinol Rev 2018;16:113–22.
[28] Albertsson-Wikland K, Aronson AS, Gutafsson J, et al. Dose-dependent effect of growth hormone o final height in children with short stature without growth hormone deficiency. JCEM 2008;93:4342–50.
[29] Quigley CA, Crowe BJ, Anglin G, et al. Growth Hormone and Low Dose Estrogen in Turner Syndrome: Results of a United States Multi-Center Trial to Near-Final Height. JCEM 2002;87(5):2033–41.

[30] Gravholt CH, Andersen NH, Conway GS, et al. Clinical practice guidelines for the care of girls and women with Turner syndrome: proceedings from the 2016 Cincinnati International Turner Syndrome Meeting. Eur J Endocrinol 2017;177(3):1–70.
[31] Gravholt CH, Viuff MH, Brun S, et al. Turner syndrome: mechanisms and management. Nat Rev Endocrinol 2019;15:601–14.
[32] Shankar RK, Backejauw PF. Current best practice in the management of Turner syndrome. Ther Adv Endocrinol Metab 2018;9(1):33–40.
[33] Bolar K, Hoffman AR, Maneatis T, et al. Long-Term Safety of Recombinant Human Growth Hormone in Turner Syndrome. JCEM 2008;93(2):344–51.
[34] Gawlik A, Hankus M, Such K, et al. Hypogonadism and Sex Steroid Replacement Therapy in Girls with Turner Syndrome. J Pediatr Adol Gynec 2016;29:542–50.
[35] O Klein K, Rosenfield RL, Santen RJ, et al. Estrogen Replacement in Turner Syndrome: Literature Review and Practical Considerations. JCEM 2018;103(5):1790–803.
[36] Mintz CS, Seaver LH, Irons M, et al. ACMG Professional Practice and Guidelines Committee. Focused Revision: ACMG practice resource: Genetic evaluation of short stature. Genet Med 2021;23(5):813–5.
[37] Rappold G, Blum WF, Shavrikova EP, et al. Genotypes and phenotypes in children with short stature: clinical indicators of SHOX haploinsufficiency. J Med Genet 2007;44:306–13.
[38] Fukami M, Seki A, Ogata T. SHOX Haploinsufficiency as a Cause of Syndromic and Nonsyndromic Short Stature. Mol Syndromol 2016;7:3–11.
[39] Vannelli S, Baffico M, Buganza R, et al. SHOX deficiency in children with growth impairment: evaluation of known and new auxological and radiological indicators. Ital J Pediatr 2020;46(163):163.
[40] Benabbad I, Rosilio M, Child CJ, et al. Growth Hormone-Treated Children with SHOX Deficiency: Data from an Observational Study and a Clinical Trial. Horm Res Paediatr 2017;87: 42–50.
[41] Genoni G, Monzani A, Castagno M, et al. Improving clinical diagnosis in SHOX deficiency: the importance of growth velocity. Pediatr Rese 2018;83:438–44.
[42] Marstrand-Joergensen MR, Jensen RB, Aksglaede L, et al. Prevalence of SHOX haploinsufficiency among short statured children. Pediatr Res 2017;81:335–41.
[43] Babu D, Vannelli S, Fanelli A, et al. Variants in the 5′UTR reduce SHOX expression and contribute to SHOX haploinsufficiency. Eur J Hum Genet 2021;29:110–21.
[44] Roberts AE, Araki T, Swanson K, et al. Germline gain-of-function mutations in *SOS1* cause Noonan syndrome. Nat Genet 2007;39:70–4.
[45] Bhambhani V, Muenke M. Noonan Syndrome. AFP 2014;89:37–43.
[46] Tafazoli A, Eshraghi P, Koleti ZK, et al. Noonan syndrome- a new survey. Arch Med Sci 2017;13:215–22.
[47] Kruszka P, Porras AR, Addissie YA, et al. Noonan syndrome in diverse populations. Am J Med Genet 2017;173(9):2323–34.
[48] Romano AA, Allanson JE, Dahlgren J, et al. Noonan Syndrome: Clinical Features, Diagnosis, and Management Guidelines. Pediatr 2010;126(4):746–59.
[49] Seo GH, Yoo H-W. Growth hormone therapy in patients with Noonan syndrome. Ann Pediatr Endocrinol Met 2018;23(4):176–81.
[50] Jeong I, Kang E, Cho JH, et al. Long-term efficacy of recombinant human growth hormone therapy in short-statured patients with Noonan syndrome. Ann Pediatr Endocrinol Met 2016;21:26–30.
[51] Siklar Z, Genens M, Poyrazoglu S, et al. The Growth Characteristics of Patients with Noonan Syndrome: Results of Three Years of Growth Hormone Treatment: A Nationwide Multicenter Study. JCRPE 2016;8(3):305–12.
[52] Malaquias AC, Noronha RM, Souza TTO, et al. Impact of Growth Hormone Therapy on Adult Height in Patients with PTPN11 Mutations Related to Noonan Syndrome. Horm Res Paediatr 2019;91:252–61.

[53] Ranke MB, Lindberg A, Carlsson M, et al. Treatment with Growth Hormone in Noonan Syndrome Observed during 25 years of KIGS: Near Adult Height and Outcome Prediction. Horm Res Paediatr 2019;91:46–55.
[54] Raman S, Grimberg A, Waguespack SG, et al. Risk of Neoplasia in Pediatric Patients Receiving Growth Hormone Therapy- A Report From the Pediatric Endocrine Society Drug and Therapeutics Committee. JCEM 2015;100(6):2192–203.
[55] Noonan JA. Noonan syndrome and related disorders: Alterations in growth and puberty. Rev Endocr Metabol Disord 2006;7:251–5.
[56] Seikaly MG, Ho PL, Emmett L, et al. Chronic renal insufficiency in children: The 2001 Annual Report of the NAPRTCS. Pediatr Nephrol 2003;18:796–804.
[57] Groothoff JW, Offringa M, Grootenhuis M, et al. Long-term consequences of renal insufficiency in children: lessons learned from the Dutch LERIC study. Nephrol Dial Transplant 2018;33(4):552–60.
[58] Mitsnefes M, Ho P-L, McEnery PT. Hypertension and Progression of Chronic Renal Insufficiency in Children: A Report of the North American Pediatric Renal Transplant Cooperative Study (NAPRTCS). J Am Soc Nephrol 2003;14:2618–22.
[59] Drube J, Wan M, Bonthius M, et al. Clinical practice recommendations for growth hormone treatment in children with chronic kidney disease. Nat Rev Nephrol 2019;15:577–89.
[60] Akchurin OM, Kogon AJ, Kumar J, et al. Approach to growth hormone therapy in children with chronic kidney disease varies across North America: the Midwest Pediatric Nephrology Consortium report. BMC Nephrol 2017;18:181.
[61] Fine RN, Kohaut E, Brown D, et al. Long-term treatment of growth retarded children with chronic renal insufficiency, with recombinant human growth hormone. Kidney Int 1996;49:781–5.
[62] Hokken-Koelega A, Mulder P, De Jong R, et al. Long-term effects of growth hormone treatment on growth and puberty in patients with chronic renal insufficiency. Pediatr Nephrol 2000;14:701–6.
[63] Norman LJ, Macdonald IA, Watson AR. Optimising nutrition in chronic renal insufficiency-growth. Pediatr Nephrol 2004;19:1245–52.
[64] Committee on Practice and Ambulatory Medicine, Bright Futures Periodicity Schedule Workgroup. 2021 Recommendations for Preventive Pediatric Health Care. Pediatr 2021;147:e2020049776.
[65] Collett-Solberg PF, Jorge AAL, Boguszewski MCS, et al. Growth hormone therapy in children: research and practice- A review. Growth Horm IGF Res 2019;44:20–32.
[66] Grimberg A. Cardiovascular Disease in Former Pediatric Recipients of Growth Hormone: Another Look at Growth Hormone Safety. JAMA Pediatr 2021;175:e205232.
[67] Souza FM, Collet-Solberg PF. Adverse effects of growth hormone replacement therapy in children. Arq Bras Endocrinol Metab 2011;55:559–65.
[68] Allen DB, Backeljauw P, Bidlingmaier M, et al. GH safety workshop position paper: a critical appraisal of recombinant human GH therapy in children and adults. Eur Soc Endocrinol 2015;174(2):1–9.
[69] Grimberg A, Kanter GP. US Growth Hormone Use in the Idiopathic Short Stature Era: Trends in Insurer Payments and Patient Financial Burden. J Endocr Soc 2019;3:2023–31.
[70] Grimberg A, Allen DB. Growth Hormone Treatment for Growth Hormone Deficiency and Idiopathic Short Stature: New Guidelines Shaped by the Presence and Absence of Evidence. Curr Opin Pediatr 2017;29:466–71.

Advances in Pediatrics 69 (2022) 219–229

ADVANCES IN PEDIATRICS

Update on Pediatric Hyperthyroidism

Priya Vaidyanathan, MD

Department of Pediatric Endocrinology, Children's National Hospital, Washington, DC 20010, USA

Keywords

• Hyperthyroidism in children • Graves' disease • Neonatal hyperthyroidism

Key points

- Hyperthyroidism is diagnosed by elevated thyroid hormones (TH), Free T4 and total T3 and suppressed thyroid-stimulating hormone (TSH).
- Graves' disease (GD), an autoimmune disorder makes up 96% of pediatric hyperthyroidism.
- Hyperthyroidism is a hypermetabolic state with cardiovascular, GI, neurologic, dermatologic, and ocular symptoms. Symptoms can also be misleading and point to other systemic disorders and delay diagnosis.
- First line of treatment of GD in children is with methimazole (MMI) while radioactive iodine (RAI) treatment and thyroidectomy offer permanent treatment and render patient hypothyroid.
- Neonates born to mothers with current or past treatment of GD are at risk for neonatal hyperthyroidism (NH).

AN UPDATE ON HYPERTHYROIDISM IN CHILDREN

Purpose of the review: This review is intended to highlight causes, enable early and accurate diagnosis and management of hyperthyroidism in children and neonates.

INTRODUCTION

Hyperthyroidism is due to increased production of thyroid hormone (TH) as noted biochemically by elevated TH, Free T4 and T3, and suppressed thyroid-stimulating hormone (TSH). The most common cause of hyperthyroidism is GD which is an autoimmune disorder from TSH receptor stimulation by TSH receptor antibody (TRAb) and makes up for 96% of pediatric

E-mail address: pvaidyan@childrensnational.org

https://doi.org/10.1016/j.yapd.2022.04.004
0065-3101/22/

hyperthyroidism [1]. GD is more common in females and may occur at any age during childhood, peaking during adolescence. A French population-based study [2] in 2015 identified a total of 670 cases of childhood hyperthyroidism for an annual incidence of 4.58/100,000 person-years showing the rarity of the diagnosis, with a 3.27 F/M ratio. Only 10% were less than 5 years of age. In a study from Sweden [3] incidence rate (IR) was higher from 2000 to 2009 versus 1990 to 1999 (2.8/100,000 vs 1.6/100,000 person-years, $P = .006$), suggesting that at least in some parts of the world the incidence of childhood hyperthyroidism is increasing. There is concern that increasing exposures to endocrine-disrupting chemicals may have caused the increase [2] Hyperthyroidism is a hypermetabolic state with cardiovascular, GI, neurologic, dermatologic and ocular symptoms [4]. Symptoms are gradual, and it may take months before families seek medical attention. Symptoms can also be misleading and point to other systemic disorders and delay diagnosis. It is important that pediatricians be aware of these diverse symptoms to facilitate early screening and referral to a pediatric endocrinologist for treatment.

CLINICAL MANIFESTATIONS OF HYPERTHYROIDISM

Hyperthyroidism has a myriad of clinical manifestations affecting multiple systems. Cardiovascular effects are pronounced due to an increase in heart rate and cardiac output leading to hyperdynamic circulation and systolic hypertension. Unintentional weight loss is noted despite an increase in appetite. Growth is often accelerated in children while puberty can be delayed and menstrual irregularities such as oligomenorrhea and secondary amenorrhea may appear. Deterioration in school performance, inability to focus, anxiety, emotional lability, and jitteriness may be mistaken for ADHD or a behavioral disorder. Fine hand tremors, brisk deep tendon reflex, and tongue fasciculations are typical signs. Due to cutaneous vasodilation, skin is moist and warm, there is heat intolerance, and hair is fine and brittle. Pretibial myxedema, a very rare Thyroid dermopathy presents as nonpitting edema or plaque-like lesions on the pretibial region due to the accumulation of glycosaminoglycans in the dermis and is thought to be mediated by TSH receptor antibodies [5] Fatigue, proximal muscle weakness, osteopenia from an increase in bone resorption are all systemic effects of hyperthyroidism [4,6,7].

A diffuse goiter is seen in most forms of hyperthyroidism, but the absence of a goiter does not rule it out. A goiter is best observed by having the patient look up at the ceiling to stretch the skin of the neck. Thyroid enlargement can sometimes be quite large leading to tracheal compression and dyspnea. Palpable nodule should raise concern for a toxic nodule. Ophthalmopathy is seen only in Graves' disease (GD) and is due to inflammatory cell infiltration in the retroocular tissue and extra-ocular muscles. TSH receptors are expressed by orbital adipose cells and fibroblasts. Elevated TSH receptor antibodies in GD not only stimulate thyroid growth and increase TH synthesis but also stimulate the secretion of glycosaminoglycan by orbital adipose cells and fibroblasts leading to proptosis seen in Graves' ophthalmopathy GO [8]. In a study from

2014, 39/80 patients with GD had GO with 81% being females [9]. In another study from i2008, 17 of the 152 children with GD were referred to ophthalmology with most noted to have only mild findings [10] Hyperthyroid symptoms and signs are further elaborated in Table 1.

DIFFERENTIAL DIAGNOSIS OF HYPERTHYROIDISM AND ITS KEY FEATURES

Aside from GD, other less common causes are autonomous toxic nodule overproducing THs, Hashitoxicosis which is a transient phase of increase in the release of THs, subacute viral thyroiditis, acute suppurative thyroiditis, McCune-Albright syndrome (MAS) as well as germline and somatic gain-of-function mutations of the TSH receptor gene, drug-induced thyrotoxicosis, pituitary TH resistance, rarely from TSH secreting pituitary adenoma, external head and neck radiation and anticancer treatment [1,4,6,7]. This is further illustrated in Table 2.

LABORATORY DIAGNOSIS OF HYPERTHYROIDISM

All patients suspected of having hyperthyroidism should have TSH, Free T4, and total T3 tested. In hyperthyroidism, TSH is very low, typically less than 0.01 mIU/mL, and Free T4 and T3 are elevated. As GD is the most common cause of pediatric hyperthyroidism, all patients must either have thyroid-stimulating immunoglobulin (TSI) or TRAb tested. TRAb has a faster turnaround time than TSI but cannot differentiate from stimulatory versus blocking antibodies and either test is acceptable. An elevated TSI/TRAb in the setting of elevated THs confirms GD. If the TSI/TRAb are negative, thyroid peroxidase (TPO) and antithyroglobulin antibody should be tested. If they are elevated, suspect Hashitoxicosis especially if hyperthyroidism is mild. Thyroid sonogram and I-123 thyroid uptake scans are reserved for the few cases with antibody-negative hyperthyroidism or if a thyroid nodule is suspected.

MANAGEMENT OF GRAVES' DISEASE

Antithyroid drug (ATD), radioactive iodine (RAI), and thyroidectomy are available treatment options for GD in children [11,12]. ATD is the preferred initial treatment with the hope that remission is achieved in a few years with the restoration of euthyroid state. Methimazole (MMI) is the drug of choice, and it inhibits the organification and coupling of iodothyronines and lowers TH synthesis. Propylthiouracil (PTU) is no longer used due to frequent side effects and severe hepatotoxicity, and it carries a US Food and Drug Administration (FDA) boxed warning against its use in children [13]. Atenolol, a cardioselective beta-blocker or propranolol can be added as an adjunct for a few weeks to offer symptomatic relief from palpitations and tremors. Propranolol has the advantage of decreasing T4 to T3 conversion but must be dosed 3 to 4 times a day.

Baseline CBC, AST, and ALT are drawn before starting MMI. Mild abnormalities can be seen in the setting of hyperthyroidism and do not exclude MMI

Table 1
Hyperthyroid symptoms and signs

Thyroid	Generally diffusely enlarged, bruit over the thyroid
Cardiovascular	Palpitations, dyspnea, systolic hypertension, wide pulse pressure, bounding pulses, carotid bruit
Gastrointestinal	Increase in bowel movements and weight loss
Neurologic	Jitteriness, restlessness, anxiety, insomnia, decline in school performance, brisk DTR, tremors, and tongue fasciculations
Ocular (Graves' ophthalmopathy)	Tearing, grittiness, photophobia, conjunctival redness, wide-eyed stare, lid lag, proptosis, exophthalmos
Muscle	Proximal muscle weakness, fatigue
Dermatologic	Heat intolerance, hair loss, friable nails, warm moist skin, rarely pretibial myxedema

treatment. While there is no evidence that neutropenia or liver disease increases the risk of complications from ATDs, the ATA task force recommends reconsidering initiating ATD if the baseline neutrophil count is < 1000 or if there is a 5-fold elevation of transaminases [12]. While less common or severe compared with PTU, idiosyncratic neutropenia and hepatitis has been reported with MMI. While on therapy, if a patient develops fever or pharyngitis, a CBC should be drawn and MMI stopped if there is agranulocytosis. If there is jaundice or clinical evidence of liver disease, AST and ALT are measured [12]. Urticaria, myalgia, and arthralgia are other known side effects of MMI.

Unlike adults, remission rates after 2 years of treatment are low, 30% versus 50% in adults, and risk of relapse after stopping therapy is high. There are emerging data over the last 10 years that suggest an increased likelihood of remission with prolonged ATD therapy [14–18]. Remission rates can be increased to 50% after 8 years of treatment and seem to plateau thereafter. It is speculated that the euthyroid state created by ATD treatment and perhaps direct immunosuppressive effect on humoral and cellular immunity may help induce remission [18]. It is also possible that long-term ATD has minimal effect in inducing remission and the remission achieved reflects natural disease progression in these patients. In any case, long-term MMI treatment is proven to be safe without any additional adverse effects noted on prolonged treatment and should be considered in patients with good compliance who can be maintained on a modest dose of MMI.

RAI and thyroidectomy offer permanent treatment of hyperthyroidism with the aim of inducing permanent hypothyroidism. It is felt that hypothyroidism is relatively easier to manage, L-thyroxine therapy for hypothyroidism has no side effects, and the course is predictable compared with hyperthyroidism from autoimmunity. Permanent treatment is considered in well-controlled patients who fail to achieve remission after long-term ATD of 6 to 8 years, are poorly compliant with ATD, have adverse effects from ATD, or are poorly controlled with ATD and remain symptomatic. The choice of RAI versus thyroidectomy depends on several factors and is a joint decision between the treating endocrinologist and the patient/family and are elaborated in detail in Box 1 under considerations for the management of GD.

MANAGEMENT OF OTHER FORMS OF HYPERTHYROIDISM

In Hashitoxicosis, hyperthyroidism is self-limiting and can be monitored if there are no significant symptoms or treated briefly with beta-blockers or MMI for symptomatic relief. Toxic thyroid nodules are treated with surgery. Hyperthyroidism from subacute thyroiditis is self-limiting as well and managed with supportive care and anti-inflammatory medications such as NSAID. Suppurative thyroiditis is treated with antibiotics and if it fails to respond to antibiotics, then with surgery. TSH receptor mutations and hyperthyroidism from MAS can be treated with MMI but will not remit and eventually will need total thyroidectomy. A heightened awareness of medications such as amiodarone, lithium, and immune check point inhibitors used in oncology patients, and even rarely external head and neck radiation inducing hyperthyroidism and screening with thyroid levels is important for effective early management of medication or radiation-induced thyroiditis which for the most part are self-limiting or reversible when the medications are stopped.

THYROID STORM

Thyroid storm is a very rare life-threatening illness in children. There is no specific laboratory or clinical abnormality that is diagnostic of thyroid storm, instead the diagnosis considers several clinical features using a scoring system. The degree of hyperthyroidism is not more severe than in patients without thyroid storm but increased sensitivity to TH and abrupt availability is thought to cause the thyroid storm. There is often a precipitating event, such as acute infection, trauma, surgical procedure, stopping ATD, or very rarely after RAI.

Although there is no pediatric scoring system, the adult clinical scoring system developed by Burch and Wartofsky is widely adopted [19]. Hyperpyrexia, mental status changes, cardiovascular decompensation, GI-hepatic dysfunction, and any precipitant history are scored. A total score greater than 45 is highly suggestive of thyroid storm, 35 to 45 supportive of diagnosis, and less than 25 thyroid storm unlikely. Pediatricians should consider thyroid storm in the differential diagnosis when a patient exhibits both CNS and GI symptoms and clinical signs of hyperthyroidism. Patients who meet the diagnostic criteria of a thyroid storm are best managed in a PICU setting and treated with beta-blockers, ATD, glucocorticoids, inorganic Iodine solutions such as SSKI which rapidly decreases TH synthesis, and supportive care.

PREDICTORS AND MANAGEMENT OF NEONATAL HYPERTHYROIDISM

It is estimated that 2% of children born to mothers with active or past GD develop transient neonatal hyperthyroidism (NH). This is due to the transplacental transfer of TSH receptor antibodies (TRAb) [20]. Elevated TRAb can persist for several years after ablation with a risk of 5.5% in the first 2 years

Table 2
Etiology of hyperthyroidism, pathogenesis and diagnostic features

Etiology	Pathogenesis	Key features	Diagnosis
Graves' disease	Autoimmune disorder due to TSH receptor antibodies stimulating thyroid hormone synthesis and thyroid enlargement	Symptomatic hyperthyroidism, Goiter, GO	TSH ↓ Free T4 and T3↑ TSI/TRAB ↑ Diffuse ↑ in thyroid uptake scan
Hashitoxicosis	Transient increase in thyroid hormone release in the setting of autoimmune thyroiditis	Asymptomatic or mildly symptomatic, Goiter, no GO, may progress t o hypothyroidism or revert to euthyroid state	TSH ↓ Free T4 and T3 mild ↑or Nl TSI/TRAB negative TPO/Anti-TG Ab ↑ ↓ uptake on thyroid scan
Toxic nodule	Autonomous hypersecretion	Asymptomatic or mildly symptomatic, +'/- palpable thyroid nodule depends on size, no GO	TSH ↓ Free T4 and T3 mild ↑ or Nl TSI/TRAB/TPO/AntiTG Ab Nl Thyroid nodule on sonogram Focal ↑uptake on thyroid scan
Subacute thyroiditis	Viral/postviral inflammation	Tender goiter, Transient hyperthyroidism (few weeks) sometimes followed by hypothyroidism before normalizing.	TSH ↓, ESR ↑ Free T4 and T3 Nl mild ↑ or Nl TSI/TRAB/TPO/Anti TG Ab Nl ↓uptake on thyroid scan
Acute suppurative thyroiditis	Bacterial infection	Fever, toxic looking, tender thyroid	Mostly euthyroid but rarely can be hyperthyroid. Sonogram shows abscess
McCune Albright Syndrome	Activating the mutation of the gene for the Gs protein	Precocious puberty, fibrous dysplasia, café au lait macules	TSH ↓ Free T4 and T3↑ TSI/TRAB Nl Diffuse ↑ in thyroid

(*continued on next page*)

Table 2
(*continued*)

Etiology	Pathogenesis	Key features	Diagnosis
		Goiter often multinodular Persistent hyperthyroidism	uptake scan Sonogram heterogenic gland with multinodularity
TSH receptor activating mutation	Autosomal dominant inheritance	Goiter, can be multinodular, permanent hyperthyroidism	TSH ↓ Free T4 and T3 ↑ TSI/TRAB negative ↑ in thyroid uptake scan
Drug-induced thyroiditis	Amiodarone induced HT type 1 from ↑ production and type 2 due to destructive thyroiditis Lithium ↑ release of TH Immune check point inhibitors cause destructive thyroiditis	Usually, no goiter and often transient	TSH ↓ Free T4 and T3 ↑ Thyroid antibodies often negative Diffuse ↑ in thyroid uptake scan in Amiodarone induced type 1 HT
Thyrotoxicosis factitia	Thyroid hormone ingestion	No goiter	TSH ↓ Free T4 ↑ Thyroglobulin ↓

Abbreviations: AntiTG, Ab; Antithyroglobulin, antibody; GO, Graves' ophthalmopathy; HT, Hyperthyroidism; NI, normal; TPO, Thyroid peroxidase antibody; TRAb, TSH receptor antibody; TSI, thyroid-stimulating Immunoglobulin.

after RAI [20]. Early diagnosis and treatment of the fetus and neonates is the key to preventing significant adverse effects in the form of premature births, IUGR, microcephaly, cardiac arrhythmias, and failure [20]. Clinical manifestations of neonatal thyrotoxicosis include irritability, poor sleep, diarrhea, and poor weight gain. Physical examination may reveal warm and moist skin, tachycardia with bounding pulses, arrhythmias, frontal bossing with triangular facies, hepatosplenomegaly, a diffuse goiter, and an adrenergic stare, and in severe cases congestive heart failure. NH typically resolves in 3 to 12 weeks [4].

Maternal TRAb levels greater than 500% of normal values in French study [21] and levels greater than 5.9 IU/L (n:<2IU/L) in another study [22] predicted NH and negative maternal TRAb is associated with no risk for NH underscoring the importance of maternal TRAb measurement and cut off values requiring close monitoring of fetus and neonates. When maternal TRAb is elevated, fetal thyroid ultrasound, fetal bone maturation, and fetal heart rate (greater than 160/min) can all be used to determine fetal

Box 1: Considerations for the management of GD

ATD is the first line of treatment

- Methimazole 0.25–1 mg/kg/d divided twice a day, first-line therapy
- Atenolol 1 to 2 mg/kg/d daily or Propranolol 0.5 to 2 mg/kg/d in 3 to 4 divided doses for a few weeks
- Thyroid function tests (free T4, total T3, TSH) are obtained at 2 to 6 weeks, the dose is adjusted if indicated, and again at 4 to 6 weeks, and then every 2 to 3 months once the dose is stabilized.
- Can be continued for up to-8 years if tolerated to increase the chance of remission
- Side effects: Urticaria, Idiosyncratic neutropenia, hepatoxicity less common

Permanent treatment with RAI with I-131

- Indication: Failure to achieve remission after prolonged ATD, side effect, poor compliance, poor control
- Contraindicated in thyroid nodule or severe GO
- Offered for children greater than 10 years of age
- Outpatient procedure
- Stop methimazole 5 days before RAI
- Posttreatment isolation for a week
- About 2 months to achieve hypothyroidism
- Persistent hyperthyroidism a year after RAI denotes treatment failure and need for repeat RAI therapy

Permanent treatment with thyroidectomy

- Indication: Failure to achieve remission after prolonged ATD, side effect, poor compliance, poor control
- Offered if there is thyroid nodule, very enlarged thyroid gland, compressive symptoms, severe GO
- Offered for Children less than 10 years of age
- Pretreatment with MMI, beta-blockers to achieve euthyroid state
- SSKI (Potassium Iodide) for 7 days before surgery
- Low complication rate in high volume centers
- Permanent hypoparathyroidism in some studies reported up to 10%
- Permanent neck scar Next line please add Immediate hypothyroidism

hyperthyroidism and the need for treatment. Fetal hyperthyroidism can be treated by administering ATDs to the mother.

Neonates at risk for NH come to medical attention at different stages and while knowing the maternal TRAb status is ideal, there are occasions when the status is not known. A 2016 review by Van der Kay and colleagues [23] gives excellent insight to the approach and management of NH when maternal TRAb levels are known and unknown. Measurement of cord or neonatal

TRAb, TSH, and Free T4 in the neonates offers additional understanding toward the risk for NH.

A SIMPLIFIED GUIDE AND INTERPRETATION ARE AS FOLLOWS

1. If maternal TRAb is unknown or positive, the neonate is considered at high risk. Check cord/neonatal TRAb. If negative, no risk for NH
2. If maternal TRAb/cord TRAb/neonatal TRAb is unknown or maternal/cord/neonatal TRAb is positive, check TSH and free T4 on days 3 to 5 of life, day 10 to 14 of life and clinical follow-up with PCP until 2 to 3 months of age. Check thyroid levels immediately at any point if neonate is symptomatic
3. If NH diagnosed at any point in time, MMI is the treatment of choice; β-blockers can be added for sympathetic hyperactivity. In refractory cases, potassium iodide may be used in conjunction with MMI

Continuation of breastfeeding is safe and should be encouraged in hyperthyroid mothers taking ATDs. Experts currently recommend using low-to-moderate MMI doses as a first-line therapy in lactating mothers. MMI dose of less than 20 mg per day, or a PTU dose of less than 300 mg per day has no adverse effects. ATD should be administered in divided doses immediately following each feeding [24,25].

SUMMARY

Hyperthyroidism leads to cardiovascular, neurologic and GI symptoms which can be misleading and point to other systemic disorders or referral to other specialists and therefore being aware of the different symptoms and early screening will facilitate prompt treatment. Hyperthyroidism is diagnosed based on suppressed TSH, elevated Free T4 and T3. TSI is elevated in GD which is an autoimmune disorder. Thyroid sonogram and I-123 thyroid uptake scan can be reserved for rare instances when a thyroid nodule is suspected. GD constitutes 96% of pediatric hyperthyroidism and is managed initially with MMI. Remission of GD in children is low at about 30% after 2 years of ATD treatment and can be improved to 50% or more after 8 years of treatment with no increase in adverse effects. Therefore, in children with good control on modest dose of MMI, long-term treatment should be offered.

RAI with I-131 offers definitive treatment and results in permanent hypothyroidism. Thyroidectomy should be offered as a definitive treatment of younger patients less than 10 years of age and those with persistently poor control and is sometimes preferred over RAI and carries the low risk of complications if conducted by high-volume surgeons.

Thyroid storm is a rare life-threatening condition and should be suspected in the presence of overwhelming cardiovascular decompensation, altered mental status, hyperpyrexia, and GI decompensation. Pediatricians and emergency medicine providers must be aware of this presentation. Neonates born to mothers with active or past GD are at risk for transient NH.

CLINICS CARE POINTS

1. Hyperthyroidism is due to increased production of thyroid hormone (TH) as noted biochemically by elevated THs, Free T4, and total T3 and suppressed thyroid-stimulating hormone (TSH). The most common cause of hyperthyroidism is GD which is an autoimmune disorder from TSH receptor stimulation by TSH receptor antibody (TRAb) and makes up for 96% of pediatric hyperthyroidism [1].
2. Hyperthyroidism is a hypermetabolic state resulting in unintentional weight loss and has cardiovascular, GI, neurologic, dermatologic, and ocular symptoms. Symptoms can be misleading and point to other systemic disorders and delay diagnosis. Pediatricians should be aware of these symptoms and signs to make an early diagnosis and referral to a pediatric endocrinologist.
3. All patients suspected to have hyperthyroidism should have thyroid-stimulating hormone (TSH), Free T4, and total T3 tested. In hyperthyroidism, TSH is very low and typically less than 0.01 mIU/mL and Free T4 and T3 are elevated. As GD is the most common cause of pediatric hyperthyroidism, all patients must either have thyroid-stimulating immunoglobulin (TSI) or TRAb tested [12]. Thyroid sonogram and I-123 thyroid uptake scans are reserved for the few cases with antibody-negative hyperthyroidism or if a thyroid nodule is suspected.
4. Methimazole (MMI) is the first line of therapy for pediatric Graves' disease (GD) [12]. Propylthiouracil (PTU) should not be used in children and carries an FDA boxed warning against its use due to hepatotoxicity (12). Long-term MMI use for up to 8 years increased the chance of remission in children. Radioactive iodine (RAI) and Thyroidectomy offer permanent treatment resulting in hypothyroidism.
5. Thyroid storm is a rare life-threatening condition resulting in hyperpyrexia, altered mental status, cardiovascular and GI decompensation and needs immediate care in an ICU setting and treated with MMI, beta-blockers, SSKI, glucocorticoids, and supportive care [19]. Pediatricians should be aware of this presentation.
6. Neonates born to mothers with active or past GD develop transient neonatal hyperthyroidism (NH), which typically self resolves in 2 to 3 months. This is due to the transplacental transfer of TSH receptor antibodies (TRAb) [20]. A robust screening of maternal TRAb and if unavailable, cord or neonatal TRAB and screening TSH and Free T4 in neonate [23] can result in proper identification and treatment of children with NH.

Disclosure

The authors have nothing to disclose.

References

[1] Leung AKC, Leung AAC. Evaluation and management of children with thyrotoxicosis. Recent Pat Endocr Metab Immune Drug Discov 2017;11(1):22–31.

[2] Simon M, Rigou A, Le Moal J, et al. Epidemiology of childhood hyperthyroidism in france: a nationwide population-based study. J Clin Endocrinol Metab 2018;103(8):2980–7.

[3] Rodanaki M, Lodefalk M, Forssell K, et al. The incidence of childhood thyrotoxicosis is increasing in both girls and boys in sweden. Horm Res Paediatr 2019;91(3): 195–202.
[4] Srinivasan S, Misra M. Hyperthyroidism in children. Pediatr Rev 2015;36(6):239–48.
[5] Kraus CN, Sodha P, Vaidyanathan P, et al. Thyroid dermopathy and acropachy in pediatric patients. Pediatr Dermatol 2018;35(6):e371–4.
[6] Hanley P, Lord K, Bauer AJ. Thyroid disorders in children and adolescents: a review. JAMA Pediatr 2016;170(10):1008–19.
[7] De Leo S, Lee SY, Braverman LE. Hyperthyroidism. Lancet 2016;388(10047):906–18.
[8] Rosenberg Bezalel S, Elbirt D, Leiba H, et al. Isr Med Assoc J 2017;19(3):188–92.
[9] Lee JH, Park SH, Koh DG, et al. Thyroid peroxidase antibody positivity and triiodothyronine levels are associated with pediatric Graves' ophthalmopathy. World J Pediatr 2014;10(2): 155–9.
[10] Goldstein SM, Katowitz WR, Moshang T, et al. Pediatric thyroid-associated orbitopathy: the Children's Hospital of Philadelphia experience and literature review. Thyroid 2008;18(9): 997–9.
[11] Kaplowitz Paul B, Priya Vaidyanathan. Update on pediatric hyperthyroidism. Curr Opin Endocrinol Diabetes Obes 2020;27(1):70–6.
[12] Ross DS, Burch HB, Cooper DS, et al. 2016 American thyroid association guidelines for diagnosis and management of hyperthyroidism and other causes of thyrotoxicosis. Thyroid 2016;26(10):1343–421.
[13] U.S. Food and Drug Administration. 2010. Available at: http://www.fda.gov/Safety/MedWatch/SafetyInformation/SafetyAlertsforHumanMedicalProducts/ucm164162.htm.
[14] Leger J, Oliver I, Rodrigue D, et al. Consensus: Graves' disease in children. Ann Endocrinol (Paris) 2018;79:647–55.
[15] Song A, Kim SJ, Kim M-S, et al. Long-term antithyroid drug treatment of graves' disease in children and adolescents: a 20-year single-center experience. Front Endocrino 2021;12: 687834.
[16] Jevalikar G, Solis J, Zacharin M. Long-term outcomes of pediatric Graves' disease. Pediatr Endocrinol Metab 2014;27(11–12):1131–6.
[17] Ohye H, Minagawa A, Noh JN, et al. Antithyroid drug treatment for Graves' disease in children: a long-term retrospective study at a single institution. Thyroid 2014;24:200–7.
[18] Azizi F, Takyar M, Madreseh E, et al. Long-term methimazole therapy in juvenile graves' disease: a randomized trial. Pediatrics 2019;143(5):e20183034.
[19] Burch 1 HB, Wartofsky L. Life-threatening thyrotoxicosis. Thyroid storm. Endocrinol Metab Clin North Am 1993;22:263–77.
[20] Léger J. Management of fetal and neonatal graves' disease. Horm Res Paediatr 2017;87(1):1–6.
[21] Banige M, Estellat C, Biran V, et al. Study of the factors leading to fetal and neonatal dysthyroidism in children of patients with Graves disease. J Endocr Soc 2017;1:751–61.
[22] Yoshihara A, Iwaku K, Noh JY, et al. Incidence of Neonatal Hyperthyroidism Among Newborns of Graves' Disease Patients Treated with Radioiodine Therapy. Thyroid 2019;29(1): 128–34.
[23] Van der Kay DC, Wasserman JD, Palmert MR. Management of newborns born to mothers with Graves' disease. Pediatrics 2016;137:e20151878.
[24] Namwongprom S, Dejkhamron P, Unachak K. Success rate of radioactive iodine treatment for children and adolescent with hyperthyroidism. J Endocrinol Invest 2021;44(3):541–5.
[25] Hudzik B. Zubelewicz-Szkodzinska B Antithyroid drugs during breastfeeding. Clin Endocrinol (Oxf) 2016;85(6):827–30.

Advances in Pediatrics 69 (2022) 231–241

ADVANCES IN PEDIATRICS

Updates on the Management of Pilonidal Disease

Amelia T. Collings, MD[a], Beth Rymeski, DO[b,*]

[a]Department of Surgery, Indiana University School of Medicine, 545 Barnhill Drive, Emerson Hall 125, Indianapolis, IN 46203, USA; [b]Cincinnati Children's Hospital Medical Center, 3333 Burnet Avenue, MLC 2023, Cincinnati, OH 45229, USA

Keywords

• Pediatrics • Pilonidal disease • Gips procedure

Key points

- Pilonidal cysts occur due to hair entering the skin in the deep intergluteal cleft, as a result of normal bodily motion, forming sinuses to the skin and a cyst in the subcutaneous tissue with hair, inflammation, granulation tissue, and possibly even infection.
- The first key to treatment is the resolution of infection including drainage of abscesses.
- Asymptomatic sinuses/pits can be managed with hygiene and hair removal.
- Current management of ongoing disease favors a minimally invasive approach, with a Gips or endoscopic procedure, in which pits/sinus tracts are excised with the removal of hair and curettage of the cavity.
- Larger excisions are reserved for when these less invasive approaches have failed.

INTRODUCTION

Pilonidal disease is a relatively common condition affecting adolescents and young adults and less commonly younger children. A spectrum of pilonidal conditions can be seen in children and adolescents including pilonidal cyst, pilonidal abscess, and pilonidal pits and sinuses (Fig. 1A, B). Pilonidal disease is classically described as involving the midline natal (gluteal) cleft and tends to affect men more than women. Pilonidal disease can also occur in the umbilicus but is far less common than in the natal cleft location.

*Corresponding author. *E-mail address:* Beth.rymeski@cchmc.org

https://doi.org/10.1016/j.yapd.2022.03.001

The pathogenesis of pilonidal disease involves ingrowth and/or injury of the skin by the hair follicle which is a structure within the dermis that produces a terminal hair. The hair follicle then creates a foreign body reaction that leads to abscess or to edema that obstructs the drainage of the hair follicle and creates a pit or sinus tract. Motion of the buttock skin then can result in continued drawing in of hair follicles into the pit [1–4]. It is the *hair shaft* itself that is the instigating factor in the development of pilonidal disease. After the hair has tunneled through the skin, due to the friction of the gluteal cleft, the body creates an epithelized tract causing a sinus to form. Oftentimes this happens continually leading to multiple sinus tracts and eventually a cyst in the subcutaneous tissue with hair, inflammation, and chronic granulation tissue. These tracts can become obstructed, creating an anaerobic environment in which bacteria can grow, causing infection and abscess formation [5].

Pilonidal disease and its complications frequently bring adolescents to primary care and surgeon offices, with a wide variety of treatment options presented based on the experience of the provider. There has been very little consensus as to the best treatment option with some providers preferring medical management options and others recommending surgery. The surgical options vary widely from minimally invasive to large resections and may also include the use of wound vac technology.

The purpose of our article is to review some of the recent advances in the management of pilonidal disease that may offer the same level of relief with less invasive procedures.

Medical management

Despite its prevalence, there is very little data or agreement on the best practice for managing pilonidal disease without surgery. Some of this may have to do with the variety of presentations (sinus/pits vs active infection/abscess) and the variety of providers seeing these patients for evaluation (primary care providers, general surgeons, colorectal surgeons, pediatric surgeons, emergency room physicians). However, some common themes have arisen from clinical practice and numerous publications, which will be further highlighted here.

Hygiene seems to play a large role in the management of patients who have pilonidal disease and is a cornerstone to almost all care algorithms described. Cleaning of the area on at least a daily basis should be encouraged to keep the surrounding skin clean and potentially wash away some of the loose hairs from the natal cleft. There is no evidence that the use of antibacterial or bactericidal soaps is more effective than traditional soap. In addition to maintaining a clean environment, removal of hair from the natal cleft and the surrounding area is central to healing and prevention of recurrence. Electric clippers should be used in the office to remove hair from the cleft and the surrounding buttock skin. Most recommend a wide area of hair removal (at least several inches on all sides from the cleft) to have the best results. Shaving with a razor is discouraged, as this can cause microabrasions to the skin and hair follicles that may actually promote infection. As regular clipping of the hair in this area is difficult

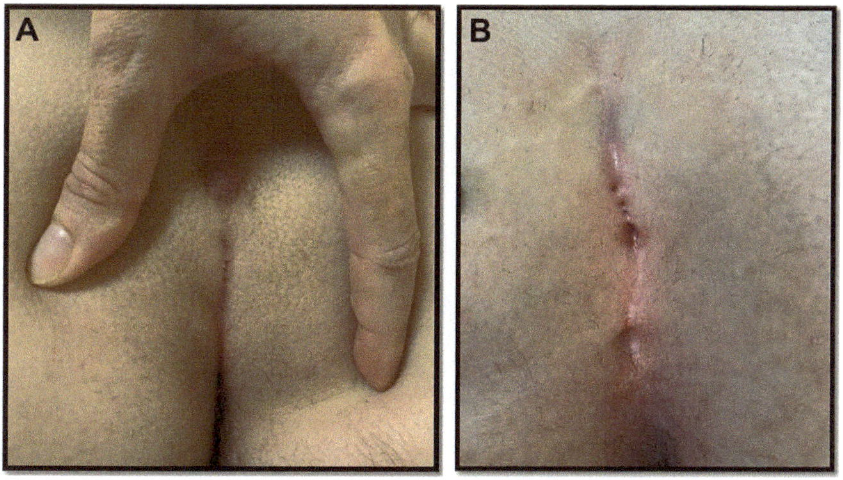

Fig. 1. (*A*) Example of pilonidal pits; (*B*) Example of pilonidal sinuses.

for a patient to do without assistance, unless a family member or friend is willing to assist, it is often not a practical home-based solution but can be performed in the provider's office with each visit. Because of the lack of practicality of routine hair clipping, many recommend the use of hair depilatory creams for home use (Nair, Veet, and others). These are easier to apply without assistance and allow for relatively quick and easy removal of hair from the area. These creams are available over the counter and are not prescribed; this can be problematic for patients with limited resources who cannot afford the out-of-pocket expense. Additionally, these products should be used with care when there is an open, nonhealed area as the application of the cream directly on wounds may lead to discomfort and burning. When possible, teaching a parent, friend, or partner how to help with hair removal is helpful.

In the office, it is common for surgeons and other providers familiar with the technique to remove hair from the sinus tracts; this technique is often described as "pit picking." Not surprisingly, there is no standard definition of what pit picking encompasses. In many instances, this may be a careful examination of sinus tracts and wounds for debris (mostly hair) that is extracted from the tract with tweezers. This technique can be easily used in the office without any anesthetic and can be taught to motivate family members to continue at home. In other instances, pit picking describes a much more involved bedside procedure conducted under local anesthesia. Mooney and colleagues described their pit picking process in adolescents as a local anesthetic followed by trephination with skin punch biopsies then debridement of the cavity. Small, angled incisions were made over exit sites to assist in debridement and then closed with suture material. Using this technique, he reports a 92% resolution of symptoms with a median follow-up of 5 months [6].

Surgical treatment

Treatment of pilonidal abscess

Oftentimes, the initial presenting symptoms of pilonidal disease are associated with its infected state. A pilonidal abscess presents as any other abscess: erythematous, painful, fluctuant, and characteristically at the natal cleft. Treatment at this stage should be focused on infection control with incision and drainage. Traditionally, further surgical control of the pilonidal disease should be deferred until it is no longer an infected field, as this will adversely affect wound healing and recurrence rates [7]. Antibiotics should be given to patients with additional complicating factors, such as associated cellulitis, systemic signs of infection, history of immunocompromise, and/or diabetes mellitus. Resolution of the infectious process should be confirmed before any definitive surgical treatment of the underlying disease is undertaken.

Traditional surgical treatment

The decision to pursue surgical management of chronic pilonidal disease is not one to be taken lightly. Historically, surgical treatments have involved extensive excisions, large, chronic wounds, and/or high rates of disease recurrence. These excisions involve a 5 to 10 cm vertical, elliptical excision of the tissue surrounding the pilonidal pits. The dissection is typically taken down to the level of the sacrum. Closure of these large wounds can be accomplished by 2 main approaches: excision with primary closure, including flap closures, and those left to heal on their own by secondary intention. There have been several randomized control trials (RCTs) comparing primary closure versus healing by secondary intention in adults. Overall, healing by secondary intention has a lower rate of recurrence, with no difference in wound complications; however, people with primary closure returned to work 10 days earlier [8,9]. In children, there is less high-quality evidence available; however, there are several small, retrospective studies that have reported shorter recovery times and lower recurrence rates in children and adolescents undergoing primary closure compared with healing by secondary intention [10–13].

Those undergoing primary closure have the option of having their wounds closed on or off the midline. The concept of closing the wound of the midline is to remove the intergluteal cleft which is thought to contribute to the hairs that irritate, enter the skin, and incite the disease. Several RCTs and systematic reviews have explored these 2 options and unequivocally off-midline closures are superior in terms of wound complications and healing time [8,9,14,15]. The three best-studied off-midline flap closures are the Rhomboid flap, the Karydakis flap, and the Bascom cleft lift (Fig. 2). These methods may be needed in patient who has extensive, chronic disease requiring large excision or those with recurrent disease. Again, most of the evidence comes from the adult literature. Fike and colleagues [16] compared midline to flap closures specifically in children undergoing excision of their pilonidal disease. There was no difference in wound breakdown, but there was a higher rate of wound infections in the midline cohort [16]. Generally, these historical surgical techniques of treating

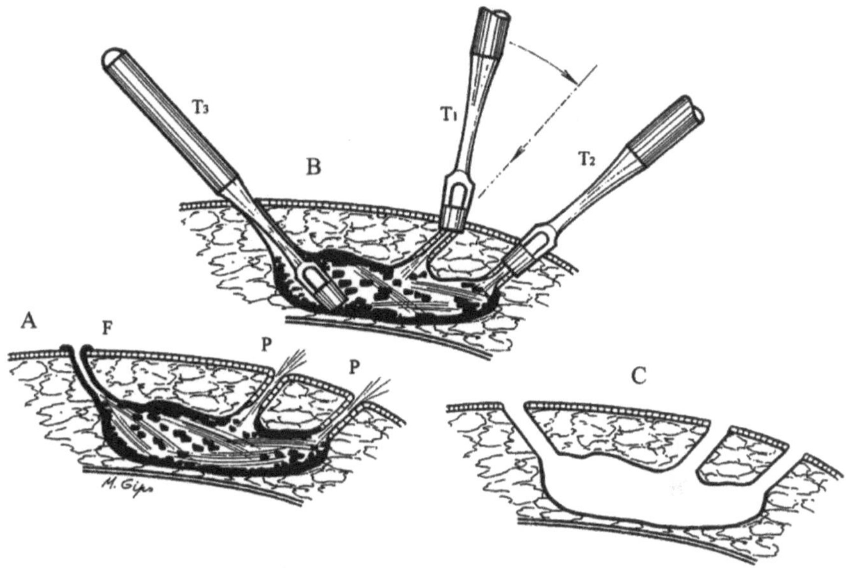

Fig. 2. Diagram of the Gips Procedure as first described by Dr Moshe Gips. (*From* Gips M, Melki Y, Salem L, Weil R, Sulkes J. Minimal surgery for pilonidal disease using trephines: description of a new technique and long-term outcomes in 1,358 patients. *Dis Colon Rectum.* 2008;51(11):1656-1663. https://doi.org/10.1007/s10350-008-9329-x.)

pilonidal disease have rates of wound complications in children ranging from 14% to 30% and can take weeks to months to heal [17]. Furthermore, the recurrence rates after wide local excision can be upwards of 30% in children [18]. Thus, these children were in desperate need of less morbid options to treat their chronic diseases.

The "Gips" procedure

In 2008, Dr Moshe Gips published a case series of more than 1300 adult patients from a military surgical clinic using a novel technique of trephination and debridement of the pilonidal cyst, all conducted under local anesthesia [19]. Trephination is a surgical procedure for creating a circular hole in tissue, often using a punch biopsy tool. The initial results of this study were excellent. They had low rates of wound complications, complete healing was seen at a mean of 3.4 weeks, and 93.5% of patients were disease free at 1 year [19]. Despite initially being described in adult patients, this innovative procedure offered the possibility of new hope for patients who historically suffered multiple recurrences often with deteriorating quality of life.

The Gips procedure is performed while the patient is in the prone position. Local anesthetic is injected into the intergluteal cleft. Then each pit is probed to investigate the depth and direction of the associated cyst. Skin trephines, or a surgical tool used to excise a circle of tissue, of various sizes depending on the

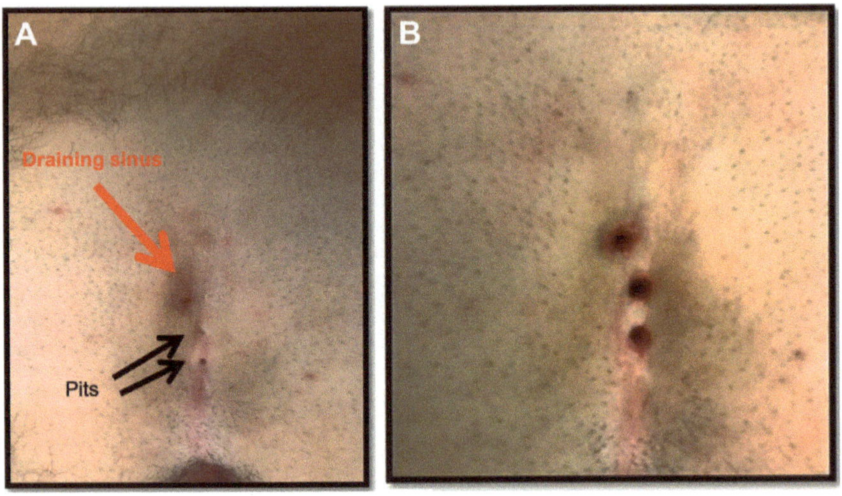

Fig. 3. Before and after trephination with Gips procedure; (*A*) before; (*B*) after.

tract length and proximity to neighboring pits, are introduced perpendicularly to the skin and advanced until it enters the pilonidal cavity (Fig. 3). Curettage is the scraping of the inside of the cavity using a tool with pointed jaws called a Rongeur device. This is performed throughout the entire cavity: removal of all hair in the cavity, an epithelialized lining and/or granulation tissue, and fistulous tracts, is important to prevent disease recurrence. This is followed by irrigation, usually with hydrogen peroxide solution, and confirmation of hemostasis. The wound cavities are not routinely packed and usually only require a dry gauze dressing on top. Patients do not require any postoperative activity limitations and may return to normal hygiene practices the following day. Additionally, no postoperative antibiotics are required and typically over-the-counter pain medicine, such as acetaminophen and ibuprofen, is all that is necessary.

Various iterations of the original Gips procedure have begun to be adopted, including within pediatric surgery. There have been several small case series in children looking at the early efficacy and safety of this innovative procedure. Metzger and colleagues reported a series of 19 children who underwent trephination and curettage. There was a 15.8% recurrence rate within the 6-month follow-up period [20]. When compared directly to wide excision, which included both open and primary midline closures, trephination and curettage had significantly fewer wound complications and postoperative visits. Trephination had an 8% recurrence rate compared with a 12% recurrence rate after excision with midline closure; however, this was not statistically significant [21]. The most significant limitation of all these studies in the pediatric population is small sample sizes and lack of long-term follow-up. The Midwest

Pediatric Surgery Consortium (MWPSC), a collaboration of surgeon investigators, has an ongoing multi-institutional, prospective study evaluating the outcomes after medical and surgical management, specifically the Gips procedure. The study (which is led by the writers) is supported by the American Pediatric Surgical Association through grant funding and recently completed patient enrollment in the fall of 2021. The patients are being followed for 1 year after enrollment so data from the study are not complete at the time of this article [22,23].

Even in the adult literature, there is a paucity of long-term data. However, early studies consistently show that the Gips procedure is safe, with low recurrence and complication rates, with shorter times to return to work [24,25]. Complication rates as low as 4.3% and a recurrence rate of 5.8% in the first year [24] were reported. Patients that underwent a Gips procedure used on average 13 less sick days when compared to wide excision [25]. Despite the nascency of the Gips procedure, early data demonstrating significantly less morbidity has led to its rapid acceptance. In addition, patients that do recur after a Gips may still undergo repeat Gips or proceed to excision, which may now be a more straightforward procedure compared with someone who has previously undergone a large excision with flap reconstruction.

Endoscopic treatment

Additional minimally invasive techniques to treat pilonidal disease include endoscopic and video-assisted ablation. The cyst space is debrided under direct visualization in both procedures. This was first described in adults in the endoscopic pilonidal sinus treatment (EPSiT) study and used a fistuloscope to debride the cyst cavity [26]. This was then adopted for the pediatric population in the pediatric endoscopic pilonidal sinus treatment (PEPSiT) study and was combined with laser hair removal as an adjunct [27]. They reported a less than 10% recurrence rate in an 18-month follow-up period with very high patient satisfaction scores [27].

Laser hair removal

Epilation has long been a mainstay in the treatment of pilonidal disease, due to the involvement of hair in the pathogenesis. Laser hair removal has been in practice for several decades, but over the last several years, it has begun to be used routinely in the treatment of pilonidal disease by many practitioners to prevent recurrence. Two of the most commonly studied lasers for this purpose are Alexandrite and neodymium-doped yttrium aluminum garnet (Nd:YAG). Typically, the hairs at the site of the pits within the intergluteal cleft along with the immediate surrounding area are ablated. This procedure is repeated at timed intervals, usually monthly, until there is no longer any hair visible. The range in the total number of treatments required was 1 to 11; however, most studies describe 3 to 5 on average [28]. It has been shown to be safe, with minimal associated pain [29]. A systematic review evaluating its use in pilonidal disease across all ages found a range of disease recurrence of 0%-28% [28]. Several studies reporting its use explicitly in children have

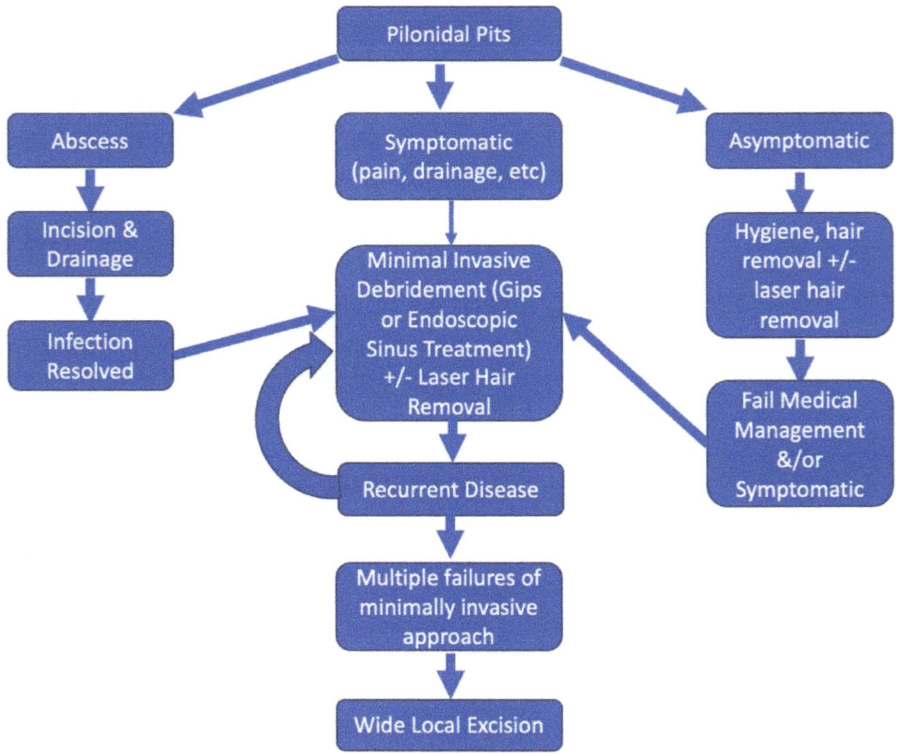

Fig. 4. Authors proposed the treatment algorithm for pediatric pilonidal disease.

reported no complications and very low rates of recurrence [29,30]. Moreover, it can be used as an adjunct after surgical intervention, to further decrease the likelihood of recurrence. When used following wide local excision, recurrence rates decline from more than 50% to less than 10% [31]. The main issue with laser treatment is that it is not broadly covered by insurance plans and results in a large out-of-pocket expense for the family; this results in laser being out of reach for many patients. Patients living in remote areas may also not have access to this treatment option because these services are not widely available and typically are clustered in urban, more heavily populated areas.

SUMMARY

Pilonidal disease can be associated with significant morbidity and decreases the child's quality of life, oftentimes impacting their social dynamics at a critical point in their psychosocial development. Treatments should be aimed at decreasing disease recurrence while not increasing the complications from the treatment itself (Fig. 4). If a patient is asymptomatic, then medical management with hygiene and hair removal; possibly even with laser hair removal; should be attempted first. If a patient presents during the acute, infective phase then incision and drainage of the abscess with additional antibiotics should be performed. Once the infection has resolved or if a patient presents with symptoms, such as pain or drainage, then a Gips or endoscopic treatment, with adjuncts such as laser hair removal, have been shown to be effective without the morbidity of traditional wide local excision. Minimally invasive approaches should still be used in recurrent disease with wide local excision reserved for severe, refractory cases, when all other modalities have been exhausted.

Acknowledgments

The authors would like to thank Dr Nelson Rosen for providing the photos in Figs. 1 and 3.

Disclosure

The authors have no disclosures.

References

[1] da Silva JH. Pilonidal cyst. Cause and treatment. Dis Colon Rectum 2000;43:1146–56 [PubMed] [Google Scholar].

[2] Bascom J. Pilonidal disease: origin from follicles of hairs and results of follicle removal as treatment. Surgery 1980;87:567–72 [PubMed] [Google Scholar].

[3] Franckowiak JJ, Jackman RJ. The etiology of pilonidal sinus. Dis Colon Rectum 1962;5: 28–36 [PubMed] [Google Scholar].

[4] Bendewald FP, Cima RR. Pilonidal disease. Clin Colon Rectal Surg 2007;20(2):86–95.

[5] Flageole H, et al. Pilonidal disease." The Pediatric surgery not a textbook (NaT) edited by Ron Hirschl, et al, Available at: https://www.pedsurglibrary.com/apsa/view/Pediatric-Surgery-NaT/829001/all/. Accessed 2022.

[6] Delshad HR, Dawson M, Melvin P, et al. Pit-picking resolved pilonidal disease in adolescents. J Pedtr Surg 2019;54:174–6.

[7] Johnson EK, Vogel JD, Cowan ML, et al. Clinical practice guidelines committee of the American society of colon and rectal surgeons. the American society of colon and rectal

surgeons' clinical practice guidelines for the management of pilonidal disease. Dis Colon Rectum 2019;62(2):146–57.
[8] Al-Khamis A, McCallum I, King PM, et al. Healing by primary versus secondary intention after surgical treatment for pilonidal sinus. Cochrane Database Syst Rev 2010;2010(1): CD006213.
[9] Grabowski J, Oyetunji TA, Goldin AB, et al. The management of pilonidal disease: a systematic review. J Pediatr Surg 2019;54(11):2210–21.
[10] Roldón Golet M, Siles Hinojosa A, González Ruiz Y, et al. Pilonidal sinus in adolescence: is there an ideal surgical approach?. sinus pilonidal durante la adolescencia: ¿existe el abordaje quirúrgico ideal? Cir Pediatr 2021;34(3):119–24.
[11] Pfammatter M, Erlanger TE, Mayr J. Primary transverse closure compared to open wound treatment for primary pilonidal sinus disease in children. Children (Basel) 2020;7(10):187.
[12] Ozcan R, Hüseynov M, Bakır AC, et al. Which treatment modality for pediatric pilonidal sinus: Primary repair or secondary healing? Asian J Surg 2018;41(5):506–10.
[13] Zagory JA, Golden J, Holoyda K, et al. Excision and primary closure may be the better option in the surgical management of pilonidal disease in the pediatric population. Am Surg 2016;82(10):964–7.
[14] Enriquez-Navascues JM, Emparanza JI, Alkorta M, et al. Meta-analysis of randomized controlled trials comparing different techniques with primary closure for chronic pilonidal sinus. Tech Coloproctol 2014;18(10):863–72.
[15] Sevinç B, Karahan Ö, Okuş A, et al. Randomized prospective comparison of midline and off-midline closure techniques in pilonidal sinus surgery. Surgery 2016;159(3):749–54.
[16] Fike FB, Mortellaro VE, Juang D, et al. Experience with pilonidal disease in children. J Surg Res 2011;170(1):165–8.
[17] Hardy EJO, Herrod PJ, Doleman B, et al. Surgical interventions for the treatment of sacrococcygeal pilonidal sinus disease in children: a systematic review and meta-analysis. J Pediatr Surg 2019;54(11):2222–33.
[18] Halleran DR, Lopez JJ, Lawrence AE, et al. Recurrence of pilonidal disease: our best is not good enough. J Surg Res 2018;232:430–6.
[19] Gips M, Melki Y, Salem L, et al. Minimal surgery for pilonidal disease using trephines: description of a new technique and long-term outcomes in 1,358 patients. Dis Colon Rectum 2008;51(11):1656–63.
[20] Metzger GA, Apfeld JC, Nishimura L, et al. Room for Improvement: the trephination procedure for pediatric patients with pilonidal disease. J Surg Res 2021;267:605–11.
[21] Prieto JM, Checchi KD, Kling KM, et al. Trephination versus wide excision for the treatment of pediatric pilonidal disease. J Pediatr Surg 2020;55(4):747–51.
[22] MidWest Pediatric Surgery Consortium. Current studies. Available at: http://www.mwpsc.org/current-studies.html.
[23] APSA Foundation Grants. American pediatric surgical association. Available at: https://apsapedsurg.org/aspa-info/apsa-foundation/awards/.
[24] Di Castro A, Guerra F, Levi Sandri GB, et al. Minimally invasive surgery for the treatment of pilonidal disease. The Gips procedure on 2347 patients. Int J Surg 2016;36(Pt A):201–5.
[25] Levinson T, Sela T, Chencinski S, et al. Pilonidal sinus disease: a 10-year review reveals occupational risk factors and the superiority of the minimal surgery trephine technique. Mil Med 2016;181(4):389–94.
[26] Meinero P, Mori L, Gasloli G. Endoscopic pilonidal sinus treatment (E.P.Si.T.). Tech Coloproctol 2014;18(4):389–92.
[27] Esposito C, Mendoza-Sagaon M, Del Conte F, et al. Pediatric endoscopic pilonidal sinus treatment (PEPSiT) in children with pilonidal sinus disease: tips and tricks and new structurated protocol. Front Pediatr 2020;8:345.
[28] Halleran DR, Onwuka AJ, Lawrence AE, et al. Laser hair depilation in the treatment of pilonidal disease: a systematic review. Surg Infect (Larchmt) 2018;19(6):566–72.

[29] Lukish JR, Kindelan T, Marmon LM, et al. Laser epilation is a safe and effective therapy for teenagers with pilonidal disease. J Pediatr Surg 2009;44(1):282–5.
[30] Braungart S, Powis M, Sutcliffe JR, et al. Improving outcomes in pilonidal sinus disease. J Pediatr Surg 2016;51(2):282–4.
[31] Kelati A, Lagrange S, Le Duff F, et al. Laser hair removal after surgery vs. surgery alone for the treatment of pilonidal cysts: a retrospective case-control study. J Eur Acad Dermatol Venereol 2018;32(11):2031–3.

Advances in Pediatrics 69 (2022) 243–257

ADVANCES IN PEDIATRICS

Current Management of Adhesive Small Bowel Obstructions in Children

Nathan S. Rubalcava, MD[a,b],
K. Elizabeth Speck, MD, MS, FACS[a,*]

[a]Section of Pediatric Surgery, Department of Surgery, University of Michigan, Mott Children's Hospital, 1540 East Hospital Drive SPC 4217, Ann Arbor, MI 48109-4217, USA; [b]Department of Surgery, Creighton University Health Science Campus, 3100 North Central Avenue, Phoenix, AZ 85012, USA

Keywords

• Pediatric small bowel obstruction • Adhesive small bowel obstruction • Adhesions • Gastrografin • Contrast challenge • SBO • Children

Key points

- Adhesions occur after abdominal surgery as a component of normal healing and are the most common cause of a bowel obstruction. Importantly, if the patient has never had surgery, they very likely have another surgical source.
- The first key is to distinguish between patients requiring urgent surgical management and those who qualify for *initial* nonoperative management.
- Adhesive bowel obstructions in children can be *safely* evaluated and possibly even treated with a contrast challenge.
- A contrast challenge guides timely decision making for patients who are initially managed nonoperatively, with high predictive value to distinguish between patients who will ultimately require surgery and those who will not.

INTRODUCTION

Although there are numerous causes of bowel obstruction, this article aims to summarize the data and provide updates on *postoperative adhesive small bowel obstruction (ASBO) in children.* Although all patients with a bowel obstruction should be evaluated by a surgeon, a bowel obstruction in a child *who has not had prior abdominal surgery* should prompt relatively urgent pediatric surgical consultation as the cause is almost certainly surgical.

*Corresponding author. *E-mail address:* speckk@med.umich.edu

https://doi.org/10.1016/j.yapd.2022.03.002

Historically, attempts were made to distinguish between a *partial* or *complete* bowel obstruction to guide the decision for immediate operation versus initial nonoperative management. Unfortunately, these clinical definitions are imprecise and, therefore, do not predict the risk for the obstruction-associated ischemia and necrosis that would require immediate operation [1]. Therefore, similar to the care of adults, management of pediatric ASBO has moved away from attempting to characterize the *degree of obstruction* and more toward *defining clinical metrics that predict failure of nonoperative management***.

INITIAL DECISION TREE

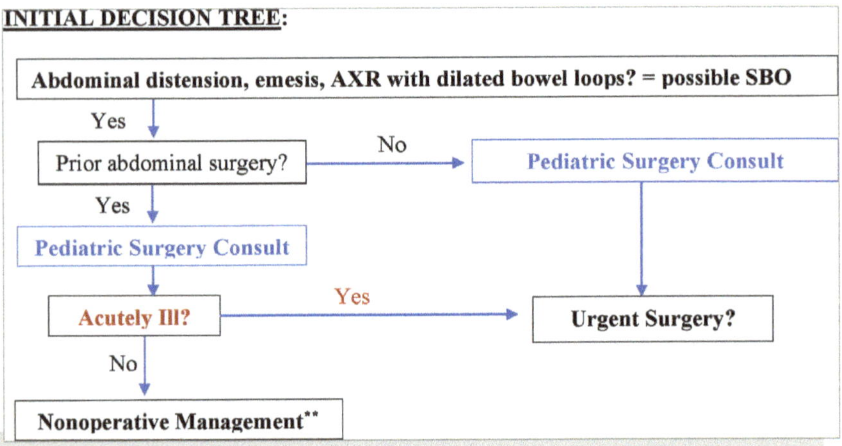

ASBOs are a significant cause of morbidity in children following abdominal operations, and a standard evaluation and management strategy has not yet been accepted across centers. As the decision tree notes, the focus of the initial evaluation of children with a suspected ASBO is to differentiate those who need urgent surgical exploration from those who are appropriate for nonoperative management. The goals are multifactorial:

- Minimize sequelae of delaying a necessary surgical intervention
- Avoid surgery if it is unnecessary
- Offer expeditious care
- Minimize length of hospitalization

Once it is determined that a patient is safe to undergo an *initial nonoperative management strategy***, a standard approach to their management would be beneficial to aid in decision making. Traditionally, nonoperative management has consisted of the following:

- Gastric decompression
- Nil per os (NPO)
- Fluid resuscitation
- Electrolyte repletion

The optimal duration of this nonoperative management continues to be poorly defined, and there are no evidence-based guidelines or best practices in children. However, there have been substantial data for decades in adults demonstrating that a water-soluble contrast challenge algorithm can decrease the need for surgery overall and decrease the hospital length of stay. Similar data are mounting in the pediatric patient population as well, and, importantly, a *contrast challenge algorithm* was recently determined to be *safe in children* [2]. Timely decision making to determine which patients will improve with nonoperative management is the key.

In this article, the authors will:

- Review the epidemiology and pathophysiology of ASBO
- Outline diagnostic modalities and key management strategies
- Discuss historic and current data regarding operative intervention
- Review the literature surrounding nonoperative management protocols, particularly contrast challenge algorithms in children
- Briefly consider prevention strategies and concerns regarding recurrence

Epidemiology

ASBOs account for 50% of all small bowel obstructions and are related to prior abdominal operations [1,3]. Although adhesions will form as a natural part of wound healing in all of the 140,000 children in the United States undergoing abdominal surgery each year, only 3% to 9% of children with adhesions will experience an ASBO [4–7]. Rates of ASBO vary based on the operative site. A population-based analysis of postoperative readmissions related to adhesions in the 5 years following surgery involving the following abdominal operations in children outlined these *incidences* [8]:

- 9.3% small bowel operation
- 5.8% laparotomy
- 2.1% large bowel operation
- 0.3% appendectomy

Notably, 55% of readmissions occurred within the first year.

These rates may be higher after *specific operations* [9]:

- 25% ileostomy creation and closure
- 24% Ladd procedure for malrotation

Over one-third of children with ASBO have at least one chronic medical condition, with many dependent on medical technology, such as a feeding tube

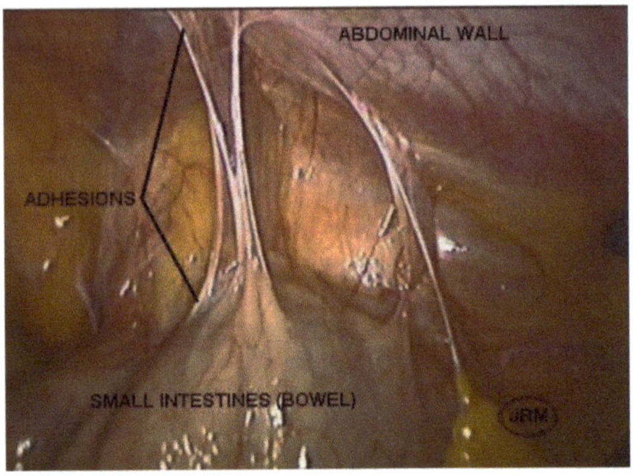

Fig. 1. Adhesions involving the small intestine to the abdominal wall. (*From* Miklos JR, Moore RD. Abdominal Adhesions. Published 2021. Accessed October 19, 2021. https://www.miklosandmoore.com/abdominal-adhesions-atlanta/.)

and/or tracheostomy [10]. ASBOs represent a significant health care problem in children and disproportionately affect children with disabilities and their families.

Pathophysiology

Adhesions can be seen in Fig. 1 and comprise the *scar tissue* that forms between the intestines, other abdominal organs, and the peritoneum of the abdominal wall [11].

The clinical presentation of ASBO is a result of these adhesions causing kinks, twists, or wrapping around the bowel, thus compromising the bowel lumen and normal intestinal transit. The obstruction of the bowel lumen results in abdominal distention, nausea, and vomiting. Ongoing peristalsis occurs both proximal and distal to the obstruction; proximal peristalsis results in vague abdominal pain, whereas distal peristalsis may allow a patient to continue to have bowel function early in the disease process.

As the obstructive process progresses, the bowel wall is stimulated to secrete fluid and electrolytes resulting in increased bowel distension upstream from the obstruction [12,13]. As the pressure of the bowel wall approaches 30 mm Hg (particularly in patients not adequately decompressed), the lacteals within the bowel wall collapse, resulting in *bowel wall edema.* With ongoing increases in luminal pressure, venous outflow obstruction and *venous hypertension* result, thereby increasing fluid filtration across the capillary bed and into the bowel lumen, resulting in *intravascular depletion* and, potentially, *metabolic acidosis. When severe distension occurs, microvascular arterial compression and, potentially, bowel wall ischemia and necrosis may ensue* [1]. Mucosal ischemia, when it occurs, also promotes *bacterial translocation*, which can result in sepsis.

DIAGNOSIS

The diagnosis of ASBO should be made primarily based on clinical presentation, physical examination, and plain radiography. Laboratory investigations help to characterize the degree of physiologic derangement. Although cross-sectional imaging is not required for diagnosis of an *adhesive* small bowel obstruction (SBO), such imaging may define the point of obstruction, reveal concerns for intestinal ischemia, and rule out other causes of SBO.

Clinical presentation

A history of prior abdominal surgery is essential for a diagnosis of ASBO. The clinical presentation of an ASBO is often a constellation of systemic and abdominal symptoms, most frequently:

- Nausea and vomiting
- Abdominal distention
- Colicky abdominal pain
- Decreased stooling or flatus

The *physical examination* is often notable for *abdominal distention, tympany, and non-focal abdominal tenderness*. In instances of bowel ischemia and perforation, more severe abdominal pain may be present, and peritonitis should prompt more urgent surgical intervention. Historically, "tinkles and rushes" heard on auscultation of the abdomen have been described as a distinguishing feature from an ileus; however, the examiner must listen for a reasonable period of time to confirm this finding. In the authors' experience, the findings on abdominal auscultation do not alter clinical management.

Laboratory investigations

Obtaining a complete blood count, basic metabolic panel, and a venous blood gas with a lactate level can assess the degree of volume depletion, guide resuscitation, and help recognize bowel ischemia. Patients with vomiting will have electrolyte imbalances, and when prolonged, present with *hypochloremic, hyponatremic, hypokalemic, metabolic alkalosis*. Both *leukocytosis* and an *elevated lactate level* are well-described markers of ischemia; however, normal values do not rule this out, and the entire clinical picture must be considered [14]. Recent studies have found elevated *procalcitonin* to be predictive of a patient who will require operative intervention, although there remains considerable heterogeneity in the cutoff value, and it has not made its way into standard clinical practice [15–17].

Imaging

An abdominal X-ray (*AXR*) is the most common imaging performed in the evaluation and diagnosis of an ASBO; however, the diagnostic accuracy is only 50% to 60% [2,18]. ASBO can be more accurately diagnosed with plain films in both *supine* (Fig. 2) and *upright* positions. Plain films cannot reliably determine the point of obstruction nor the presence of bowel ischemia.

Although computed tomography (CT) scans are well established in the clinical evaluation of ASBO in the adult literature, the risk-benefit analysis of CT in children with ASBO remains controversial. The main benefits of CT are its ability to identify a transition point; to evaluate for the presence of bowel ischemia, necrosis, or perforation; and to assess for other nonadhesive causes

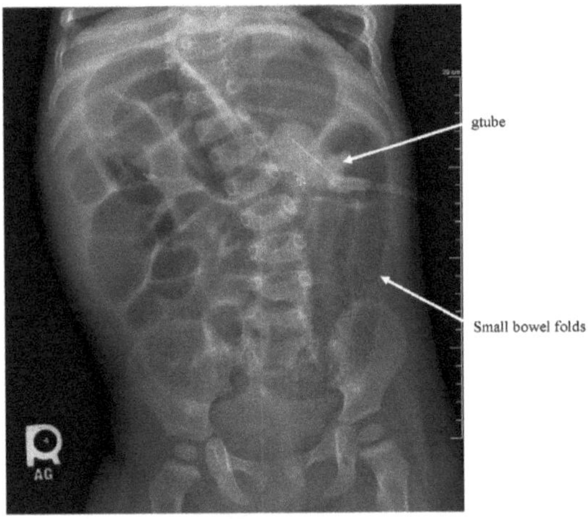

Fig. 2. *Supine* AXR demonstrating distended loops of air-filled small intestine and stomach with a gastrostomy tube (G-tube) present in the left upper quadrant. Note the visible small bowel folds on the patient's left side with more dilated small bowel on the right side.

of obstruction. Wang and colleagues [19] reported that the use of CT is highly sensitive (91.5%) for diagnosing SBO in children with a 78.7% accuracy rate in identifying the site of obstruction. Similarly, Halepota and colleagues [20] reported a sensitivity of 97.4% and specificity of 81.8% in diagnosing an SBO. Findings that correlate with bowel ischemia include free intraperitoneal fluid, mesenteric edema, pneumatosis, and portal venous gas [14,21].

The National Cancer Institute acknowledges that children are more sensitive than adults to radiation. Given their longer life expectancy and the higher than necessary radiation doses when protocols are not adjusted for their smaller size, their risk for developing cancer related to radiation exposure over their lifetime presents a concern [22]. As with any tool, CT scans have their utility in patient-specific situations; hence, *individualized decision making to minimize radiation exposure* should be a priority when evaluating children with a possible bowel obstruction. The *Image Gently* initiative created in 2007 has protocols to adjust radiation dosing and specifics to protocolize imaging studies for children [23]. In 2013, Linden and colleagues [24] demonstrated a decrease in CT scan utilization in children from 79% to 17% without an increase in complications when a contrast challenge protocol for ASBO was implemented, whereby they individually determined the need for a CT scan. This supports the reality that with a concerted effort, radiation exposure in children can be decreased (Table 1).

MANAGEMENT

Resuscitation and initial management

While the diagnostic workup is underway, the initial management of any patient presenting with an ASBO involves *correction of their dehydration and electrolyte*

Table 1
The workup summary

History	Physical examination	Laboratory tests	Imaging
Nausea Vomiting Abdominal pain Decreased stooling or flatus	Abdominal distension Tympany Dehydration Peritonitis → OR	CBC (WBC) BMP (dehydration) VBG with lactate	AXR upright & supineNote: *Cross-sectional imaging only if clinically warranted*

Abbreviations: BMP, basic metabolic panel; CBC, complete blood count; OR, operating room; VBG, venous blood gas.

derangements related to the obstructive process. The endpoints of resuscitation for uncomplicated ASBO include normal blood pressure and heart rate, and adequate weight-based urine output. All patients with an ASBO should have their stomach decompressed, via either a nasogastric (NG) or orogastric tube, or via a previously placed gastrostomy tube. Importantly, a low-profile button-type gastrostomy tube does not decompress as well as a standard (longer type) gastrostomy tube or an NG tube placed through the gastrostomy site; hence, the gastrostomy button can be exchanged for one of these at the time of presentation.

Resuscitation:
- Correct electrolytes
- 20 mL/kg bolus isotonic fluid (lactated Ringers or 0.9% normal saline)
  - → Reassess based on urine output (~ 1 mL/kg/hr)

Gastric decompression:
- Helps relieve symptoms
- Minimizes the risk of aspiration
- Provides access for subsequent contrast administration

Operative management

The outdated adage "never let the sun rise or set on a small bowel obstruction" was based on the idea that a delay to the operating room increased the risk of bowel ischemia. A recent Pediatric Health Information System (PHIS) review demonstrated wide interhospital variability in the likelihood of surgical intervention (median 51%; range 35%–75%) in PHIS-participating US children's hospitals, independent of patient and hospital characteristics [10]. Although there are clear indications for immediate operative exploration (ie, evidence of bowel compromise, perforation, nonadhesive bowel obstruction), the data are mixed concerning timing of operation and risk for bowel resection. An analysis of more than 27,000 adult patients from the National Inpatient Sampling database found no association between delay in management of SBO with complication or bowel resection [25]. In contrast, a study of more than 2000 children from the Kid's Inpatient Database found that children had similar odds of bowel resection (odds ratio = 1.40; $P = 0.01$) whether they underwent operation on day 1 when compared with day 2 following admission; however, the incidence of bowel resection increased when their operation was performed on days 3 to 14 (odds ratio = 1.67; $P = 0.003$) [26]. In a recent pediatric study by Hyak and colleagues [27–29], bowel resection was found to be more common when nonimmediate surgery was delayed by more than 48 hours, particularly in children less than 1 year of age (36.6% vs 15.3%; $P = 0.04$).

Historically, adhesive disease requiring surgery has been addressed through a laparotomy. In recent years, *laparoscopic lysis of adhesions* (LOA) has been introduced with several potential benefits [30,31]:

- Reduced new adhesion formation
- Decreased postoperative pain
- Quicker return of bowel function
- Shorter hospital length of stay

However, a recent population-based study found an increased rate of bowel intervention (enterotomy with repair or resection) in those undergoing laparoscopic LOA versus open LOA (53.5% vs 43.4%; $P < 0.0001$) [32]; this may speak to the learning curve given the rate of laparoscopic LOA was 4.3% in 2005 and only increased to 14% at the end of the study period (2014). In a review of 34 children, Aguayo and colleagues [5] found that laparoscopic LOA was safe with 32% requiring conversion to an open approach.

Importantly, the historic data regarding incidence of bowel resection, timing to surgery, and even need for surgical intervention should be taken with a degree of skepticism, as contrast challenge algorithms in children have only been described in the literature since 2011 and still have not been standardized in the pediatric patient population. For example, in 2013 Linden and colleagues [24] described a decrease in the incidence of surgery from 45% to 17% ($P = 0.04$) after implementation of a contrast challenge in children who qualified for nonoperative management.

Nonoperative management

Once a patient has been deemed appropriate for a *trial of nonoperative management*, serial clinical examinations should be closely followed for signs of clinical deterioration. Importantly, the optimal duration of nonoperative management and criteria for operative intervention are not well defined.

Over the last 3 decades, water-soluble contrast agents, such as methylglucamine diatrizoate (Gastrografin) and diatrizoate meglumine (Cystografin 30%), have been used successfully in the nonoperative management of ASBO in the adult population [5,33–39]. These contrast agents are high osmolar agents commonly used in gastrointestinal radiographic studies, and when given to patients with a bowel obstruction, are termed a "*contrast challenge*." Overall, data on the effectiveness of a contrast challenge in the setting of ASBO demonstrate a decreased need for operation and a decrease in hospital length of stay [3,4,40]. Although there remains methodologic variability across institutions (ie, different agents, doses, and duration from administration to assessment), ongoing prospective research is underway to standardize this approach in children.

A *contrast challenge* is performed as follows:

- A period of gastric decompression
  - At least 1 hour, up to 48 hours; varies by study [4–6]
- Water-soluble contrast administration via the gastric tube
  - Gastrografin (often diluted in water), Cystografin 30%, or Omnipaque 240 [1,3,7]
- Abdominal plain films to evaluate transit of the contrast (typically 2 AXRs)
  - The first at 4 to 10 hours; varies by study [1,8]
  - The second at 24 hours Figs. 3 and 4

Transit, or lack thereof, of contrast into the colon (or the ileostomy bag in patients who are diverted) is of *diagnostic benefit* in predicting which patients will need an operation.

Recent studies have shown promising results of water-soluble contrast challenge protocols in the *pediatric* population [2,24,41]:

- Linden and colleagues [24] reported benefit of a contrast challenge protocol where Cystografin 30% was given to children with an ASBO early in their admission, without the typical 48 hours of decompression described in adults. Outcomes were reviewed retrospectively before (n = 26) and after (n = 11) protocol initiation, and they concluded that contrast administration may provide a diagnostic and therapeutic benefit with decreased incidence of operative intervention (45% to 17%), length of stay (6.2–3.6 days), and cost.
- Bonnard and colleagues [41] reviewed 8 children who received a contrast challenge and 16 controls that did not and found the addition of a Gastrografin contrast challenge increased the rate of successful nonoperative management from 50% to 75%.

Despite these promising findings, pediatric studies have been limited by the small sample size of patients who received a contrast challenge.

- More recently, the authors of this review retrospectively evaluated *82 children* diagnosed with ASBO receiving a contrast challenge at 5 children's hospitals [2]. *As this was the largest pediatric study to date*, the purpose of the study was to evaluate the *safety and efficacy* of a contrast challenge for children presenting with ASBO.
  - With *zero* complications related to contrast administration, including children with neurologic and pulmonary comorbidities, a contrast challenge for children with an ASBO is *safe*.
  - The study also confirms that a contrast challenge is *highly reliable* for predicting patients who will resolve their ASBO nonoperatively.
  - Based on these findings, a multi-institutional observational prospective study is underway evaluating an algorithm for pediatric ASBO that incorporates a consistent protocol for assessing contrast transit (Fig. 5). Given the variability of the contrast agents (Gastrografin, Cystografin 30%, Omnipaque 240) in the literature and across sites, and the variable age-based dosing recommendations, the authors have also created a dosing table that accounts for weight and age and dilution of the Gastrografin to maintain consistency of osmolality across the various agents.

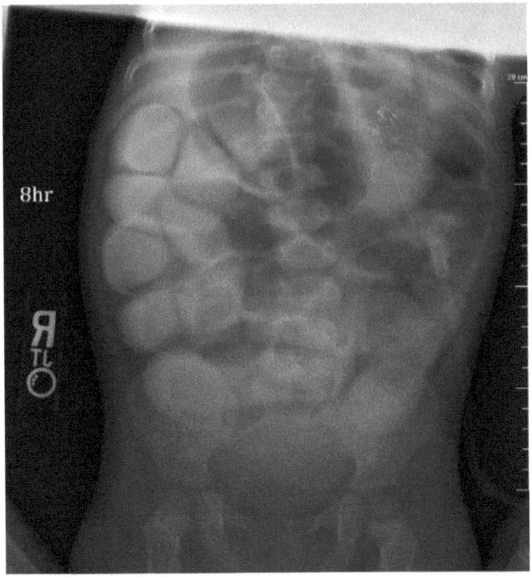

Fig. 3. Lateral AXR demonstrating dilated loops of small bowel filled with contrast at 8 hours after administration of contrast. In a standard contrast challenge algorithm, this patient would get another AXR at 24 hours to assess for transit of contrast into the colon.

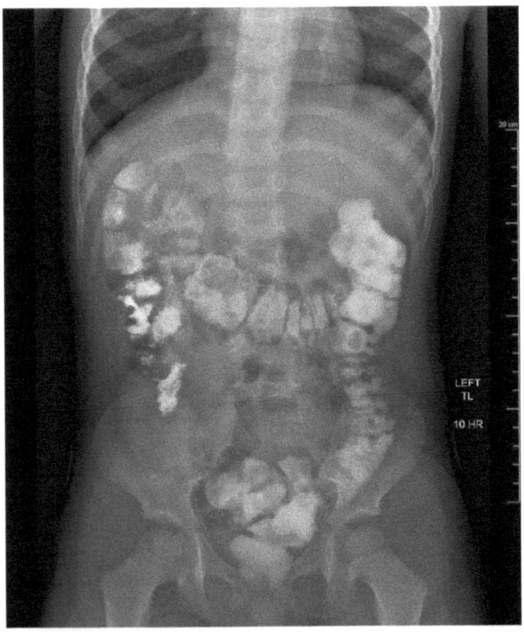

Fig. 4. Upright AXR at 10 hours from contrast administration, demonstrating contrast filling the colon with resolution of dilated loops of small bowel.

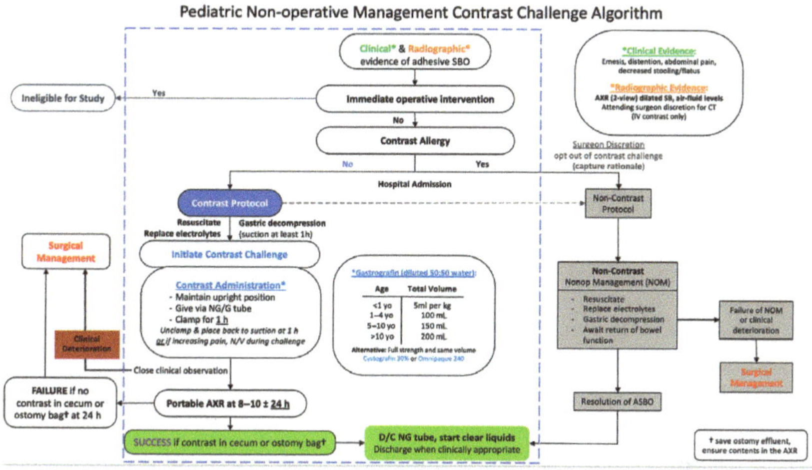

Fig. 5. Management algorithm for a contrast challenge currently under prospective study for children with an ASBO. The green* indicates clinical findings of an ASBO. The orange* indicates radiographic findings of an ASBO. The blue* indicates concentration, dosing, and type of contrast used in the algorithm.

Other considerations: Prevention

Given that adhesions are a result of the mesothelial lining being disrupted during surgical exploration, fibrin creation, and ultimate collagen deposition and remodeling, several adjunct therapies, including nonsteroidal anti-inflammatory medications, modified adenoviruses, and manual manipulation therapy, have been studied to reduce adhesion formation [42–46]. Although these agents have been shown to diminish the development of adhesions in animal models, their effect in humans is limited.

Of the multiple products developed, the use of hyaluronate carboxymethylcellulose (Seprafilm) not only decreases adhesion formation but also decreases the incidence of early postoperative obstruction [46,47] and is cost-effective when used in the setting of open colorectal surgery [48]. Similarly, a large study in ~850 children showed a decreased incidence of ASBO in the Seprafilm group (2.0%) versus controls (4.9%) after laparotomy ($P = 0.015$) [49]. These studies suggest that there may be options for decreasing the morbidity associated with postoperative ASBO.

Other considerations: Recurrence

The management of recurrent ASBO remains another point of ongoing discussion, and again, data are limited in children. Miller and colleagues [50] found a 5% risk of readmission in 50 days in their study of 552 adults. Importantly, they found those treated nonoperatively did not experience less favorable outcomes than those undergoing operative intervention with regards to symptom resolution, length of stay, or risk of recurrence or operation. Nevertheless, with a 15% 5-year risk of recurrent ASBO [51], balancing the risks of immediate operative intervention with the potential long-term risks associated with recurrent ASBO remains challenging. In a recent longitudinal propensity-matched cohort study of 27,904 patients, Behman and colleagues [52] showed a reduced risk (hazard ratio, 0.59; 95% confidence interval, 0.54–0.65) of recurrent bowel obstruction when the first episode of ASBO was managed operatively. However, a significant limitation of this study using administrative data was a lack of information related to perioperative complications. Also, they assessed survival benefit in adults (mean age 61 years), and extrapolated data to mean surgery may have prevented bowel obstructions. More data will be forthcoming in the aforementioned prospective, multi-institutional study that will help elucidate the long-term risks and benefits of nonoperative versus operative management of ASBO in children.

SUMMARY

ASBOs in children remain a common and significant cause of morbidity after abdominal surgery. The concept of partial versus complete bowel obstruction is outdated and imprecise with minimal clinical utility. Rather, what is important is the recognition of patients who require immediate surgical exploration versus those who can be managed nonoperatively.

In patients who do not require urgent operation, predicting which patients will successfully resolve their obstruction with nonoperative management remains challenging. For decades, adult data have supported use of a contrast challenge to decrease the need for surgery and to determine those requiring operative intervention, and similar data are mounting in children. Recently, a *contrast challenge* has been demonstrated to be *safe in children* and can both decrease the likelihood of operation and expedite decision making in those patients who ultimately will require an operation. It is likely that such an approach will decrease length of stay and hospital cost for children with ASBO. In addition, laparoscopic LOAs have been shown to minimize postoperative recovery, reduce hospital length of stay, reduce development of future adhesions, and possibly prevent recurrent ASBO.

Future efforts should focus on improving predictive models and incorporating them into standardized protocols to reduce interpractitioner variability and to ultimately improve clinical outcomes.

CLINICS CARE POINTS

- If a patient has never had abdominal surgery and appears to have a bowel obstruction, operation is likely warranted.
- Children with a bowel obstruction require fluid resuscitation, electrolyte repletion, and gastric decompression, and their care should be driven by or in conjunction with a pediatric surgeon.
- A water-soluble contrast challenge can decrease the need for operative intervention and/or determine the need for operation in a more timely fashion.

Disclosure

The authors have nothing to disclose.

References

[1] Zielinski MD, Bannon MP. Current Management of Small Bowel Obstruction. Adv Surg 2011;45(1):1–29.
[2] Rubalcava NS, Bence CM, Jensen AR, et al. Contrast Challenge Algorithms for Adhesive Small Bowel Obstructions Are Safe in Children. Ann Surg 2021; https://doi.org/10.1097/SLA.0000000000005159.
[3] Mucha P. Small Intestinal Obstruction. Surg Clin North Am 1987;67(3):597–620.
[4] Festen C. Postoperative small bowel obstruction in infants and children. Ann Surg 1982;196(5):580–3.
[5] Aguayo P, Ho B, Fraser JD, et al. Bowel Obstruction after Treatment of Intra-Abdominal Tumors. Eur J Pediatr Surg 2010;20(04):234–6.
[6] Menzies D, Ellis H. Intestinal obstruction from adhesions - How big is the problem? Ann R Coll Surg Engl 1990;72(1):60–3.
[7] Ellis H, Moran BJ, Thompson JN, et al. Adhesion-related hospital readmissions after abdominal and pelvic surgery: A retrospective cohort study. Lancet 1999;353(9163):1476–80.
[8] Grant HW, Parker MC, Wilson MS, et al. Population-based analysis of the risk of adhesion-related readmissions after abdominal surgery in children. J Pediatr Surg 2006;41(8):1453–6.
[9] Grant HW, Parker MC, Wilson MS, et al. Adhesions after abdominal surgery in children. J Pediatr Surg 2008;43(1):152–7.
[10] Apfeld JC, Cooper JN, Gil LA, et al. Variability in the management of adhesive small bowel obstruction in children. J Pediatr Surg 2021; https://doi.org/10.1016/j.jpedsurg.2021.11.006 S0022-3468(21):00775-2.
[11] Attard JAP, MacLean AR. Adhesive small bowel obstruction: epidemiology, biology and prevention. Can J Surg 2007;50(4):291–300. Available at: http://www.ncbi.nlm.nih.gov/pubmed/17897517.
[12] Shields R. The absorption and secretion of fluid and electrolytes by the obstructed bowel. Br J Surg 1965;52(10):774–9.
[13] Wright HK, O'Brien JJ, Tilson MD. Water absorption in experimental closed segment obstruction of the ileum in man. Am J Surg 1971;121(1):96–9.
[14] Zielinski MD, Eiken PW, Bannon MP, et al. Small bowel obstruction-Who needs an operation? A multivariate prediction model. World J Surg 2010;34(5):910–9.
[15] Bracho-Blanchet E, Dominguez-Muñoz A, Fernandez-Portilla E, et al. Predictive value of procalcitonin for intestinal ischemia and/or necrosis in pediatric patients with adhesive small bowel obstruction (ASBO). J Pediatr Surg 2017;52(10):1616–20.
[16] Cosse C, Regimbeau JM, Fuks D, et al. Serum procalcitonin for predicting the failure of conservative management and the need for bowel resection in patients with small bowel obstruction. J Am Coll Surg 2013;216(5):997–1004.
[17] Al-Nawas B, Krammer I, Shah PM. Procalcitonin in diagnosis of severe infections. Eur J Med Res 1996;1(7):331–3. Available at: http://www.ncbi.nlm.nih.gov/pubmed/9364034.
[18] Maglinte DD, Reyes BL, Harmon BH, et al. Reliability and role of plain film radiography and CT in the diagnosis of small-bowel obstruction. AJR Am J Roentgenol 1996;167(6):1451–5.
[19] Wang Q, Chavhan GB, Babyn PS, et al. Utility of CT in the diagnosis and management of small-bowel obstruction in children. Pediatr Radiol 2012;42(12):1441–8.
[20] Halepota HF, Khan MAM, Shahzad N. Sensitivity and specificity of CT scan in small bowel obstruction among children. J Pakistan Med Assoc 2018;68(5):744–6.
[21] Zielinski MD, Eiken PW, Heller SF, et al. Prospective, observational validation of a multivariate small-bowel obstruction model to predict the need for operative intervention. J Am Coll Surg 2011;212(6):1068–76.

[22] National Cancer Institute. Radiation Risks and Pediatric Computed Tomography (CT): A Guide for Health Care Providers. 2018. Available at: https://www.cancer.gov/about-cancer/causes-prevention/risk/radiation/pediatric-ct-scans.
[23] The Image Gently Alliance. Pediatric Radiology and imaging I radiation safety - Image Gently. 2014. Available at: https://www.imagegently.org/. Accessed January 2, 2022.
[24] Linden AF, Raiji MT, Kohler JE, et al. Evaluation of a water-soluble contrast protocol for nonoperative management of pediatric adhesive small bowel obstruction. J Pediatr Surg 2019;54(1):184–8.
[25] Schraufnagel D, Rajaee S, Millham FH. How many sunsets? Timing of surgery in adhesive small bowel obstruction : A study of the Nationwide Inpatient Sample. J Trauma Acute Care Surg 2012;74(1):181–9.
[26] Lautz TB, Raval Mv, Reynolds M, et al. Adhesive small bowel obstruction in children and adolescents: Operative utilization and factors associated with bowel loss. J Am Coll Surg 2011;212(5):855–61.
[27] Hyak J, Campagna G, Johnson B, et al. Management of Pediatric Adhesive Small Bowel Obstruction: Do Timing of Surgery and Age Matter? J Surg Res 2019;243:384–90.
[28] Lautz TB, Barsness KA. Adhesive small bowel obstruction-Acute management and treatment in children. Semin Pediatr Surg 2014;23(6):349–52.
[29] Akgür FM, Tanyel FC, Büyükpamukçu N, et al. Adhesive small bowel obstruction in children: The place and predictors of success for conservative treatment. J Pediatr Surg 1991;26(1):37–41.
[30] Nakamura T, Sato T, Naito M, et al. Laparoscopic surgery is useful for preventing recurrence of small bowel obstruction after surgery for postoperative small bowel obstruction. Surg Laparosc Endosc Percutaneous Tech 2016;26(1):e1–4.
[31] Grafen FC, Neuhaus V, Schöb O, et al. Management of acute small bowel obstruction from intestinal adhesions: Indications for laparoscopic surgery in a community teaching hospital. Langenbeck's Arch Surg 2010;395(1):57–63.
[32] Behman R, Nathens AB, Byrne JP, et al. Laparoscopic Surgery for Adhesive Small Bowel Obstruction Is Associated with a Higher Risk of Bowel Injury: A Population-based Analysis of 8584 Patients. Ann Surg 2017;266(3):489–98.
[33] Mulder MB, Hernandez M, Ray-Zack MD, et al. A significant proportion of small bowel obstructions require >48 hours to resolve after gastrografin. J Surg Res 2019;233:408–12.
[34] Baghdadi YMKK, Choudhry AJ, Goussous N, et al. Long-term outcomes of gastrografin in small bowel obstruction. J Surg Res 2016;202(1):43–8.
[35] Ceresoli M, Coccolini F, Catena F, et al. Water-soluble contrast agent in adhesive small bowel obstruction: A systematic review and meta-analysis of diagnostic and therapeutic value. Am J Surg 2016;211(6):1114–25.
[36] Zielinski MD, Haddad NN, Cullinane DC, et al. Multi-institutional, prospective, observational study comparing the Gastrografin challenge versus standard treatment in adhesive small bowel obstruction. J Trauma Acute Care Surg 2017;83(1):47–54.
[37] Goussous N, Eiken PW, Bannon MP, et al. Enhancement of a Small Bowel Obstruction Model Using the Gastrografin® Challenge Test. J Gastrointest Surg 2013;17(1):110–7.
[38] Loftus T, Moore F, VanZant E, et al. A protocol for the management of adhesive small bowel obstruction. J Trauma Acute Care Surg 2015;78(1):13–9.
[39] Trevino CM, VandeWater T, Webb TP. Implementation of an adhesive small bowel obstruction protocol using low-osmolar water soluble contrast and the impact on patient outcomes. Am J Surg 2019;217(4):689–93.
[40] Branco BC, Barmparas G, Schnüriger B, et al. Systematic review and meta-analysis of the diagnostic and therapeutic role of water-soluble contrast agent in adhesive small bowel obstruction. Br J Surg 2010;97(4):470–8.
[41] Bonnard A, Kohaut J, Sieurin A, et al. Gastrografin for uncomplicated adhesive small bowel obstruction in children. Pediatr Surg Int 2011;27(12):1277–81.

[42] Montz FJ, Monk BJ, Lacy SM, et al. Ketorolac tromethamine, a nonsteroidal anti-inflammatory drug: ability to inhibit post-radical pelvic surgery adhesions in a porcine model. Gynecol Oncol 1993;48(1):76–9.
[43] Atta HM, Al-Hendy AA, Abdel Raheim SR, et al. Modified Adenovirus Reduces De Novo Peritoneal Adhesions in Rats and Limits Off-Target Transfection. Role of EZH2 in Adhesion Formation. J Invest Surg 2017;30(2):78–87.
[44] Wei G, Chen X, Wang G, et al. Effect of Resveratrol on the Prevention of Intra-Abdominal Adhesion Formation in a Rat Model. Cell Physiol Biochem 2016;39(1):33–46.
[45] Bove GM, Chapelle SL, Hanlon KE, et al. Attenuation of postoperative adhesions using a modeled manual therapy. PLoS One 2017;12(6):1–18.
[46] Fazio VW, Cohen Z, Fleshman JW, et al. Reduction in Adhesive Small-Bowel Obstruction by Seprafilm® Adhesion Barrier After Intestinal Resection. Dis Colon Rectum 2006;49(1): 1–11.
[47] Vrijland WW, Tseng LNL, Eijkman HJM, et al. Fewer intraperitoneal adhesions with use of hyaluronic acid-carboxymethylcellulose membrane: A randomized clinical trial. Ann Surg 2002;235(2):193–9.
[48] Krielen P, Grutters JPC, Strik C, et al. Cost-effectiveness of the prevention of adhesions and adhesive small bowel obstruction after colorectal surgery with adhesion barriers: A modelling study. World J Emerg Surg 2019;14(1):1–9.
[49] Inoue M, Uchida K, Otake K, et al. Efficacy of Seprafilm for preventing adhesive bowel obstruction and cost-benefit analysis in pediatric patients undergoing laparotomy. J Pediatr Surg 2013;48(7):1528–34.
[50] Miller G, Boman J, Shrier I, et al. Readmission for small-bowel obstruction in the early post-operative period: Etiology and outcome. Can J Surg 2002;45(4):255–8.
[51] Foster NM, McGory ML, Zingmond DS, et al. Small Bowel Obstruction: A Population-Based Appraisal. J Am Coll Surg 2006;203(2):170–6.
[52] Behman R, Nathens AB, Mason S, et al. Association of Surgical Intervention for Adhesive Small-Bowel Obstruction with the Risk of Recurrence. JAMA Surg 2019;154(5):413–20.

Advances in Pediatrics 69 (2022) 259–271

ADVANCES IN PEDIATRICS

Postoperative Opioid Prescribing, Use, and Disposal in Children

Marjorie Odegard, MD[a,*],
Lorraine I. Kelley-Quon, MD, MSHS[a,b,c]

[a]Division of Pediatric Surgery, Children's Hospital Los Angeles, 4650 Sunset Boulevard, Mailstop #100, Los Angeles, CA 90027, USA; [b]Department of Surgery, Keck School of Medicine of the University of Southern California, Los Angeles, CA 90033, USA; [c]Department of Population and Public Health Sciences, University of Southern California, Los Angeles, CA 90033, USA

Keywords

• Opioid • Safety • Disposal • Postoperative • Prescribing

Key points

- Opioids are frequently prescribed to children undergoing surgery, but most families report unused prescription opioid pills.
- Providers must be aware of unconscious bias in pain management strategies when caring for minority children and families.
- Education about safe prescription opioid storage and disposal should be provided to all families receiving opioids and coupled with easily available means of disposal.
- Procedure-specific data about actual opioid consumption after discharge could help providers tailor their practices.

INTRODUCTION

As the opioid epidemic continues in the United States, physicians are increasingly aware of their role in responsible opioid stewardship, defined as minimizing opioids prescribed while continuing to provide adequate analgesia. Most of the children who receive an opioid prescription after surgery only use a fraction of their prescription [1–4]. This can contribute to excess unused

*Corresponding author. Division of Pediatric Surgery, Children's Hospital Los Angeles, 4650 Sunset Boulevard, Mailstop #100, Los Angeles, CA 90027. *E-mail address:* modegard@chla.usc.edu

https://doi.org/10.1016/j.yapd.2022.03.003
0065-3101/22/

opioids in a child's home, thereby increasing the risk of poisoning, accidental ingestion, and diversion to other family members or friends [5–7]. There are increasing published guidelines and resources emerging to inform and engage providers in opioid stewardship efforts both during hospitalization and after discharge home [8–11]. In this review, we will summarize current evidence regarding postoperative opioid prescription, use, storage, and disposal in children undergoing surgery and highlight gaps in knowledge requiring further study.

OPIOID PRESCRIBING PATTERNS

There is ample evidence that excess opioids are typically prescribed after surgery in both adults [12–14] and children [1–4], with as much as 71% of opioid pills left unused [15]. Many possible contributing factors have been identified including wide variation in prescribing habits due to the lack of consensus in terms of need [4,16–19], lack of prescription of multi-modal pain medication regimens [1,2], and lack of knowledge about the actual postoperative consumption of opioids [2]. In addition, it can be difficult to assess pain in children [1], and the total number of opioid pills used after surgery is largely associated with a child's procedure such as tonsillectomy or open reduction with internal fixation [2,20] and older age is associated with higher opioid consumption [21]. Chua and colleagues recently showed that 61% of pediatric opioid prescriptions in the United States were from dentists and surgeons. Notably, 46% were found to be high risk by at least one of 6 metrics of high risk prescribing including codeine and tramadol prescriptions dispensed to children 11 years old or younger that were for codeine and proportion of those prescriptions that were for tramadol [22]. In response, many targeted efforts to reduce the amount of excess opioids have been implemented including changes in local laws [23] and institutional adoption of consistent prescribing methods [9,23–26].

Efforts to develop evidence-based, procedure-specific opioid prescribing guidelines for children undergoing surgery are underway. Cravero and colleagues recently published guidelines regarding perioperative opioid use in hospitalized children and conclusions included that providers should follow age-appropriate guidelines for opioid dosing, and use multi-modal methods of pain control [11]. The first postoperative opioid prescription guidelines for children undergoing surgery generated 20 evidence-based protocols highlighting the risks associated with prescription opioid use, emphasized the importance of using nonopioid alternatives for pain management and underscored the need for family education before and after surgery. Furthermore, these guidelines identified many outpatient and minimally invasive surgical procedures which may not require postoperative opioids, though the levels of evidence vary for the procedure-specific guidance [8]. Currently, several single- and multi-center procedure-specific projects to expand principles of opioid stewardship have been successfully implemented for appendectomy [27], umbilical hernia repair [25], and tonsillectomy [24,26], with a reduction of prescribed opioids and no evidence for an increase in adverse events.

Expanding evidence-based, procedure-specific guidelines for opioid prescribing after common pediatric surgical operations could significantly reduce variability in prescribing practices and, therefore, reduce excess opioid prescribing.

Another method to constrain opioid prescribing is to limit prescriptions to the total amount of opioids used during hospitalization. In adult surgery, an example of this includes the "5x Multiplier" method for which the provider prescribes 5x the amount of opioids taken in the last 24 hours of hospitalization (eg, 2 pills $\times$ 5 = 10 pills; 0 pills $\times$ 5 = 0 pills) [10]. In a single-center study of children with cancer, Mansfield and colleagues demonstrated a significant correlation between the amount of opioids a child used in the last 24 and 48 hours of hospitalization and the amount of opioids used after discharge [23]. The authors proposed a procedure-specific algorithm to minimize opioid prescribing which was subsequently validated in a later study [28]. This seems to be a promising method to help reduce the over-prescription of opioids, but larger studies in diverse pediatric surgical populations need to be evaluated. Furthermore, it is unclear whether such a strategy would be applicable to the ambulatory surgical setting.

Provider-level interventions aimed at reducing opioid prescriptions are also promising and are summarized in Table 1. For example, a randomized controlled trial performed by Docter and colleagues demonstrated that informing clinicians when their adult patient dies from a fatal overdose decreases opioid prescribing by 10% [29]. The findings of this study demonstrate that providers will change their practice when receiving real-time data reflecting actual patient prescription opioid use resulting in poor outcomes. Howard and colleagues studied the state-wide effect of an insurance provider offering 35% more reimbursement to surgeons who followed opioid reduction guidelines published by the University of Michigan to counsel patients about pain expectations, side effects of opioids, alternative medications, and safe opioid disposal. They found an increase in the rate of utilization from 38.1% to 60.7% over the course of 8 months, suggesting that financial incentives at the provider level could be a useful tool in reducing excess opioid prescriptions [30]. In addition, Kelley and colleagues are performing a randomized controlled trial in primary care clinics in 2 states using "nudges" from the electronic health record as an intervention to address prescribing behaviors [31]. Similar provider-level interventions have yet to be performed in pediatric populations but do seem to be a promising avenue for expanding opioid stewardship efforts.

Finally, the influence of local, state, and federal laws and regulations to reduce the prescription of opioids have also contributed to curtailing unsafe opioid prescribing in children. In 2013, the Food and Drug Administration's (FDA) issued a black box warning for use of codeine in children as it was associated with severe adverse events including death in children who had undergone tonsillectomy or adenoidectomy. In addition, in 2017 the FDA issued a warning and restrictions on the postoperative use of tramadol in children again citing several reported adverse events [32]. In both cases, many of the adverse

Table 1
Behavioral interventions for providers and caregivers to improve pain control and reduce opioid consumption

	Informed of patient overdose	EMR "nudges"	Standardized pain scales	Drug information sheet	STOMP
Target	Provider	Provider	Caregiver	Caregiver	Caregiver
Purpose	Reduce unnecessary opioid prescribing	Reduce unnecessary opioid prescribing	Improve pain control and patient satisfaction	Improve patient pain control	Improve caregiver education about opioid safety
Result	Decreased opioid prescribing	Randomized-controlled trial in progress	No change vs increased number of analgesics given	Improved patient pain control	Caregivers less likely to give opioids high-risk situations
Evidence	Doctor et al.	Kelley et al.	Unsworth et al., Vincent et al.	Bailey et al.	Voepel-Lewis et al.

Abbreviations: EMR, electronic medical record; STOMP, scenario tailored opioid messaging program.

events were thought to be attributable to genetic mutations causing alterations in drug metabolism [24,32,33]. These warnings resulted in a significant reduction in codeine and tramadol prescribing overall, but unfortunately its use has not been completely eliminated [24,33,34]. In addition, state laws, such as a 2018 Tennessee law that prohibited opioid prescriptions greater than 3 days or 180 morphine equivalents without documented medical need, have also driven work to reduce opioid prescribing [23,28]. Quality improvement efforts implemented due to this law have shown a reduction in opioids prescribed at discharge without decreases in patient satisfaction [23,28]. Laws and FDA recommendations aimed at curtailing unsafe opioid prescribing can be an important impetus to changing provider behaviors, but additional hospital and patient-level efforts continue to be needed to fully expand opioid stewardship efforts.

PRESCRIPTION OPIOID USE

Understanding the factors that influence prescription opioid use after discharge could enable prescribers to tailor their practices in a data-driven way. Studies show that the total number of opioid pills prescribed after surgery is positively associated with patient consumption [35,36]. In other words, the greater the number of pills prescribed, the greater the number of pills that will be consumed by a patient and vice versa. Conversely, recent research demonstrates that patients can be prescribed and consume fewer doses of opioids without a decrease in patient satisfaction [23,28], increase in refill requests [9], or increase in emergency department visits [24]. These studies demonstrate that it is possible to not only decrease unused opioids in the community, but to decrease postoperative opioid consumption overall without compromising functional recovery or patient satisfaction.

Several patient-level factors are associated with increased postoperative opioid consumption. Female sex [21,37,38], higher patient pain scores [37,39], higher in-hospital opioid consumption [39,40], and previous opioid consumption [37] are associated with higher opioid use after discharge in addition to the previously mentioned factors of age [20,21] and surgery type [2,20]. The incidence of opioid prescription refills, which infers prolonged use, tended to be increased when the initial prescription was for higher amounts of opioids, but these findings are inconsistent [17,20]. For example, Meza and colleagues showed that among children who underwent orthopedic surgical procedures and received hydromorphone or methadone, the amount of opioid consumption during inpatient recovery was associated with the likelihood of seeking a prescription opioid refill after surgery [40]. There are certainly multiple drivers of refill behavior and future studies evaluating specifically how caregiver and patient attitudes, perceptions, and education influence refill behaviors are much needed.

One additional area in need of further study involves pain management and prescription opioid use in minority children. Previous studies have shown that Black patients are less likely to receive analgesia in the emergency department, the outpatient setting, and overall [41–45]. In some studies, white patients are more likely to fill prescriptions while in other studies no difference across race was noted [46,47]. One multi-center study evaluating children after tonsillectomy/adenoidectomy showed that Hispanic/Latino parents perceived their children to have higher pain levels compared with non-Hispanic/Latino parents, but that did not change the amount of opioids administered [48]. Overall, little literature exists assessing prescription opioid use and effectiveness in minority children. More research is needed to develop targeted educational tools addressing the biopsychosocial differences, including cultural beliefs and perceptions, around pain and opioid medications in minorities [49]. Such interventions could assist providers in providing culturally competent care and in optimizing postoperative pain control for minority children.

Several studies have examined the role of family education in minimizing postoperative opioid use while still providing appropriate analgesia (see Table 1). The utility of standard pain scales is variable with some studies showing no benefit and others observing an increase in opioid use when pain scales were used [50,51]. Bailey and colleagues found that providing an oxycodone information sheet to the caregiver improved patient postoperative pain control when compared with verbal communication from the surgeon [52]. It has been demonstrated that with appropriate education, caregivers will recognize the risks and appropriately manage opioid administration in children [53]. Voepel Lewis and colleagues specifically developed and compared the value of a series of interactive educational videos [the Scenario Tailored Opioid Messaging Program (STOMP)] to an educational pamphlet [54]. Parents in the STOMP group were less likely to give their children opioids in high-risk situations [54]. These results highlight the necessity for effective caregiver education on both appropriate and safe opioid administration.

PRESCRIPTION OPIOID DISPOSAL

When a family has unused prescription opioids in the home, there is an increased risk of diversion and misuse [7,55]. In McCabe and colleagues' analysis of the diversion of controlled substances among adolescents in 2 school districts, they found that 1 in 7 adolescents had diverted their medications [7]. Current literature demonstrates that families infrequently report safely disposing of unused opioid pills, with rates as low as 19% without intervention [2,3,56–58]. While it is important to reduce the amount of opioids prescribed and thereby reduce the amount of unused opioids in the home, concurrent efforts should be undertaken to encourage safe opioid storage in a locked and/or latched location and proper, prompt disposal preferably in a Drug Enforcement Agency (DEA) bin or via an authorized take-back event/program [59–61]. The options, benefits, and limitations of disposal options are summarized in Table 2. All of these disposal options have potential drawbacks. Though the DEA has a website for people to locate opioid disposal sites, events, and mail back programs [62,63], these resources may not be readily accessible for patients depending on where they live [64], though the DEA has targeted take back

Table 2
Opioid disposal methods

	DEA bin	DEA takeback event	DEA mail-in program	Disposal kit	Household garbage	Flushing
Definition	DEA receptacle at an approved location, typically a pharmacy or police station	DEA approved event whereby patients/caregivers can return controlled substances	Mailing back medications to a DEA approved drug return site	An envelope containing drug deactivating chemicals that are mixed with prescription opioids before disposing in the garbage	Mixing opioids with undesirable substances such as coffee grounds or cat litter before disposing in the garbage	Flushing unused opioids down the toilet
Benefits	Security, ease of use	Security, ease of use	Convenience	Convenience	Convenience	Convenience, ease
Limitations	Not all sites accept liquid opioids, accessibility	Accessibility	Accessibility, unable to use for liquid opioid prescriptions	Cost, unable to use for liquid opioid prescriptions	Risk of accidental ingestion or diversion	Possible environmental impact
Security	Secure	Secure	Secure	Secure	Not secure	Secure
Evidence	Gray et al., White and Triboleti	Gray et al.	Adler et al.	Lawrence et al., Brummett et al.		Khan et al.

Data From 1. https://www.fda.gov/consumers/consumer-updates/where-and-how-dispose-unused-medicines; and 2. https://www.deadiversion.usdoj.gov/drug_disposal/.

events [65] and disposal bins to rural areas with high rates of prescription opioid abuse [66]. If such disposal options are not accessible, properly disposing opioids in the trash or flushing approved medications down the toilet is a low effort option for families which can lead to higher rates of safe disposal [56,58,67–69]. But, not every drug is approved for these approaches by the Food and Drug Administration (FDA) and disposing opioids in the garbage by mixing them with undesirable materials instead of a deactivation kit can still lead to diversion and potential ingestion. Also, even though the FDA's own study asserts that the flushing of these drugs has negligible effects on the environment and low risk of toxic exposure [70], questions still remain about the long-term effects of this type of disposal. Drug disposal kits and the cost of postage may be cost-prohibitive if they aren't provided to the patient by their health care provider. The brand used in 2 randomized controlled trials which demonstrated enhanced safe disposal when provided to caregivers [58,68] currently costs $20 USD for a pack of 3 pouches [71]. Overall, the low rates of safe disposal reflect a need for better, more cost-effective options for disposal along with patient and caregiver education regarding the safe disposal and the risk of unused opioids in the home.

Many caregivers do not know how to properly dispose of opioids or the risks of improper retention and/or disposal [72]. The prevalence of postoperative parent and child education about the safe disposal of opioids varies. In a survey of the American Pediatric Surgery Association (APSA) membership, 65% of pediatric surgeons responding reported that they did not educate their patients about how to properly dispose of opioids and 29% reported not knowing how to properly dispose of opioids themselves [73]. Other studies report that between 19% and 50% of caregivers and/or patients receive education about safe opioid storage and disposal [2,3,57]. Even among those who do receive education, reports of the effectiveness of that education on increasing safe storage and disposal are variable. Some studies report that education increases safe opioid disposal behaviors [74] while others find that education does not have an impact, perhaps because of ineffective educational approaches or lack viable disposal options [57]. Health care provider education coupled with easily accessible disposal approaches would be most effective, although under the best of circumstances the overall rate of disposal was still 72% [56,58,68].

SUMMARY

Expanding the principles of opioid stewardship for children undergoing surgery continues to be a goal for pediatric surgeons and other health care providers. Prescribers must balance the need to effectively treat pain, which may require prescribing opioids, with minimizing the risk of increased opioid consumption in children and excess opioids in the community. Provider-level interventions and education are much needed as is procedure-specific data on actual opioid use and need in pediatric surgical populations. Further investigation into the postoperative opioid use patterns of minority patients and their perceptions of opioid use is also necessary to enable culturally competent care. Finally, health care providers must engage families and educate caregivers both before and after surgery about safe prescription opioid use, storage, and disposal.

CLINICAL CARE POINTS

- Children frequently receive more prescription opioids after surgery than are used.
- Early and multimodal pain control is important for reducing opioid consumption after discharge.
- Opioid prescription amounts should be tailored to actual patient use by the procedure.
- Outpatient opioid prescribing that reflects in-hospital opioid use may ensure appropriate amounts of opioids are given to meet patient needs.
- Education about safe postoperative opioid use, storage, and disposal needs to be delivered to families both before and after surgery.
- An effective means of safe disposal must be provided to families receiving a prescription opioid.

Disclosure

The authors have nothing to disclose.

References

[1] Horton J, Munawar S, Corrigan C, et al. Inconsistent and excessive opioid prescribing after common pediatric surgical operations. J Pediatr Surg 2019;54(7):1427–31.
[2] Pruitt LCC, Swords DS, Russell KW, et al. Prescription vs. consumption: Opioid overprescription to children after common surgical procedures. J Pediatr Surg 2019;54(11):2195–9.
[3] Garren BR, Lawrence MB, McNaull PP, et al. Opioid-prescribing patterns, storage, handling, and disposal in postoperative pediatric urology patients. J Pediatr Urol 2019;15(3):260.e1-7.
[4] Anderson K, Bartz-Kurycki M, Ferguson D, et al. Too much of a bad thing: Discharge opioid prescriptions in pediatric appendectomy patients. J Pediatr Surg 2018;53(12):2374–7.
[5] Lovegrove M, Mathew J, Hampp C, et al. Emergency hospitalizations for unsupervised prescription medication ingestions by young children. Pediatrics 2014;134(4):e1009–16.
[6] Burghardt LC, Ayers JW, Brownstein JS, et al. Adult Prescription Drug Use and Pediatric Medication Exposures and Poisonings. Pediatrics 2013;132(1):18–27.
[7] McCabe S, West B, Teter C, et al. Characteristics associated with the diversion of controlled medications among adolescents. Drug Alcohol Depend 2011;118(2–3):452–8.
[8] Kelley-Quon LI, Kirkpatrick MG, Ricca RL, et al. Guidelines for Opioid Prescribing in Children and Adolescents After Surgery: An Expert Panel Opinion. JAMA Surg 2021;156(1):76–90.
[9] Howard R, Waljee J, Brummett C, et al. Reduction in Opioid Prescribing Through Evidence-Based Prescribing Guidelines. JAMA Surg 2018;153(3):285–7.

[10] Day R, Newhook T, Dewhurst W, et al. Assessing the 5×-Multiplier Calculation to Reduce Discharge Opioid Prescription Volumes After Inpatient Surgery. JAMA Surg 2020;155(12):1166–7.
[11] Cravero J, Agarwal R, Berde C, et al. The Society for Pediatric Anesthesia recommendations for the use of opioids in children during the perioperative period. Paediatr Anaesth 2019;29(6):547–71.
[12] Hill M, McMahon M, Stucke R, et al. Wide Variation and Excessive Dosage of Opioid Prescriptions for Common General Surgical Procedures. Ann Surg 2017;265(4):709–14.
[13] Chen EY, Marcantonio A, Tornetta P. Correlation Between 24-Hour Predischarge Opioid Use and Amount of Opioids Prescribed at Hospital Discharge. JAMA Surg 2018;153(2): e174859.
[14] Neuman MD, Bateman BT, Wunsch H. Inappropriate opioid prescription after surgery. Lancet 2019;393(10180):1547.
[15] Bicket MC, Long JJ, Pronovost PJ, et al. Prescription Opioid Analgesics Commonly Unused After Surgery: A Systematic Review. JAMA Surg 2017;152(11):1066–71.
[16] Raney E, van Bosse H, Shea K, et al. Current State of the Opioid Epidemic as it Pertains to Pediatric Orthopaedics From the Advocacy Committee of the Pediatric Orthopaedic Society of North America. J Pediatr Orthop 2018;38(5):e238–44.
[17] Cartmill R, Yang D, Fernandes-Taylor S, et al. National variation in opioid prescribing after pediatric umbilical hernia repair. Surgery 2019;165(4):838–42.
[18] Denning N, Kvasnovsky C, Golden J, et al. Inconsistency in Opioid Prescribing Practices After Pediatric Ambulatory Hernia Surgery. J Surg Res 2019;241:57–62.
[19] Van Cleve W, Grigg E. Variability in opioid prescribing for children undergoing ambulatory surgery in the United States. J Clin Anesth 2017;41:16–20.
[20] Wetzel M, Hockenberry J, Raval M. Opioid Fills in Children Undergoing Surgery From 2011 to 2014: A Retrospective Analysis of Relationships Among Age, Initial Days Supplied, and Refills. Ann Surg 2021;274(2):e174–80.
[21] Harbaugh C, Lee J, Hu H, et al. Persistent Opioid Use Among Pediatric Patients After Surgery. Pediatrics 2018;141(1); https://doi.org/10.1542/PEDS.2017-2439.
[22] Chua K, Brummett C, Conti R, et al. Opioid Prescribing to US Children and Young Adults in 2019. Pediatrics 2021;148(3); https://doi.org/10.1542/PEDS.2021-051539.
[23] Mansfield SA, El Gohary Y, Kimble A, et al. A quality improvement intervention to decrease postoperative opioid prescriptions in pediatric oncology patients. J Pediatr Hematol Oncol 2019; https://doi.org/10.1097/MPH.0000000000001641.
[24] Luk L, Mosen D, MacArthur C, et al. Implementation of a Pediatric Posttonsillectomy Pain Protocol in a Large Group Practice. Otolaryngol Head Neck Surg 2016;154(4):720–4.
[25] Piper K, Baxter K, Wetzel M, et al. Provider education decreases opioid prescribing after pediatric umbilical hernia repair. J Pediatr Surg 2020;55(7):1319–23.
[26] Horton JD, Corrigan C, Patel T, et al. Effect of a Standardized Electronic Medical Record Order Set on Opioid Prescribing after Tonsillectomy. Otolaryngol Head Neck Surg 2020;163(2):216–20.
[27] Freedman-Weiss M, Chiu A, Worhunsky D, et al. An Evidence-Based Guideline Supporting Restricted Opioid Prescription after Pediatric Appendectomy. J Pediatr Surg 2020;55(1): 106–11.
[28] Mansfield SA, Kimble A, Rodriguez L, et al. Validating an opioid prescribing algorithm in postoperative pediatric surgical oncology patients. J Pediatr Surg 2021;56(1):110–4.
[29] Doctor JN, Nguyen A, Lev R, et al. Opioid prescribing decreases after learning of a patient's fatal overdose. Science 2018;361(6402):588–90.
[30] Howard R, Hallway A, Santos-Parker J, et al. Optimizing Postoperative Opioid Prescribing Through Quality-Based Reimbursement. JAMA Netw Open 2019;2(9):e1911619.
[31] Kelley M, Persell S, Linder J, et al. The protocol of the Application of Economics & Social psychology to improve Opioid Prescribing Safety Trial 1 (AESOPS-1): Electronic health record

nudges. Contemp Clin Trials 2021;103; https://doi.org/10.1016/J.CCT.2021.106329.
[32] FDA Drug Safety Communication: FDA restricts use of prescription codeine pain and cough medicines and tramadol pain medicines in children; recommends against use in breastfeeding women I FDA. Available at: https://www.fda.gov/drugs/drug-safety-and-availability/fda-drug-safety-communication-fda-restricts-use-prescription-codeine-pain-and-cough-medicines-and. Accessed November 4, 2021.
[33] Chua KP, Shrime MG, Conti RM. Effect of FDA Investigation on Opioid Prescribing to Children After Tonsillectomy/Adenoidectomy. Pediatrics 2017;140(6):e20171765. Available at: https://publications.aap.org/pediatrics/article/140/6/e20171765/38185/Effect-of-FDA-Investigation-on-Opioid-Prescribing.
[34] Kohler JE, Cartmill RS, Kalbfell E, et al. Continued Prescribing of Periprocedural Codeine and Tramadol to Children after a Black Box Warning. J Surg Res 2020;256:131–5.
[35] Howard R, Fry B, Gunaseelan V, et al. Association of Opioid Prescribing With Opioid Consumption After Surgery in Michigan. JAMA Surg 2019;154(1):e184234.
[36] Larach DB, Sahara MJ, As-Sanie S, et al. Patient Factors Associated With Opioid Consumption in the Month Following Major Surgery. Ann Surg 2021;273(3):507–15.
[37] Monitto CL, Hsu A, Gao S, et al. Opioid Prescribing for the Treatment of Acute Pain in Children upon Hospital Discharge. Anesth Analg 2017;125(6):2113.
[38] Harbaugh C, Nalliah R, Hu H, et al. Persistent Opioid Use After Wisdom Tooth Extraction. JAMA 2018;320(5):504–6.
[39] Owusu-Agyemang P, Cata J, Meter A, et al. Perioperative factors associated with persistent opioid use after extensive abdominal surgery in children and adolescents: A retrospective cohort study. Paediatr Anaesth 2018;28(7):625–31.
[40] Meza B, Swarup I, Woodard T, et al. Refilling Opioid Prescriptions After Pediatric Orthopaedic Surgery: An Analysis of Incidence and Risk Factors. J Pediatr Orthop 2021;41(3):e291–5.
[41] Hoffman K, Trawalter S, Axt J, et al. Racial bias in pain assessment and treatment recommendations, and false beliefs about biological differences between blacks and whites. Proc Natl Acad Sci U S A 2016;113(16):4296–301.
[42] Green C, Anderson K, Baker T, et al. The unequal burden of pain: confronting racial and ethnic disparities in pain. Pain Med 2003;4(3):277–94.
[43] Johnson T, Weaver M, Borrero S, et al. Association of race and ethnicity with management of abdominal pain in the emergency department. Pediatrics 2013;132(4); https://doi.org/10.1542/PEDS.2012-3127.
[44] Goyal M, Kuppermann N, Cleary S, et al. Racial Disparities in Pain Management of Children With Appendicitis in Emergency Departments. JAMA Pediatr 2015;169(11):996–1002.
[45] Groenewald CB, Rabbitts JA, Hansen E, et al. Racial differences in opioid prescribing for children in the United States. Pain 2018;159(10):2050.
[46] Chavez L, Cooper J, Deans K, et al. Evaluation of racial disparities in postoperative opioid prescription filling after common pediatric surgical procedures. J Pediatr Surg 2020;55(12):2575–83.
[47] Kim H, Heard K, Heard S, et al. Opioid prescription fill rates after emergency department discharge. Am J Health Syst Pharm 2016;73(12):902–7.
[48] Donaldson C, Jenkins B, Fortier M, et al. Parent responses to pediatric pain: The differential effects of ethnicity on opioid consumption. J Psychosom Res 2020;138; https://doi.org/10.1016/J.JPSYCHORES.2020.110251.
[49] Campbell CM, Edwards RR. Ethnic differences in pain and pain management. Pain Manag 2012;2(3):219–30.
[50] Vincent C, Chiappetta M, Beach A, et al. Parents' management of children's pain at home after surgery. J Spec Pediatr Nurs 2012;17(2):108–20.

[51] Unsworth V, LFranck L, Choonara I. Parental assessment and management of children's post-operative pain: a randomized clinical trial. J Child Health Care 2007;11(3):186–94.
[52] Bailey L, Sun J, Courtney M, et al. Improving postoperative tonsillectomy pain management in children–a double blinded randomised control trial of a patient analgesia information sheet. Int J Pediatr Otorhinolaryngol 2015;79(5):732–9.
[53] Voepel-Lewis T, Zikmund-Fisher B, Smith E, et al. Parents' Analgesic Trade-Off Dilemmas: How Analgesic Knowledge Influences Their Decisions to Give Opioids. Clin J Pain 2016;32(3):187–95.
[54] Voepel-Lewis T, Zikmund-Fisher B, Boyd C, et al. Effect of a Scenario-tailored Opioid Messaging Program on Parents' Risk Perceptions and Opioid Decision-making. Clin J Pain 2018;34(6):497–504.
[55] Boyd C, McCabe S, Cranford J, et al. Prescription drug abuse and diversion among adolescents in a southeast Michigan school district. Arch Pediatr Adolesc Med 2007;161(3): 276–81.
[56] Voepel-Lewis T, Farley FA, Grant J, et al. Behavioral Intervention and Disposal of Leftover Opioids: A Randomized Trial. Pediatrics 2020;145(1); https://doi.org/10.1542/PEDS.2019-1431.
[57] Sloss K, Vargas G, Brummett C, et al. Association of caregiver-reported education with locked storage and disposal of prescription opioids after children's surgery. J Pediatr Surg 2020;55(11):2442–7.
[58] Lawrence AE, Carsel AJ, Leonhart KL, et al. Effect of Drug Disposal Bag Provision on Proper Disposal of Unused Opioids by Families of Pediatric Surgical Patients: A Randomized Clinical Trial. JAMA Pediatr 2019;173(8):e191695.
[59] McDonald EM, Kennedy-Hendricks A, McGinty EE, et al. Safe Storage of Opioid Pain Relievers Among Adults Living in Households With Children. Pediatrics 2017;139(3); https://doi.org/10.1542/PEDS.2016-2161.
[60] How to Safely Dispose of Drugs I HHS.gov. Available at: https://www.hhs.gov/opioids/prevention/safely-dispose-drugs/index.html. Accessed October 14, 2021.
[61] Drug Disposal Information. Available at: https://www.deadiversion.usdoj.gov/drug_disposal/. Accessed October 14, 2021.
[62] Controlled Substance Public Disposal Locations - Search Utility. Available at: https://apps2.deadiversion.usdoj.gov/pubdispsearch/spring/main?execution=e1s1. Accessed October 14, 2021.
[63] National Prescription Drug Take Back Day. Available at: https://www.deadiversion.usdoj.-gov/drug_disposal/takeback/index.html. Accessed October 14, 2021.
[64] Steiger R, Khalsa C, Schwartz A, et al. 144 Access to permanent opioid disposal sites in the state of michigan. Inj Prev 2017;23(Suppl 1):A53–4.
[65] Gray JA, Hagemeier NE. Prescription Drug Abuse and DEA-Sanctioned Drug Take-Back Events: Characteristics and Outcomes in Rural Appalachia. Arch Intern Med 2012;172(15):1186–7.
[66] Gray J, Hagemeier N, Brooks B, et al. Prescription Disposal Practices: A 2-Year Ecological Study of Drug Drop Box Donations in Appalachia. Am J Public Health 2015;105(9): e89–94.
[67] Where and How to Dispose of Unused Medicines I FDA. Available at: https://www.fda.-gov/consumers/consumer-updates/where-and-how-dispose-unused-medicines. Accessed October 14, 2021.
[68] Brummett CM, Steiger R, Englesbe M, et al. Effect of an Activated Charcoal Bag on Disposal of Unused Opioids After an Outpatient Surgical Procedure: A Randomized Clinical Trial. JAMA Surg 2019;154(6):558–61.
[69] Drug Disposal. FDA's Flush List for Certain Medicines I FDA. Available at: https://www.fda.gov/drugs/disposal-unused-medicines-what-you-should-know/drug-disposal-fdas-flush-list-certain-medicines. Accessed October 14, 2021.

[70] Khan U, Bloom R, Nicell J, et al. Risks associated with the environmental release of pharmaceuticals on the U.S. Food and Drug Administration "flush list. Sci Total Environ 2017;609: 1023–40.
[71] Deterra SP - Drug Deactivation & Disposal System (Small Stand-Up Pouch – Deterra Systems. Available at: https://shop.deterrasystem.com/products/deterra-sp-drug-deactivation-disposal-system-small-stand-up-pouch-3-pack. Accessed November 5, 2021.
[72] Garbutt JM, Kulka K, Dodd S, et al. Opioids in Adolescents' Homes: Prevalence, Caregiver Attitudes and Risk Reduction Opportunities. Acad Pediatr 2019;19(1):103.
[73] Hunsberger JB, Monitto CL, Hsu A, et al. Pediatric surgeon opioid prescribing behavior: A survey of the American Pediatric Surgery Association membership. J Pediatr Surg 2021;56(5):875–82.
[74] Buffington DE, Lozicki A, Alfieri T, et al. Understanding factors that contribute to the disposal of unused opioid medication. J Pain Res 2019;12:725.

FSC
www.fsc.org
MIX
Papier | Fördert gute Waldnutzung
FSC® C083411

Kolibri 360 GmbH
Ferdinand-Jühlke-Straße 7
99095 Erfurt, Deutschland
produktsicherheit@kolibri360.de